THE MAPLE LEAF
AND THE WHITE CROSS

*A History of St. John Ambulance and the
Most Venerable Order of the Hospital of
St. John of Jerusalem in Canada*

CHRISTOPHER MCCREERY
PRIORY HISTORIAN

Copy-editor: Nigel Heseltine
Proofreader: Ellen Ewart
Designer: Heidy Lawrance, WeMakeBooks.ca
Printer: Friesens

Library and Archives Canada Cataloguing in Publication

McCreery, Christopher
    The maple leaf and the white cross : a history of the Venerable Order of the Hospital of St. John of Jerusalem in Canada / Christopher McCreery.

ISBN 978-1-55002-740-2

    1. St. John Ambulance—History. I. Title.

HV593.C3M32 2007   362.18'06071   C2007-904667-3

1   2   3   4   5   12   11   10   09   08

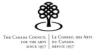

THE CANADA COUNCIL | LE CONSEIL DES ARTS
FOR THE ARTS | DU CANADA
SINCE 1957 | DEPUIS 1957

ONTARIO ARTS COUNCIL
CONSEIL DES ARTS DE L'ONTARIO

Canada

We acknowledge the support of the **Canada Council for the Arts** and the **Ontario Arts Council** for our publishing program. We also acknowledge the financial support of the **Government of Canada** through the **Book Publishing Industry Development Program** and **The Association for the Export of Canadian Books**, and the **Government of Ontario** through the **Ontario Book Publishers Tax Credit** program and the **Ontario Media Development Corporation**.

Printed and bound in Canada
www.dundurn.com

Dundurn Press
3 Church Street, Suite 500
Toronto, Ontario, Canada
M5E 1M2

Gazelle Book Services Limited
White Cross Mills
High Town, Lancaster, England
LA1 4XS

Dundurn Press
2250 Military Road
Tonawanda, NY U.S.A.
14150

Dedication

To those who have selflessly served in the cause of humanity

Pro Fide
Pro Utilitate Hominum

AUTHOR'S NOTE

In the writing of this book the author, by the terms of his commission, was given full access to all relevant documents extant, in the possession of the Priory of Canada, and those documents related to Canada held at St. John's Gate in London. The facts and figures used by him have been verified from official sources, but he was left free to select and arrange material. The inferences drawn and the opinions expressed are those of the author himself.

CONTENTS

COLOUR PLATES

Section I

Section II

ABOUT THE AUTHOR

Christopher McCreery has served as the priory historian for the Order of St. John since 2005. His previous works, *The Canadian Honours System* and *The Order of Canada: Its Origins, History, and Development*, are the main works on the history of honours in Canada. A respected institutional historian, McCreery holds a doctorate in Canadian history from Queen's University, is a Fellow of the Royal Canadian Geographic Society, and has been the recipient of a number of awards for his work on honours. A highly regarded expert on honours and the role of the Crown in Canada, McCreery is a frequent commentator in the press on such matters.

PREFATORY MESSAGE

HRH The Duke of Gloucester KG, GCVO

KENSINGTON PALACE

For one hundred and twenty five years, the Order of St. John, and its operating arm St. John Ambulance, have been active in Canada. From its modest beginnings in Quebec City and Kingston, St. John Ambulance has grown to become the leading provider of first aid training in the Country.

I am proud that one of my forbears, HRH Prince Arthur Duke of Connaught, Governor General from 1911 to 1916 and long serving Grand Prior of the Order, played such an important role in promoting the work of the Brigade and Association, now combined at the St. John Ambulance Foundation, in a then youthful Canada.

That St. John first aid instruction was provided to so many of those who served in the Canadian Expeditionary Force during the First World War, is a testament to the value of such training, both at home and on the battlefield. The work of St. John in Canada during the Second World War was best personified by Katherine "Kay" Gilmour and her Voluntary Aid Detachments. The thousands of Canadian women and men who served in times of conflict and peace afforded St. John Ambulance a firm and highly respected foundation in Canada, and throughout the Commonwealth.

St. John Ambulance has played an important role in the wellbeing of countless thousands of Canadians through the provision of first aid training. From the training of railway men of the CNR and CPR, and the special centres set up by Bell Telephone and many other industries, to the relationship that has developed with the Canadian Forces and Royal Canadian Mounted Police, the Order has continued to grow in many fields.

My own impression of St. John in Canada is the way it has had the flexibility to react to the various needs of the communities it serves, particularly in the remote parts.

As Grand Prior of the Most Venerable Order of the Hospital of St. John of Jerusalem, I am pleased that Dr. McCreery's book captures the role of St. John Ambulance in the history of Canada. I am certain that the reader will find much of the previously unpublished information contained in the book to be of great interest, and that it will help Canadians better understand the long and proud roots that St. John has in this Country.

FOREWORD

THE GOVERNOR GENERAL
LA GOUVERNEUR GÉNÉRALE

There is a great history behind the special ties that unite the Order of St. John and St. John Ambulance in Canada, and I would like to take this opportunity to wish them my very best on the occasion of their 125th anniversary.

Since the very beginning of New France and Acadia, a number of representatives of the Crown have had a special bond with the White Cross in Canada. Notably, Field Marshal, Earl Alexander of Tunis was named the first Prior of the Priory of Canada, a responsibility that continues to be associated with the Governor General today. Vincent Massey, who would later become Governor General, served in the Order for almost his entire life. He and his wife Alice were ardent supporters of the St. John Ambulance Brigade during the Second World War.

St. John Ambulance also played a pioneering role in recognizing the contribution women make to society, as it encourages women to participate in the organization. The Order of St. John was also the first honour bestowed upon both men and women.

Aware of the needs of the workplace and skillfully adapting to these needs, St. John Ambulance started providing training to workers at the beginning of the 20th century. The organization then began a strong relationship with the Armed Forces and the country's protective services, all the while continuing to provide essential services from one ocean to the other, which continues to include first aid training.

It gives me great pride to join the long line of those who have been part of the organization's history. I encourage all Canadians to join the tradition and help St. John Ambulance celebrate many more milestone anniversaries.

Michaëlle Jean

2008

PREFACE

As a foundation of the Order of St. John, St. John Ambulance — originally know as the St. John Ambulance Association and the St. John Ambulance Brigade — has been providing first aid training programs throughout Canada for the past 125 years. From the rail yards of the Edwardian era and military hospitals of the First World War to a modern-day volunteer organization devoted to the service of humanity, this history recounts the remarkable story of the Order's contribution to our country and those who made it possible.

With its connection to the hospitaller tradition of the 10th and 11th centuries, the Order of St. John finds its modern roots in the English revival of this charitable work in 1831. The 1883 inauguration of the Order in Canada signalled the beginning of a long and distinguished history of service to Canadians and people around the globe. As a nationwide volunteer organization involving more than 25,000 Canadians, St. John Ambulance continues to be the principal provider of first aid training in Canada.

The Most Venerable Order of the Hospital of St. John of Jerusalem makes up the oldest continuously bestowed element of Canada's national honours system and is Canada's only order of chivalry. Her Majesty The Queen is sovereign head, HRH The Duke of Gloucester is grand prior of the Order, while the governor general serves as prior of the Priory of Canada. Each lieutenant-governor holds office as vice-prior during their time in vice-regal office, reflecting the historic connection between the Crown and the work of the St. John Ambulance.

Made up of provincial and territorial councils, St. John Ambulance has been federal in nature since its founding as a branch in Canada; thus reflecting the diversity of Canada's various regions and peoples.

The Order's eight-pointed white cross continues to be an internationally recognized symbol. Found on everything from Police uniforms and first aid kits to the St. John Eye Hospital in Jerusalem, St. John Ambulance continues to play a role in the everyday lives of many Canadians and people around the globe.

Strongly linked to the Christian foundations of the Order and its hospitaller work, the Order of St. John has grown to encompass people of all faiths, maintaining that timeless commitment to helping people in need.

Pro Fide
Pro Utilitate Hominum

Acknowledgements

It has been an honour to undertake this project. The role that the Most Venerable Order of the Hospital of St. John of Jerusalem and its operating arm, St. John Ambulance, has played in the fostering of charity and kindness towards our fellow humankind is an inspiring testament to the goodness of the human spirit. The Order has shown its versatility over the centuries, evolving from a Christian military order that undertook charitable works into an organization that today is open to citizens of all faiths and backgrounds who wish to help those in need. The attention given to the historical roots and foundations of the Most Venerable Order has helped serve as a touchstone for countless generations of members who have sought to carry forth the motto *pro fide, pro hominum.*

Following in the footsteps of Sir Edwin King and Sir Harry Luke has been a humbling experience. If this work has a fraction of the influence that *The Knights of St. John in the British Realm* had in helping members of the Order and broader society to understand its foundations and development then my task will not have been in vain.

This book is not an attempt to update *The White Cross in Canada,* the work of Colonel G.W.L. Nicholson and Colonel Strome Galloway. It is intended to provide a new examination of the history of the Most Venerable Order of the Hospital of St. John of Jerusalem — St. John Ambulance Brigade, and St. John Ambulance Association — in Canada; what is today known as St. John Ambulance.

I am grateful to His Royal Highness, The Duke of Gloucester, grand prior of the Order for providing a prefatory message for this book. I am equally grateful to Her Excellency the Right Honourable Michaëlle Jean, prior of the Priory of Canada, for including the foreword. The interest shown by these two senior officials of the Order speaks to the high regard with which the Order is held by our sovereign and her representatives.

The noted Acadian historian, Robert Pichette's advice was of great assistance in helping me to navigate the history of the Sovereign Military Order of Malta in Canada and the development of relations between it and the Most Venerable Order.

As with all of my previous works, I am indebted to two members of the Most Venerable Order: Bruce Patterson, Saguenay Herald, and Captain Carl Gauthier. Their friendship, editorial skills, and critical advice significantly improved the quality of this work. Through their advice and often entertaining marginalia the laborious task of editing the early drafts of this work was made more tolerable.

Thanks are owed to Judge René Marin, past chancellor of the Most Venerable Order for allowing me the opportunity to undertake this project. Never one to shy away from distributing tasks, Judge Marin's interest in this work and confidence in my abilities has been greatly appreciated. Similarly, Daniel Bellemare's persistent interest and desire to assist should not go without thanks and recognition. The present chancellor of the Order, John Mah has also shown an active interest in this work, which helped push it to completion.

At St. John national headquarters thanks are owed to the priory secretary, Dawn Roach, and to Patricia Kearney. Their tolerance of my work habits, sense of humour, and office tomfoolery has played no small role in the success of this history. From collaborating on such projects as national investitures in the Senate chamber to the logistical work behind getting a book to press their support has been crucial.

In the United Kingdom three individuals were particularly helpful to the author in navigating through a variety of sensitive issues. Rear-Admiral Andrew Gough, Professor Anthony Mellows, and Professor Jonathan Riley-Smith each provided important advice on content and proposed a number of important revisions.

Various friends encouraged me as I researched and wrote this work. Father Jacques Monet, Rev. Dr. Peter Galloway, Joyce Bryant, Robert Watt, Kevin MacLeod, Sean Morency, Lieutenant-Colonel Dan MacKay, Patrick Crocco, Vicken Koundakjian, and Charles Maier. Richard Brabander, delegate in Canada for the Johanniter Orden was most helpful in explaining the history of that noble order in Canada and its relationship with the Most Venerable Order.

My former employer the Honourable Noël Kinsella, Speaker of the Senate of Canada, a member of both the Order of St. John and Order of Malta was most supportive, as was my co-worker, Janelle Feldstein. Without their subtle support this project would not have come to fruition. The Honourable Marilyn Trenholme-Council, former vice prior of the Order in New Brunswick was also most supportive of my labours.

This is the first major historical project that I have undertaken with the support of a broader organization. My previous works on the Canadian honours system, Order of Canada, and Royal Victorian Order in Canada were all completed without support from the institution charged with their promotion and administration. Indeed, on occasion seemingly insurmountable obstacles were erected to hinder my progress in completing these earlier books. That some of those same officials who once busied themselves with games of circumlocution now see some value in recording the history of honours in Canada, beyond a colour pamphlet, is reassuring. Throughout the research and writing of this work, it has been an enjoyable experience to work with the various parts of St. John Ambulance. I have not forgotten the interest shown by members of the Order in my earlier works.

Lastly thanks are owed to my parents Paul and Sharon. Without their support for my various and many projects words would never reach the paper. During visits home to Kingston or while on holiday at the cottage their genuine interest in my endeavours is the fuel that powers my desire to write and research. As the descendant of a long line of eye care specialists, and the son of two optometrists it is a privilege to have been given the opportunity to recount the Canadian contribution to the St. John Eye Hospital in Jerusalem.

It is hoped that in these pages the reader will find that the Most Venerable Order is less a shiny piece of tinsel hung from black silk, than a living organization that has enhanced our national life here in Canada and in places all around the world.

Christopher McCreery, SBStJ, PhD, FRCGS
Priory Historian
Ottawa

SOURCES

This work draws heavily upon the annual reports of the Canadian branch of the St. John Ambulance Association, Commandery in Canada, and Priory of Canada. As a complete record of the state of the Order in Canada prior to 1911 does not exist, the annual reports of the St. John's Ambulance Association and St. John Ambulance Brigade Overseas have also served as an invaluable resource. Until 1980 these "British" annual reports of the Grand Priory, which should more correctly be recognized as "International" in scope, included summary reports from each priory and commandery.

The archives held at St. John's Gate in Clerkenwell, London, were also useful in tracing the development of St. John Ambulance in Canada. Similarly the archives maintained by St. John's Ambulance at its national headquarters in Ottawa were an invaluable resource. Nevertheless the archives are far from complete. As a non-governmental organization and charity, there has not been a strong focus on the preservation of documents related to the history of St. John Ambulance in Canada. Although inexcusable, it is understandable that St. John Ambulance in Canada chose not to focus any significant resources on the preservation of its documentary history. The provision of first aid training and first aid has always been the driving purpose of the organization, and in this context it is easy to see why resources were focused more on outreach and the provision of aid than on dusty documents. Any organization that losses track of its history is without a viable future.

As with any historical project such as this the author is faced with a dilemma as there is, and can never be, a complete set of documents detailing every aspect of an organization such as St. John Ambulance. A notable example of such gaps is found in the development of the brigade and association in Newfoundland before the province's entry into Confederation in 1949. Once situated in an independent dominion, equal in status to Canada, both the association and the brigade had some success on the island in the days leading up to the First World War. Although the inaugural meeting of the association was held in April 1910, other than the details held in the various British annual reports there is no wealth of information that can fully illuminate the history of St. John's Ambulance in Newfoundland. We know that first aid training courses were held sporadically between 1910 and 1949, and that at its height there were three brigade units on the island, but more concrete details are scarce. Indeed when the colony joined the Dominion of Canada in 1949, officials at St. John's Gate asked that all documents related to the association and brigade in the newly formed province be transferred to St. John's House in Ottawa. Whether the documents did not arrive or were simply discarded at some point is not known, but they do not seem to have survived in any quantity. We have lost a bit of who we are as an organization by not preserving our heritage. In the electronic age it is more important than ever to ensure that an accessible record is maintained for future generations.

It is hoped that this book will provide the reader with an engaging history of St. John Ambulance in Canada and the role that the Order has played in this country over the past century-and-a-quarter. The service rendered to countless fellow citizens through the provision of first aid training and first aid itself has and continues to be of immeasurable value. Like all organizations, the Order in Canada has experienced difficult times and — with the benefit of hindsight — made errors in judgment, but the positive contributions made by the individual members who make up St. John Ambulance have more than outweighed the missteps along the way.

INTRODUCTION

It is often difficult for some to understand that the Most Venerable Order of the Hospital of St. John of Jerusalem is both an honour, being an order of chivalry, and a charitable organization. While the honour side of the Order is self-evident, the charitable organization originally had three parts: the St. John Ambulance Association, the St. John Ambulance Brigade, and the St. John Eye Hospital in Jerusalem. Since 1974 the association and brigade have been combined into what is known as St. John Ambulance. Thus the term "Order" in the broadest sense refers to all the parts, while in the more narrow sense it refers to the order of chivalry that is an element of Canada's national honours system; St. John Ambulance being the operating arm of the Order. It is the modern day hospitaller work, which is first aid, that has given the Order its meaning and purpose. In the period immediately after the reactivation of the Order in England the membership was little more than a social dining club, with a marginal charitable purpose, for gentlemen interested in the concept of chivalry and honour. This would change through the vision of Sir Edmund Lechmere, Sir John Furley, Colonel Francis Duncan, and the Duke of Manchester. These four men worked in various ways to give the Order of St. John a modern charitable purpose, through the teaching and administration of first aid. While the Order had been transported to Canada in 1842, when Sir Allan Napier MacNab, premier of the Province of Canada, was made a Knight of Justice, it was not until the inaugural first aid class was held in Quebec City during the winter of 1882–1883 that the Order's first aid work began in this country. By the late Edwardian era, the value of first aid training was being more fully realized by members of the general public, labourers, and employers. In 1909 the first Canadian ambulance division of the St. John Ambulance Brigade (SJAB) was established, and in 1910 the Canadian branch of the St. John Ambulance Association (SJAA) was created, although there had been earlier incarnations of this body.

As an official history, this work seeks to provide members of the Most Venerable Order of the Hospital of St. John of Jerusalem and those interested in the work of St. John Ambulance with an accessible history of the overall organization in Canada. Despite being an official history, this work is not a hagiography, void of criticism or reflection. Such a work would be of little value other than as a pleasant story about the provision of first aid and an important element of the national honours system. To fully understand the growth and development of St. John Ambulance in Canada, both the successes and failures have to be revealed.

Other histories of the St. John Ambulance in Canada have been written. Most notably

G.W.L. Nicholson's *The White Cross in Canada,* published in 1967 and Colonel Strome Galloway's revision of this work, which was printed in 1983 for the centenary of St. John Ambulance in Canada. The present work is not an attempt to update or edit *The White Cross in Canada,* but to build upon the work undertaken by Nicholson and Galloway and provide a new perspective on the history of St. John Ambulance in Canada.

Sir Edwin King and Sir Harry Luke's *The Knights of St. John in the British Realm,* first published in 1924 and followed by a multiplicity of editions and revisions is a solid resource and immensely readable. *Hospitallers: The History of the Order of St. John* by Jonathan Riley-Smith is another useful resource for those wishing to learn about the Hospitallers and their early work. H.J.A. Sire's *The Knights of Malta* is a similarly accessible book, which provides a history of the Knights of Malta. For those seeking to learn about other priories with histories comparable to the Canadian Priory there is perhaps no better work than Ian Howie-Willis's *A Century For Australia: St. John Ambulance in Australia, 1883–1983.* Guy Stair Sainty's *The Orders of Saint John,* offers an excellent overview of not only the Most Venerable Order, but also the Order of Malta, and Johanniter Orden, along with the myriad of unrecognized Order's of St. John that have emerged over the past century.

The first two chapters of this work examine, in broad terms, the development of the Order of St. John and the association and brigade before the present organization was established in Canada. These chapters are intended to provide historical background related to the Order's early history, its development in England and eventual propagation throughout what is today know as the Commonwealth of Nations. It is within this context that St. John Ambulance was established and has flourished in Canada. The focus of this work is thus decidedly on the role of St. John Ambulance in Canada.

As integral components of the Order, the history of the association and brigade have been intermingled throughout, as it did not make sense to separate each of them; they are the component parts of modern day St. John Ambulance. Admittedly, less attention has been paid to the St. John Eye Hospital in Jerusalem. While Canadians have been involved in this foundation of the Order, it is St. John Ambulance that has been the primary and driving focus in Canada. Towards the end of the book, three separate chapters have been devoted to the Order and the awards of St. John Ambulance in Canada. These chapters examine the honours system side of the Most Venerable Order of the Hospital of St. John of Jerusalem and how the Order is the oldest continuously awarded element of our national honours system.

Similarly, the role and development of the various provincial and territorial councils has not been separated — other than in the case of Newfoundland — as this would require a separate chapter on each individual body. While the detailing of the most minute development at the provincial or even local level might provide some insight into the development of St. John Ambulance in Canada, it would fail to illuminate the national role that the organization has played. This being said, the provincial councils and the work done at the provincial and local level is the most important work undertaken by St. John. Specific provincial achievements and contributions are highlighted throughout.

Although we trace the founding of St. John Ambulance in Canada to the date when the inaugural first aid courses were offered, in 1882–83 in Quebec City and in 1883–84 at the Royal Military College in Kingston, St. John Ambulance has only been active in Canada without interruption since 1907. The period preceding this was one of sporadic operation, mostly centred in Toronto. St. John Ambulance has been active in peace and in war and it has been present at most of the great public events in our nation's history. It has also been present, along with other organizations such as the Red Cross, to help citizens in distress in some of the great disasters. From the Regina Cyclone of 1912 and the 1917 Halifax Explosion, to the Manitoba Floods of 1950 and the 1998 Ontario–Quebec Ice Storm, St. John Ambulance has been an active force for good.

One of the principal purposes of St. John Ambulance has been to impart knowledge of first aid and to provide first aid. Through these contributions St. John Ambulance has been at the leading edge, developing some of the first instructive silent films, with English and French subtitles — a real innovation in the early 1920s, as well as providing first aid manuals and classes in both official languages, at a time when the French language was marginalized. The training of Canadians in first aid, whether it be members of the Canadian Forces or various protective services, or to students at all levels of education, remains the most important asset and service that St. John Ambulance provides. The work of community volunteers in both traditional brigade activities, such as providing first aid services at public events, and non-traditional services such as the therapy dog program compose an important outreach component of St. John Ambulances continuing services to the Canadian public.

The effect of first aid training is immeasurable, because it often results in the saving of a human life.

ONE

ANCIENT AND HISTORICAL ORIGINS OF THE ORDER

Establishment of the Hospital of St. John of Jerusalem

Pro Fide, Pro utilitate hominum
Mottoes of the Order of St. John

Through the hospitaller tradition, initiated by the Blessed Gerard, the modern day Most Venerable Order of the Hospital of St. John of Jerusalem finds its guiding purpose and ethos. The work undertaken at the Hospital of St. John in Jerusalem nearly a millennium ago served as the foundation of the Hospitallers who would endure many privations, invasion, and exile, while always maintaining their commitment to serve humankind through the provision of care. This work has continued through the ages, in times of great wealth and, most important, in periods of despair. The eight-pointed white cross has, over nine centuries, come to be recognized as the symbol of the Knights Hospitaller and their devotion to treating the sick and injured.

The Hospital of St. John of Jerusalem, what would become the Sovereign Military Order of Malta (SMOM), began as a monastic community that ran a hospice in Jerusalem; founded as a religious order devoted to the treatment of pilgrims making the journey to the Holy Land. By 1160 the Order adopted a dual function of both hospitaller and defender of the faith, although the "process by which the hospital of St. John became a military order remains a mystery."[1] With this the Order "gained the unusual function of contributing to the physical defence,"[2] while simultaneously maintaining a "responsibility of caring for the sick and poor."[3] The principal role of the Hospitallers was to treat the sick and never to forget the paramountcy of Christian charity. Raymond de Puy, second master of the Order, best defined the military part of the Hospitaller's existence:

> never draw the sword except when the standard of the cross was displayed, either for the defence of the Kingdom of Jerusalem or in the siege of some enemy city.[4]

Other religious orders such as the Knights Templar existed for a sole military purpose, yet it was the dual purpose of the Hospital of St. John that would offer the Hospitallers great longevity, stretching into the modern age. Given the turbulence of the Holy Land and frequency with which Jerusalem was attacked, it was a practical development that the Hospitallers gained a military role. First located in Jerusalem (1099–1187), the Hospitallers then moved to Margat and Acre (1188–1291), then to the island of Cyprus (1291–1309), then to the island of Rhodes (1309–1522), and eventually to Malta (1530–1798), where they were expelled by Napoleon Bonaparte.

The number of Hospitallers in Jerusalem, Margat, Acre, Cyprus, Rhodes, and Malta was never large. In 1291 it is estimated that there were 300 brothers, during the period in Rhodes (1310–1523) there were between 250 and 450 brothers, we know there were 540 brothers defending Malta during the Great Siege in 1565, and that there were 332 present on the island when it fell in 1798. There were however a significant number of knights who lived on the continent.

Christian pilgrims began making their way to the Holy Land shortly after the death of Christ, and the tradition of travelling to Christendom's holiest places continues to this day. These early pilgrims were met with danger and disease in an unfriendly and foreign environment.

By 638 Jerusalem fell to the Muslims, who had a much more favourable attitude towards the Christian presence and allowed the hospice to operate unmolested. During the reign of Haroun al-Raschid as Caliph, the Emperor Charlemagne rebuilt and enlarged the hospice, which was destroyed in 1010 by the fanatical Muslim Caliph al-Hakim. Following the death of al-Hakim the hospice was restored by the citizens of Amalfi, the conditions in Jerusalem no longer being so hostile towards Christians. Located south of Naples, the city republic of Amalfi was an influential naval power in the region, holding a near monopoly on Egyptian and Syrian trade with Europe. By the middle of the eleventh century a group of Amalfi merchants revived the hospice to provide assistance to pilgrims and traders travelling through the Holy Land; the land on which Charlemagne's hospital and church was acquired and a new hospice was constructed. The hospice was dedicated to St. John the Almoner and was directed by the Benedictine Order, which had a history of ministering to the sick. For more than half a century the hospice operated without incursion from the non-Christian population. During this period the abbot of St. Maria Latina had appointed Brother Gerard to be rector of the pilgrim's hospice in Jerusalem.

The Hospitallers were not limited to ministering to the sick and injured in their hospital alone. They also possessed a mobile tent hospital that was used during the Crusades.[5] It is interesting to consider the similarities between the treatment of sick and injured soldiers throughout the Crusades and the treatment of wounded soldiers during the First and Second World Wars, treatment that was often dispensed in the field.

The period of relative tranquility came to an end when Palestine was conquered by Turcoman Muslims, who required payment of an admission fee in order to gain entry into the Holy City. The increasing difficulty that met pilgrims at they attempted to discharge their holy duty of travelling to Jerusalem was the principal cause behind the First Crusade which commenced in 1097.

Jerusalem was captured during the First Crusade on 15 July 1099. The hospice and Gerard worked ministering to the sick and injured Crusaders, and eventually annexed the old Orthodox monastery of St. John the Baptist, and the entire square below the Church of the

Holy Sepulchre was acquired. As a result of this move St. John the Baptist, "naturally became the patron saint of the new Order in place of the original patron and the old hospice."[6] Gerard separated the hospice from the Benedictines and adopted the Augustinian Rule to further demonstrate the independence of the new Order. Members of the Order wore a black *cappa clausa* (a long cloak) defaced with the white Amalfi cross on the breast. The members of the Order became known as Hospitallers and took three vows, of chastity, poverty, and obedience. Through a papal bull issued on 13 February 1113, Pope Paschal II put the hospital under his protection and allowed the Hospitallers to elect their own superior, thus making them an independent order. The Blessed Gerard, as he became known, was succeeded by Raymond du Puy in 1120. Du Puy would take the title of "Master" and guide the Order for the next forty years, building upon the solid foundations laid by his venerated predecessor.

As Master du Puy gave the Order its military dimension, the hospitaller responsibilities of the Order were retained. Sir Edwin King, the celebrated twentieth century historian of the Order in the British Realm noted that "if Gerard was the founder of the Order, none the less Raymond du Puy was its real maker."[7] He transformed a small community of monks ministering to the sick and injured into a powerful institution. A great builder, du Puy also permitted the establishment of priories throughout Europe. These semi-autonomous entities were responsible to the Grand Master. The move towards decentralized growth would be one of du Puy's greatest innovations as it provided the Order with increased strength through diversity and subordinate institutions that would become so widely spread that an attack on the Order as a whole was made nearly impossible. It was in this period that the Knights Hospitaller took the style Ordo (Order), "to describe their confraternity … future religious-military confraternities were described as such."[8]

Another improvement pioneered by du Puy was to divide the Order into different levels. At the top there were "Knights of Justice," men of noble birth who already held a secular knighthood and thus were armigerous (entitled to a coat of arms). On rare occasions men whose lineage was not noble, and therefore unable to hold a coat of arms, were admitted as "Knights of Grace." The second class was populated by monks and conventual chaplains who discharged ecclesiastical duties of the convent and priories. Lastly there were "Serving Brothers," who composed the largest number of members, being divided into servants of arms, who acted as esquires to knights, and servants of office who performed administrative duties.

The Holy Land was never free from threat and in 1187 the Sultan Saladin captured Jerusalem. In the battle that preceded the city's fall Roger Des Moulins, master of the Order, was killed and many Knights Hospitaller were captured, subsequently being dispatched for their refusal to renounce the Christian faith. The principal residency of the Hospitallers was then moved to Margat, north of Jerusalem. Here it remained for ten years when it was moved, this time to Acre, the main port of Palestine. Ever industrious, the Hospitallers constructed another large hospital. They would remain in Acre until 1291, when it fell to the Muslims. The Order was decimated during the defence of Acre, with only seven of the 140 defenders surviving.[9] The remaining knights fled to Cyprus where they would set up yet another hospital.

As the Knights Templar went into decline their order was abolished in 1312 by papal bull. Much of their property was absorbed by the Hospitallers and this greatly increased the wealth of the Order. In England, the Templars had long maintained the Commandery of Egle in Lincolnshire, which was duly absorbed into the Priory of England in 1340.

A new hospital was established at Limassol in Cyprus and the Order set about rebuilding and expanding. Here the Hospitallers formed a squadron of galleys becoming an important sea power in the eastern Mediterranean. Finding difficulties in Cyprus, the Order moved to Rhodes at the insistence of Pope Clement V. Rhodes was a notorious haven for Mediterranean marauding pirates who made travel and commerce highly dangerous. Rhodes was captured in 1310. The Hospitallers founded a convent there and were, at this time, given jurisdiction over the island. Knights from each kingdom formed separate parts of the convent known as Langues or Tongues. All the eight tongues were represented:

Table 1

Tongues of the Order of St. John[10]

Tongue	Priories
Provence	St. Giles and Toulouse
France	France, Aquitaine, and Champagne
Germany	Germany, Bohemia, Dacia (Scandinavia), Hungary, and the Bailiwick of Brandenburg
England	England and Ireland (including the commanderies of Scotland and Wales)
Aragon	Navarre, Catalonia, and the castellany of Amposta
Castile	Castile-Leon and Portugal
Italy	Lombardy, Venice, Pisa, Rome, Capua, Barletta, and Messina

The Order would remain in Rhodes for 200 years, constructing a cathedral, an impressive palace for the grand master, and a fortress that included a hospital, which was built in 1440. It was here that the Order gained great wealth, in part through its acquisition of the properties of the Knights Templar, and it became a prominent supporter of the arts. The island was attacked by the Turks in 1480, but after three months and significant losses to both sides the attackers retreated. The final blow came in 1522 when the tiny island was attacked by a force of 200,000 Turks under Sultan Suleiman the Magnificent. A six-month siege ensued, which resulted in heavy casualties on both sides. Grand Master Philippe Villiers de l'Isle Adam surrendered to the Turks to avoid the slaughter of the civilian population. So impressed was the Sultan with the Order's defence of the island, that he allowed the members to leave the island without let or hindrance. This was the second great crisis in the history of the Order. The previous loss of Acre two centuries earlier had nearly brought about the extinction of the Hospitallers, as had been the fate of the Knights Templar. The loss of Rhodes also posed another problem, as once again "it was possible for unsympathetic governments [...] to allege that the Order was failing to justify its existence."[11] Without territory and a hospital the Hospitallers lacked an ability to fulfill their purpose.

The surviving knights went first to Crete and then to southern Italy. Although the Grand Master had attempted to raise support for an expedition to recapture Rhodes he was unsuccessful. In 1530, the Holy Roman Emperor Charles V granted the Order sovereign power in Malta. After eight years without a permanent home the Order was finally able to focus on its good works.

One of the first projects undertaken was the construction of extensive fortifications to defend the island from invasion. In 1565 Suleiman the Magnificent laid siege to Malta with 180 ships and a landing force of 30,000. The defenders of Malta numbered approximately 8,000 and would put up a valiant defence, ultimately driving off the Turks. The presence of the Knights Hospitaller in Malta had the effect of securing the Mediterranean for Christian ships and commerce.[12] With the return of peace a new city was built, carrying the name Valetta in honour of the Grand Master who had directed the defence of the island. This would be the last time that the Turks would attack the island. The ensuing years were filled with prosperity and advances for the Order. A hospital had been constructed at Birgu in 1533 and yet another was erected in Valetta in 1575, known as the Grand Hospital/Sacred Infirmary. The move to Malta signalled the beginning of a golden age for the Hospitallers, who would more than exceed the successes they achieved in Rhodes. Yet, although the Order was flourishing in Malta and many other parts of Europe one of the wealthiest tongues, that of England, was soon to meet with disaster.

The care rendered to the sick by the Order became renowned throughout Europe. In the eyes of the Hospitallers, every patient or poor person in need of aid was Christ and required treatment of the highest standard, as though the Lord himself was receiving the care. Patients were given separate beds, in a time when only the wealthiest noble possessed such luxury. Silver utensils and plate were used for feeding the sick, along with a regimented diet of white bread, meat, and a wide variety of fruits and vegetables. Bed clothes and sandals were also provided and the bed linens were changed every fortnight. In an age when there was little understanding of the importance of cleanliness and a high quality diet for the sick, it is obvious that the Hospitallers were at the leading edge of medical care. By 1682 the Hospitallers began regulating medical practice through the development of strict requirements that had to be met before an individual could receive a medical licence.[13]

Throughout the Order's history the Hospitallers made no distinction on the basis of religion. "Knowing that the Lord, who calls all to salvation, does not want anyone to periods, mercifully admits men of the Pagan faith [Muslim] and Jews ... because the Lord prayed for those afflicting him ... 'love your enemies and do good to those who hate you.'"[14]

Malta provided an ideal home for the Order, as the fortress island was well suited to the Hospitaller's endeavours and, although not as fertile as Rhodes, it had the advantage of location and size. The golden age of the Hospitallers in Malta came to an end in 1798, not on account of incursion by the traditional adversary, the Muslims, but through the invasion of Napoleon Bonaparte. Indeed relations with the Ottoman Turks had improved so considerably that in the two decades preceding the fall of Malta, the Hospitallers, and Ottomans began exchanging diplomatic envoys.[15] That a French general not yet a ruler would effect the removal of the Hospitallers from the island of Malta was full of irony, especially given the high proportion of Frenchmen who were members of the Order.

The Order in England

The role of the Order in England is of particular interest as the Priory of Canada of the Most Venerable Order of the Hospital of St. John of Jerusalem was established as a branch of its English parent in the 1880s. The Knights of Malta were also active in New France and Acadia. This Canadian connection is examined in Chapter Two.

In the 1140s a commandery was established at Clerkenwell, which was dependent on the Priory of St. Gilles. It would not be until 1185 that the English estates were organized into a priory. The first known Knight Hospitaller in England was Gerard Jebarre, "who in 1135 was sent on a secret mission to the country to bring back Raymond of Poitiers."[16] Upon ten acres were constructed what would become St. John's Gate and the Priory Church, the latter being dedicated by the Patriarch of Jerusalem in 1185. The Order was also active in Scotland, where David I granted it the house of Torphichen sometime between 1143 and 1153, and Malcolm IV granted it "a house in every burgh in the kingdom."[17] A priory was established in Ireland outside Dublin at Kilmainham near Dublin in 1174. Scotland operated as a semi-independent commandery and was subordinate to the grand prior in England, and although Ireland had its own grand prior, it formed part of the Tongue of England in the organization of the Order. Given that England and Scotland were independent kingdoms these arrangements may seem odd, but they speak to the transnational character of the Order and its work.

The Hospitallers received gifts of land in Scotland and England beginning in the twelfth century, growing in influence and wealth through political connections and services rendered to the Crown. A number of priors held office as treasurers of the Crown and were active in English politics. Such political involvement was occasionally costly to the Order. The priory's buildings, including a hospital and church were destroyed during the Peasant Revolt/Wat Tyler's Revolt of 1382. The rebellion had broken out over the issue of taxation, and the wealthy priory was an easy target for the disgruntled peasantry.

By 1389 the establishment of the Order consisted of thirty-seven commanderies housing thirty-four brother knights, thirty-four chaplains, and forty-eight sergeants. This did not include Buckland, the Hospitaller nunnery that even as late as 1539 housed fifty sisters. In 1350 the estates of the Knights Templar were absorbed by the Order and the number of commanderies grew to thirty seven. Some historians have suggested that by the end of the thirteenth century the Hospitallers were the largest ecclesiastical land owners in all England.[18]

The Dissolution and Decline of the Order in England

Following the loss of Rhodes, Henry VII was of great assistance to the Order and a strong relationship was fostered between the English Crown and the priory in England.

The Priory of England and King had a close relationship; this was fully realized in 1506 when Sir Thomas Docwra, grand prior of England, arranged for the title "Protector of the Order" on Henry VII. The King took an active interest in the affairs of the Order and Docwra became a confidant of the King who paid regular visits to Clerkenwell.[19] Henry VII died in 1509 and was succeeded by his son Henry VIII. As a gesture of friendship the grand prior conferred the title "Protector of the Order" on the new King, and Docwra would go on to become close to the Henry VIII, who sent him on a number of diplomatic missions. Most significantly he participated in the meeting in the *Field of the Cloth of Gold* between the Kings of England and France. Despite holding the title of protector, following his break with Rome, Henry VIII felt no such compunction to actually protect the Order. Instead he repressed its operation, confiscated its holdings, and persecuted its members.

To some extent the priory was a victim of its own success. The building now known as St. John's Gate was completed in 1504, paid for through the immense wealth of the Grand Priory of England. After the dissolution of the Knights Templar, the priory in England consisted of 37 commanderies throughout the kingdom. Holder of more than 1,900 separate properties, in 1535 the priory headquarters at Clerkenwell had an annual revenues of £2,385 and the priory properties beyond had annual revenues of £3,206, both immense sums of money.[20] Of the other religious houses closed down under Henry VIII, only the monasteries at Westminster and Glastonbury had higher incomes. Sir Edwin King noted that Henry VIII was covetous of the wealth and properties of the Grand Priory of England. Always faced with financial difficulties, in 1527 Henry attempted to transfer responsibility of the English fortress at Calais to the Grand Priory. There is evidence to suggest that Henry intended to constitute the Tongue of England as a separate state military order, with the principal purpose of maintaining the Fortress at Calais.[21] Relations between the King and the Order deteriorated in the years leading up to England's break with the Roman Catholic Church. Following the death of Grand Prior Docwra, Henry VIII nominated a "court favourite" to become grand prior of the Priory of England, but another man, William Weston, had been chosen by the grand master. The situation was not helped by the fact that the King of France and the Holy Roman Emperor had both been consulted on issues related to the future of the Order, although Henry VIII was not. In an effort to placate the irascible Henry VIII, Grand Master de L'Isle Adam travelled to England to meet with the King. Upon his arrival in London he lodged at Clerkenwell, and then with great ceremony was processed to stay with the King. The meeting was convivial; Henry donated nineteen bronze cannon and more than 1,000 cannon balls as a contribution towards the defence of Malta. It was also agreed that Weston could become grand prior of the Priory of England, while the King's candidate John Rawson was reappointed prior of Ireland. L'Isle Adam departed England in early June 1528 and died six years later.

The story of Henry VIII's break with the Roman Catholic Church over the issue of the dissolution of his marriage is well known. Henry VIII's Queen, Katherine of Aragon failed to bear the King a son over their 24 years of marriage. The King became enamoured with Anne Boleyn, who regularly attended court. In an effort to divest himself of Katherine, Henry requested Pope Clement VII to dissolve his marriage on the grounds that he had married the widow of his deceased elder brother Arthur — a considerable sin. The Pope refused to grant the dissolution partly for religious reasons, but primarily because Katherine was the aunt of Emperor Charles V, Holy Roman Emperor. The situation escalated further when in 1534 the Pope excommunicated the King. Henry VIII retaliated by denying the Pope supremacy over the Church in England and thus appointed himself Supreme Head of the Church of England. With this England formally broke with the Roman Catholic Church. The newly elected Pope Paul III published a bull (papal letter) in 1536 calling on Charles V, Holy Roman Emperor to depose Henry VIII.

Institutions that were loyal to the Rome were dissolved over the next five years. As one of the staunchest supporters of papal supremacy, the wealthy religious orders were included. The Grand Priory of England was dissolved along with the other religious orders in 1540 by an act of Parliament. Knights who remained loyal to their respective orders were deemed to be acting:

> unnaturally and contrary to the duty of their allegiance sustained and maintained the usurped power and authority of the Bishop of Rome [Pope] and have not only adhered themselves to the said Bishop, being common enemy to the King our Sovereign Lord and to his realm, untruly upholding, knowledging and affirming maliciously and traitorously the same Bishop to be the supreme head of Christ's Church by God's holy words, intending thereby to subvert and overthrow the good and godly laws and statues of this realm their natural country, made and grounded by the authority of the holy Church by the most excellent wisdom and policy and goodness of the King's Majesty.[22]

The act transferred to the Crown all properties of the Grand Priory of England and also prohibited the wearing of the white cross of the Order. Henry VIII had been reluctant to attack the Order, which he held in high regard. The King gave members of the Order one chance to survive; in a patent dated 7 July 1538 he authorized Grand Prior William Weston to admit subjects of the Crown providing they agreed to take the oath to the King, and required that appointees to commanderies be confirmed by the King and pay their first year of revenues to the Royal Treasury. It is likely that the English knights could have accepted these regulations, however Henry VIII also required them to refuse to "recognize the jurisdiction or authority of the Pope."[23] The King was to have jurisdiction over appeals from the Order's provincial chapter and tithes were to be paid directly to the King. Given that the knights were sworn to defend and uphold papal supremacy such demands were unacceptable. Writing to the grand master in July 1539, Henry VIII demanded that "Papal supremacy should cease to be recognized by the Order in England."[24] Grand Master Juan de Homedes dispatched a special delegation to London in an attempt to reason with the King, but with no positive result.

Grand Prior Weston died on 7 May 1540 from a "broken heart," the same day that the Act of Dissolution came into force. Some knights renounced their vows, others fled to Malta, but three in particular remained and continued to profess their loyalty to their faith. For refusing to deny the Pope's supremacy over the Church the Blessed Adrian Fortescue, Brother Thomas Dingley and Brother David Gunstone were martyred. Fortescue and Dingley were beheaded on 10 July 1539 at Tower Hill, while Gunstone suffered a more brutal fate, being drawn and quartered at St. Thomas Waterings on 1 July 1541.

The Grand Priory of England had thus been dissolved by an act of Parliament, but this did not prevent the grand master of the Order in Malta from gathering together ten English Knights to prepare for the Order to return to England in the future.[25] The religious troubles being viewed as "temporary," it was decided not to fill the various posts of the Priory of England as they became vacant. Thus no new grand prior, turcoplier, and bailiff of Egle were filled following the death of their incumbents. So that the Tongue of England did not go without representation in the Order, Brother Oswald Massingberd was elected lieutenant-turcopolier, which now became the premier post within the Priory of England in the absence of more senior officials.

With Henry VIII's death in January 1547 there was hope that the King's policy towards the Order would be overturned. There was no immediate change until the death of King Edward VI and the accession of Queen Mary, wife of King Philip of Spain. One of the new Queen's driving ambitions was to see her country return to the fold of the Roman Catholic Church and to mend relations with Rome. Early in her reign, Mary dispatched Captain Ormond to Malta to enter into negotiations to effect the restoration of the priories of England and Ireland.[26] On 2 April 1557 letters patent were issued in the name of Philip and Mary authorizing Reginald Cardinal Pole, who was now archbishop of Canterbury, to restore the Order to its pre 1540 position and return all properties that had not yet been liquidated. Cardinal Pole subsequently issued a decree recognizing the Grand Priory of England and it appeared as though the Order would once again be able to flourish in England after more than a decade of uncertainty and despair.

Hope evaporated in November 1558 following the death of Mary. The new Queen, Elizabeth I, did not expend great efforts to suppress the Order, her "imposition of royal supremacy was less bloody than her father's"[27] but the remaining commanderies were confiscated, depriving the Order of any financial base, and making it impossible to undertake their traditional work. Likewise the Priory of Ireland became dormant in 1559. The Commandery of Torphichen did not become dormant, its commander converted to Protestantism and was granted the lands of the commandery as a Barony. Grand Master de la Valette sent a mission to England in the hopes of protecting the Order, but "in the prevailing atmosphere of the English court, no possibility of success existed."[28]

True to their faith and ever hopeful that God would deliver a revival of the Grand Priory of England, the Order in Malta continued to appoint knights to the various senior positions of the Priory of England. James II showed an interest in restoring the Order, but was only on the throne for three years, hardly enough time to take meaningful action, especially given the turbulent nature of the period. After James was deposed by William and Mary, hope for a revival of the Order was once again dashed. From 1689 to 1701, James's illegitimate son, Henry FitzJames held the position of grand prior of England, a title that would eventually pass to another illegitimate son of the King, Lord Peter FitzJames, for the year 1733, being succeeded by his younger bother Lord Anthony Bonaventure FitzJames, who served in this post until 1755.

There was a subsequent, and highly unusual, attempt to revive the Grand Priory of England in the late eighteenth century. The Elector of Bavaria, Charles Theodore, wished to see a tongue of the Order established in his principality. As a devout Roman Catholic, the possibility of becoming part of the Lutheran Bailiwick of Brandenburg was unfeasible. Charles Theodore approached Grand Master de Rohan in Malta and a plan was devised to incorporate Bavaria into the dormant Grand Priory of England as the Anglo-Bavarian Tongue of the Order. The consent of Pope Pius VI was obtained in 1782, and in an effort not to upset the King of Great Britain, George III was approached through the Neopolitian envoy to the Court of St. James to ensure that the revival of the old Grand Priory, albeit beyond the seas, was acceptable to him. As the creation of the Anglo-Bavarian Tongue was purely an administrative arrangement that had no effect on the affairs of Britain, George III consented to allow the name of the Grand Priory to be used. His interest in the matter "could hardly have been slighter."[29] The Anglo-Bavarian Tongue of the Order was established with the Grand Priory of Ebersburg and the Bailiwick of Neuberg, joined, on paper at least, with the Grand Priory of England, the Priory of Ireland and the Bailiwick of Egle. In 1785 the Grand Priory of Poland was added, but this was removed in 1797 following Russia's partition of the country. This highly unusual arrangement came to an end when King Maximilian Joseph of Bavaria, which had been erected into a kingdom in 1805, became embroiled in a series of disputes surrounding the Grand Priory of Poland. The King of Bavaria abolished the Priory in 1808 and the Anglo-Bavarian Tongue, which had become known as the Bavaro-Russian Tongue following the Treaty of Amiens 1801, vanished from existence.[30]

As we will see, Protestantism was not, as a rule, antagonistic towards the Order and this would play a significant role in the nineteenth century revival of the Order in England. The Hospitallers had operated in northern Germany beginning in the first half of the fourteenth century. Like the Priory of England their wealth and estates increased with the acquisition of Templar properties. In the Protestant German state of Brandenburg the local branch of the Order had remained in operation following the Reformation, as many brothers adopted Lutheranism and even married. These Lutheran Hospitallers were separated from the Order until the branch was officially recognized as a bailiwick by Grand Master Pinto in 1763. The bailiwick paid dues to Malta and even sent delegates to the Order's chapter general in 1776.

The Order was subsequently suppressed in Germany only to be re-established as the Bailiwick of Brandenburg by King Frederick William IV of Prussia in 1852. It was established as an independent protestant order, which is today known as the Johanniter Orden. The German example provided the template that Protestants in England hoped could be applied to the re-establishment of the Order in the British Isles.[31]

TWO

THE LONG ABSENCE

The White Cross Revived in England

The old Hospitaller Order of St. John revived in England half a century
ago has pursued a course of undemonstrated practical philanthropy
in the spirit of its founders, and in a way adapted to the
changes and changing circumstances of the 19th century.[1]
Major Francis Duncan, 1881

The history of the founding and flourishing of the Most Venerable Order of the Hospital of St. John of Jerusalem in Canada began across the Atlantic in England. It is through the attempted revival of the English tongue of the Order of Malta and the subsequent constitution of the Most Illustrious Order of St. John in England, that the modern Most Venerable Order was brought to Canada.[2] Certainly, without Royal patronage and formal recognition by the Crown in 1888, the Order would have been little more than a philanthropic club. Today it is accepted that the Most Venerable Order (Order of St. John) continues its "commitment to the traditions established by *The Order of the Hospital of St. John of Jerusalem* in the middle ages."[3] The Sovereign Military Order of Malta (the Order of Malta) is unquestionably the original order, while the Order of St. John, along with the other three members of the Alliance of the Orders of St. John of Jerusalem[4] stem from the same roots "and are orders of chivalry as well as being Christian confraternities."[5]

The establishment of the Most Venerable Order of the Hospital of St. John of Jerusalem in England was done under the rubric of reviving the English priory, often called the English tongue or langue — of the Order of Malta. The subsequent establishment of the Order of St. John is integrally tied to the failing fortunes of the Order of Malta and a series of conflicts that ravaged Europe in the later half of the eighteenth century. After the capture of Malta by Napoleon in 1798 the Order of Malta entered a period of nearly "forty years of stagnation."[6] Added to this situation were a number of opportunistic Frenchmen and an honour covetous group of Englishmen.

Following the restoration of the French monarchy, a number of Knights of Malta who resided in France offered knighthoods to various British subjects without any authority of the lieutenant-grand master. The actions of the French Knights of Malta in the 1820s provided the Order of St. John in England with an illegitimate continuity with the original Order of the Hospital of St. John of Jerusalem. This illegitimate continuity was legitimized by the Crown in 1888 when the Order was granted a Royal Charter and made an order of chivalry under the Crown.[7]

England comprised one of the Order's tongues before the dissolution of the Grand Priory of England by Henry VIII. The English tongue had been dormant for more than two hundred years as had the Order's Scottish commandery at Torphichen and the priory in Ireland both of which had been suppressed in the late 1550s.[8]

In the minds of those who reactivated the English tongue — which in their view had only been dormant and not abolished — the constitution of the English tongue was a reactivation, and not the creation of a new entity. While the reactivation of the English tongue was intended to be a revival of the Grand Priory of England, the subsequent refusal of the lieutenant-grandmaster of the Order of Malta to recognize the English priory resulted in the establishment of the Order of St. John as an entirely separate organization.

To fully understand how the Order came to England we must travel across the channel to examine events occurring in France and throughout Europe. While the Order had been dormant in England since 1558 following its suppression by Henry VIII, a brief revival by Queen Mary, and dormancy under Elizabeth I, it continued to exist in the abstract in the kingdom. There was also the brief revival of the Priory of England through the establishment of the short lived Anglo-Bavarian tongue of the Order between 1782 and 1808.

Despite the Reformation and the religious upheaval experienced throughout Western Europe, the Order remained very active in Malta, having been given sovereignty over the island by the Holy Roman Emperor, Charles V, in 1530 in his capacity as King of Sicily, and this was subsequently recognized by Pope Clement VII in a papal bull of 7 May 1530. It was the fall of Malta that brought about one of the greatest calamities in the history of the Order of Malta and played a major role in the revival of the Order in England.

Napoleon Bonaparte is an unusual figure to credit for the revival of the Order in England, but his invasion and conquest of Malta resulted in the dispersion of the knights throughout Europe. As a general, Napoleon was sent by the French government to capture Egypt, to protect France's trading interests in the area; the capture of Malta was a by-product of this expedition. Ignoring the neutrality of the Order, France invaded the island. On 12 June 1798 Malta fell to Napoleon, in part through the incompetence of Grand Master Ferdinand von Hompesch, who showed no aptitude for defending the island from foreign invaders, despite having 18,000 men at his disposal. Malta was, after all, one of the most heavily fortified citadels in Europe and could have in theory "held out for months even against a force as large as Napoleon's."[9] In his defence, the men were not highly trained, and the fact that the weapons and fortifications were ridiculously old is often overlooked.[10] The cannon in particular would have likely proven more deadly to their operators than as a weapon against the invaders.

Undoubtedly von Hompesch was aware that Lord Nelson and the Royal Navy were in the vicinity and certain to aid in the defence of the island from the French invaders. Scarcely seven weeks after the capitulation of Malta, Nelson destroyed the French fleet at the Battle of the Nile. This only had the effect of highlighting the feebleness of the grand master, who would retire to die in obscurity and poverty. Seven days after the fall of Malta von Hompesch fled the island along with many knights who returned to their native lands. Some however made their way to Russia to become part of the grand priory that had been set up there in 1782 as part of the Anglo-Bavarian tongue.

Czar Paul of Russia had been appointed Protector of the Order in 1799 and would go to some lengths to assist the Order.[11] The enthusiastic czar even contemplated sending the Russian Imperial Navy, under the Order's flag, to recapture Malta. It is difficult to account for his interest in the Order. It may well have been inspired by a desire to become more involved in Malta so the Russian empire could have a Mediterranean base, with protection of the island for the Order of Malta serving as convenient cover.[12]

It was well known that who controlled Malta was in a position to control most of the Mediterranean.[13] In spite of his earlier comment that "I would rather see the English on the heights of Montmartre than on Malta,"[14] by 1800 Napoleon's military fortunes had deteriorated and he was looking to divest himself of Malta. On 5 September 1800 Britain took control of Malta after the Maltese people asked the British to rid them of the French. The takeover was formally recognized by the *Treaty of Paris*, and the British would retain sovereignty over the island until 1964.[15] Although it was agreed in 1802 under the *Treaty of Amiens* that Britain would return the island to the Order, the island was never turned over: it was too valuable a strategic point to relinquish. The disastrous capitulation of the Order to the French in 1798 and failure to provide a meaningful defence of the island gave the British government no confidence in the Order's ability to prevent the islands from falling into unfriendly hands once again.

The Russian interference in the Order reached a peak. Czar Paul succeeded in having von Hompesch abdicate as grand master in July 1799, and subsequently had himself elected as the new grand master. This was a highly unusual move and against the statutes of the Order given that Paul was not a Roman Catholic. This further reveals the demoralizing effect of von Hompesch's surrender to Napoleon that a hitherto sovereign order was willing to elect a grand master who was in his own right an emperor, with interests that were not necessarily symbiotic with the Order itself. It can be speculated that members of the Order felt that in Paul they had the most realistic possibility of returning to Malta. Pope Pius VII opposed the election of the new grand master on the grounds that he was married and an Orthodox Christian who happened to be the head of a non-Roman Catholic state, in a position that had historically been held by a celibate Roman Catholic who owed allegiance to the Order and no specific nation.

Paul was furious with the British for refusing to immediately turn over the islands to the Order, and thus he imposed an embargo on all British ships entering Russian ports. His foreign policy became fixated on regaining Malta for the Order, and Russian authorities began impounding British vessels and burning those that attempted to evade the embargo. Given the recently proven prowess of the Royal Navy, this was a brazen act, one that in other circumstances would have probably lead to a complete deterioration in relations between Britain and Russia. Paul's assassination on 12 March 1801 brought an end to his antagonistic policy towards Britain, and the embargo was subsequently lifted.

Paul was succeeded by his son Alexander I, who assumed the title of Protector of the Order but refused to become grand master. Alexander was more practical and conservative when it came to Russia's position in world affairs and knew that it would do his country little good to become embroiled in conflict with Britain at this time. The subsequent deterioration in relations between Britain and France further prevented any discussion of returning Malta to the Order. It is interesting to note that many of the "unrecognized" orders of St. John claim to trace their lineage to the Russian period of the Order.[16] Not emanating from a legitimate head of state or sovereign authority they are little more than private clubs.

Pope Pius VII was requested to name Bailiff John Baptist Tommasi di Cortona as the new grand master. Tommasi di Cortona was charged with setting up a convent at Catania, only 86 kilometres south of Messina on the coast of Sicily, in close proximity to Malta. Sadly Tommassi di Cortona, who had made progress in rebuilding the Order, died in 1805 after only two years in office. He was replaced by Bailiff Innico-Maria Guevara Suardo who was styled lieutenant-master: no new grand master would be appointed until 1879.[17] The Order moved from Catania in 1826 to Ferrara in the Papal States and most recently to Rome in 1834, Pope Gregory XVI "Summoned the Convent from Ferarra to take up a new residence in the old Embassy of Malta in Rome ... the Pope's act had been that not of a despot but of a friend."[18]

The period following the capitulation of Malta and expulsion from the island was perhaps the most tumultuous in the Order's history; "the worst twenty years in the Order's history."[19] Out of this great calamity came the revival of the Priory of England. It became obvious to the Order that Britain intended to retain Malta and the island was eventually made a Crown colony.[20] With Malta out of their reach, the Order began looking for other territories. King Gustav IV of Sweden offered the Order the island of Gothland, which is located in the Baltic sea. This was graciously refused out of a fear that if they ensconced themselves in Gothland, a return to Malta would be prevented, their search for a home having been completed. During the Peace of Paris negotiations of April 1814, King Louis XVIII, the recently restored Bourbon monarch of France, proposed that the Order be given the Adriatic island of Corfu, but this suggestion was overtaken by events when Napoleon returned from Elba and once again Europe was thrust back into war.

The Congress of Vienna began meeting in September 1814 to decide on what the post-Napoleonic map of Europe would look like. Although the knights were party to these negotiations, they had little hope of influencing the transactions of the conference. They may have been sovereign in name, "but it was an impoverished body controlling no territory."[21] There was the additional fact that the knights of the various tongues were now widely dispersed throughout Europe.

The second restoration of the Bourbon dynasty in France brought new hope to the Order. During the French Revolution, all orders of chivalry, including the Order of Malta, were abolished by an act of the national assembly on 30 July 1791. The French tongues of Auvergne, Provence, and France were thus officially outlawed by the revolutionary government. Prince Camille de Rohan, grand prior of Aquitaine, convened a chapter general of the Order in 1814 to consider what future direction the Order should take. This chapter general transpired in Paris and would result in the election of a capitular commission, which consisted of the prince and six senior knights, two from each of the French tongues of the Order. Through a misinterpretation of a papal letter from Pope Pius VII dated 10 April 1814, the commission "arrogated to themselves the right to manage the order's affairs."[22] The commission viewed the convent at Catania as being devoid of authority and thus decided to take on the role of managing the French tongues and the affairs of the whole Order throughout Europe. The lieutenant-grand-master had little choice but to recognize the authority of the commission, as did Louis XVIII.[23] France after all held the largest number of living knights and according to the noted scholar Géraud-Marie Count Michel de Pierredon, the commission functioned *de facto* if not *de jure*.[24]

The commission was primarily concerned with protecting the interests of the Order at the Congress of Vienna. They hoped to obtain a Mediterranean island in compensation for their loss of Malta. The congress merely confirmed that Malta was a British possession, and little attention was given to the desire of the Order to re-establish itself. The commission then entered into negotiations with the Greeks, who were fighting in a war of independence from the Ottoman Empire. Greece proclaimed itself independent in 1822, and in July 1823 the Order signed a treaty with Greece in which it was agreed that the islands of Sapienza and Cabrera would be ceded to the Order with a proviso that Rhodes would be given to the Order if it were captured from the Ottomans. All that was required of the Order and the capitular commission was to raise £640,000 in bonds redeemable at the lucrative interest rate of 5 percent over twenty years. It was a tremendous amount of money for the period.[25] All of these large scale real estate deals came to naught, the Austrians disapproving of such transactions in their sphere of influence, and because the lieutenant-master of the Order, Anthony Busca, did not agree with the proposed deals. Indeed Busca worked to have the Commission disbanded, which occurred in 1824. Nevertheless the commission continued to operate without the sanction of the French Crown or lieutenant-master; even trying to raise the £640,000 after its disbandment.

Given the virtual successes encountered by the capitular commission, they refused to dissolve having spent more than a decade working towards gaining a new home for the Order, while the lieutenant-master merely administered the convent at Catania. The commission thought of itself as an effective body that was ensuring the longevity of the Order. The three French tongues of the Order were much more influential and powerful than the convent at Catania, and they were under the protection of Louis XVIII and had done more to preserve and enlarge the Order than had been achieved by any group or single person since the capitulation of Malta.

To enhance their base of support, the capitular commission began seeking help from abroad. The grand chancellor of the Order, the self-styled Marquis Pierre-Hippolyte de

Sainte-Croix-Molay, who was by this point leader of the commission, had the idea of reviving the English tongue of the Order. Britain was unquestionably the wealthiest and most powerful Empire in the world, commanding the seas, with colonies on every continent, and as pre-eminent leader in international trade, had the potential to be a valuable ally and supporter for the Order. It was also widely known that the properties of the Order in England had been among the most profitable and influential before being dissolved by Henry VIII. The Marquis de Sainte-Croix Molay was a shadowy figure and we know relatively little about him. He has been accused by some of staging an elaborate confidence trick that resulted in the false reactivation of the English tongue through exploiting the interpretation of Pope Pius VII's letter of 1814.[26]

One of the positive actions taken by the disgraced Grand Master von Hompesch, before the fall of Malta, was to appoint a number of influential English gentlemen into the Order. This, coupled with the fact that Czar Paul had freely admitted a number of British subjects into the Order, provided a ready-made group of supporters for the revival of the English tongue. This list even included Lady Emma Hamilton, Lord Nelson's paramour.

The Marquis de Sainte-Croix-Molay engaged in a series of discussions with members of the Order in England. Through these discussions, articles of convention were drawn up over the period of June 1826 to October 1827 that delineated how the tongue of the Order would function as the revival of the Grand Priory of England. One of the main obstacles was the fact that most Britons were Protestant; and not even of one denomination; from Anglicans and Presbyterians to Methodists and Baptists, there was a great diversity of religion accepted in England, unlike most other European countries.

There were however other precedents for the admission of non Roman Catholics. Both the Lutheran Bailiwick of Brandenburg and the Orthodox Grand Priory of Russia, admitted non-Roman Catholic adherents to the local religion. In a detailed letter of instruction, the grand chancellor laid out that "candidates might be admitted and received according to the mode and form used by the Bailiwick of the Reformed religion,"[27] but he also stipulated that Roman Catholic brothers of the Priory of Ireland would have to follow the statutes of the Order in their entirety. The "Articles of Convention" clearly set out that the English tongue was being revived with the approval of the three French and two Spanish tongues of the Order.

To oversee the reactivation of the English Priory Philippe de Chastelain, a French knight, represented the capitular commission and Donald Currie represented the British membership.[28] Currie set about raising the £640,000 that had been promised to leaders of the Greek War in Independence in August 1827. All this despite the fact that the lieutenant-master had published a disavowal of the attempt to raise the money in 1824 and had also dissolved the capitular commission. Sainte-Croix-Molay who refused to acknowledge the actions of the lieutenant-master continued to raise money. He commissioned Currie to raise £240,000 in donations to hire men and buy the necessary arms, ammunition, and ships for a Mediterranean expedition. It was an extraordinary fanciful plan, one that never left paper. Currie was unable to raise any significant amount of money, although he had successfully recruited a few hospitallers, who "formed the basis of the new [English] langue."[29] Of course, without recognition by the lieutenant-master of the Order of Malta in Rome the English tongue was an entirely private organization.

The reactivation of the Priory of England was lethargic, there being a significant delay between the decision of the Capitular Commission and events in London. Finally on 29 January 1831 the Reverend Dr. Robert Peat,[30] a former chaplain to King George IV was elected as the first active grand prior *as interim* in England in nearly 300 years.[31] The English tongue was thus revived in law. With this, the English tongue believed itself to be fully legitimate, with the support of the French and Spanish tongues, and thus began to solicit support from eminent men of social standing. Peat and other officials of the Order expected that the dormant, but still extant, Royal Letters Patent of Mary I, which had reconstituted the Order in 1558 after the death of Henry VIII provided all the legitimacy of a connection to the original English tongue of the Order. Peat took the grand prior's oath, as required under the Royal Letters Patent of Queen Mary before the Lord Chief Justice of England at the Court of King's Bench at the Guildhall on 24 February 1834.[32] The revival of the Order through Queen Mary's dormant letters patent was legal in the eyes of the English judiciary, but not in the eyes of the lieutenant-master of the Order in Italy. One noted historian of the Order of St. John observed that "without recognition of the Lieutenancy in the early 19th century the English Priory was a purely private organization."[33]

Following Peat's death in 1837, he was replaced by Sir Henry Dymoke. The other great supporter of the revival, Sainte-Croix-Molay, had died in 1841 and this would lead to further complications as the Capitular Commission had been abolished. The purpose of the Order in England had been delineated in the Nine Declaratory Resolutions published on St. John's Day 1841, and this would become the cornerstone of the constitution of the Order of St. John. The 1849 statutes of the Order sought to explain the revival of the English tongue:

> in the RECLAMATION preferred to the Congress of Sovereigns, at Verona, in 1822, by Count Achille de Jouffroy, as the accredited Envoy of the three Langues of France, and those of Castille and Aragon — through the instrumentality of which five important branches of the Order the LANGUE OF ENGLAND was formally reorganized between 1826 and 1831 — it is set forth that the Order of St. John is necessarily a rallying point throughout Europe for all friends of religion, reason and good will, without inconvenience of government, cost to people or irritation of opinions.[34]

The statues went further, explaining that

> the Order of St. John being the sole POINT d'APPUI in all Europe for gentlemen of high chivalrious sentiment, active benevolence, and social virtue; it needs but such an accession to its ranks as what the gentiticial families in England, Scotland, Ireland, Wales and the races sprung from their blood, can well supply to make its trophied and time-venerated

banner once again the "LAUS ET TUTAMEN" of all who in their respective birthlands fear God, honor their sovereign and love their fellow kind.[35]

The French tongues of the Order returned to the control of the lieutenant-master who was now resident in Rome. The lieutenant-master was increasingly reluctant to admit Protestants to a Roman Catholic order and he advised that unlike the Bailiwick of Brandenburg, every English Protestant put forward for appointment to the Order would have to receive a special dispensation.[36] Admission to the Order was further restricted in 1843 when Lieutenant-Master Charles Candida refused to admit any person from the English tongue other than Roman Catholics. Members of the English tongue of the Order attempted to open negotiations with the lieutenant-master in Rome, but they met little success.

Again, events in France would play a role in the future of the English tongue. The three French tongues of the Order had returned to the control of the lieutenant-master in Rome following the downfall of the French monarchy in 1848. The overthrow of King Louis-Philippe and the events of 1848 lead to the near extinction of the French tongues of the Order. They were thus no longer in a position to support the fledgling Grand Priory of England that they had played such a central role in reactivating.

Authorities in Rome had never been enthralled with the inclusion of so many Protestants in the Order from the English tongue[37] and continued to have difficulty with the mode by which the Grand Priory of England was revived by the questionable Marquis de Sainte-Croix-Molay. Literally "the possibility of another non-Roman Catholic branch of the Order was no longer viewed with sympathy."[38] Thus the final act of Fra Philip von Colloredo, lieutenant-master of the Order in relation to the English tongue, came in 1858. He informed members of the English tongue that the actions of the Capitular Commission and the three French tongues of the Order in reviving the English tongue were illegitimate, just as Rome now considered the English tongue of the Order.

The English tongue of the Order was initially re-established as a tongue of the Order of Malta, and regarded the lieutenant-master in Rome as its superior, even if the Order of Malta did not recognize it. Although they "sought only to conform to the general policy of the Sovereign Military Order of Malta,"[39] questions about the legitimacy of the actions of Sainte-Croix and the involvement of Protestants were clearly a great concern for the authorities in Rome.

Disowned and declared illegitimate by the Order of Malta, the English tongue had few options, not surprisingly it took the boldest of those available and set out to ignore the lieutenant-master in Rome and declare its independence. With this the Most Illustrious Order of St. John of Jerusalem; England, sometimes known as the "Illustrious and Sovereign Order of the Knights Hospitallers of Saint John of Jerusalem, Venerable Langue of England, Comprehending the Grand Priories, Bailiwicks and Commanderies in England, Scotland, Ireland and Wales," was established in 1858. This title was changed in 1871 to the Order of the Hospital of St. John of Jerusalem in England, and the Order adopted a new constitution at the same time.

The lieutenant-master and officials of the Order of Malta in Rome likely assumed that without their support and approval that the English tongue would simply wither and fade into the scenery. Given the extremely lethargic growth of the English tongue and collection of questionable characters that it encompassed through the 1820s and 1830s it is understandable that the lieutenant-master in Rome came to this conclusion. Nevertheless, the establishment of an entirely separate order had the opposite effect, though it would take some time for the organization to fully flower. With Royal patronage and a newfound purpose in first aid training, the lack of recognition from Rome and the Order of Malta was of little concern as the Order of St. John grew from an organization fixated on the theatrical side of the Knights of Malta, to the relief of human suffering and first aid training.

A Christian Order

That the English tongue of the Order was from its inception open to Christians of all adherences was a novelty, one that helped to ensure, unintentionally, the split from the Order of Malta. The Order of Malta was limited in membership to Roman Catholics alone. Non-Roman Catholics had to seek a special and individual dispensation from the Pope to become a member of the Order.

In the early stages following the reactivation of the English tongue the Order was open to both Roman Catholics and Protestants. That the Order admitted any Christian who ascribed to its Christian purpose, was in many ways the product of Victorian liberalism and a "greater concern with society as a whole ... and how the good of the individual was to be promoted."[40] The same liberalism that played an important role in the granting of responsible government to residents of British North America and eventually lead to Confederation and the establishment of the Dominion of Canada.

Although England, like most European countries of the period, had a state church, the Church of England, the unique structure of the United Kingdom and broader Empire prevented the restriction of the Order to Anglicans alone. Scotland was predominantly Presbyterian, Ireland Roman Catholic, and the various colonies and dominions were even more diverse in their religious composition. The issue of religious affiliation was particularly important, "the Ancient Statutes of the Order in general are acknowledged in so far as they are compatible with the principles of the Church of England allegiance to the reigning Sovereign and the existing state of British society."[41]

Beyond Dreaming: First Aid and the Order of St. John

The transformation of the Order from a group of men who wanted to don the costumes of knights from days of yore and learn about the principles of chivalry, into a broad-based civic organization promoting the Christian values of faith, hope, and charity was not instant. The Victorian concept of civic responsibility, public education, and self help played a significant role in making the Order into a working order and more than just an honour. Before the 1870s the Order of St. John was, to put it kindly, a "backward-looking body of dreamers,"[42] with no purpose other than to hold fancy dress parties and attend social engagements. It was a relatively easy way for an individual to obtain a grandiose title and set of insignia for a modest donation and token involvement. If the Order was to gain legitimacy, it required a driving purpose.

It was a quartet of adept administrators and promoters who fashioned the Order into the charitable organization that we are familiar with today. Sir William Drogo Montague 7th Duke of Manchester, Sir Edmund Lechmere, Sir John Furley, and Colonel Francis Duncan would energize and build the Order of St. John into the foremost first aid training organization in the world. Duncan was an Army colonel who had served in Canada from 1857 to 1862 and later in Egypt. A gunnery instructor in the Royal Artillery, he did not limit his zeal for education to military matters alone, this largely explains his involvement with St. John and the important role he played in establishing a centre at Woolwich. Another person who would offer legitimacy was Prince Arthur Duke of Connaught, who maintained a near lifelong connection to the Order. Manchester was elected as grand prior of the English tongue of the Order in 1861, a post he would serve in until 1888 when the office was assumed by Albert, Prince of Wales, the future Edward VII.

While the interest of the Order in hospitaller work was natural given the historic disposition to such endeavours, it was the series of conflicts that ravaged Europe and the resulting conferences that helped to push the Order towards undertaking work in the first aid field. During the brief Schleswig-Holstein War of Succession of 1864,[43] Furley served on the senior staff of the Danish Army and was exposed to the horrors of armed conflict and the resulting suffering of the injured on both sides. Furley became particularly concerned by the treatment of the wounded and the haphazard way in which medical attention was dispensed.[44] He reported that the war "opened our eyes to the fact that in such matters [first aid and relief] we were lamentably behind the rest of Europe."[45]

As a result of his observations, Furley came to work with Henri Dunant and the Red Cross Societies. Dunant had been greatly influenced by the innovations in treatment made by Florence Nightingale during the Crimean War. Aside from the use of statistics to evaluate treatment methods and conditions, something that had hitherto never been employed, Nightingale's the most significant discovery was that improving sanitary conditions of hospitals greatly reduced the mortality rate.

The First Geneva Convention was held in 1864 and was attended by leaders from fourteen European nations. The conference was in large part organized by Dunant, who ensured that the Order of St. John was present.[46] Furley would attend subsequent Red Cross conferences in Paris, 1867 and Berlin, 1869. This would mark the beginning of a long association between St. John and the Red Cross in times of armed conflict. The potential for the Order to take on a leading role in first aid training was made clear by the extent of suffering experienced by the wounded on the battlefield and the lack of organized training or relief for those in need.

The Franco-Prussian War, which broke on 19 July 1870, provided an opportunity for the

Order to become directly involved in relief work. Early in the conflict, the Order acted as the British branch of the Red Cross Society. The Duke of Manchester headed up a group of members of the Order, including Furley and Lechmere to help found the British National Society for the Sick and Wounded, the forerunner of the British Red Cross Society. The Society sent an Anglo-American Ambulance Unit to provide battlefield service during the Franco-Prussian War, and Furley served as one of the joint commanders. The unit employed a staff of just over 200 surgeons, nurses, and orderlies who supplied both sides with medical supplies and hospital related equipment. Furley and other members of the Order who witnessed the war and participated in the work of the ambulance unit were dissatisfied with the aid that the Red Cross was providing, which was simply delivering supplies, although under difficult circumstances. They saw that there was great opportunity for the provision of treatment and healing — much in the vein of the hospitallers during the crusades — and they wanted to help the individual casualties, not simply deliver bandages and blankets.

In a limited sense, what today we would call humanitarianism was simply seen as part of the broader progressive social reforms of the Victorian era. The Order of St. John took on its devotion to first aid training and to the treatment of suffering in the context of other humanitarian organizations that grew out of nineteenth century British society; the Red Cross, Elizabeth Fry Society, John Howard Society, Royal Society for the Protection of Animals, the Royal Society for the Protection of Life from Fire, the various Temperance Unions, and even religious organizations such as the Salvation Army owe their founding to this period.

Lechmere, who became secretary-general of the Order in 1866, had been trying to define what precise charitable work the Order should undertake.[47] In addition to the work undertaken as part of the Anglo-American Ambulance unit, meetings of the Order increasingly became places for the discussion of sanitary education, diets for the poor, how to treat the ill, and how to effectively transport the sick. Out of these discussions the medical committee was formed to refine first aid techniques and teaching methods.

The Franco-Prussian War was a turning point, because for the first time the organization was actually involved in relieving suffering. The war also forced Lechmere, Furley, and other senior leaders of the Order to consider how to efficiently transport the wounded and injured. To this end, it contributed £100 towards the first British ambulance transport unit in 1872. By 1876 the Order had developed its own vehicle for the conveyance of the sick and by 1890, they were selling them all over Britain. This was followed by instructional classes held for members of the public on how to carry the ambulances, and with this the "Ambulance Department" of the Order was created in 1875.

War between Turkey and Serbia broke out in 1876 and the Order sprung into action, founding the Eastern War Sick and Wounded Fund "for the purpose of affording such aid as is possible to sufferers in the conflict raging in the East."[48] This fund was eventually merged with the British National Society for Aid to the Sick and Wounded. A group of thirty five surgeons, nurses, and orderlies were dispatched to serve in tent hospitals set up on the conflict region, St. John medical supplies being provided to both sides. The fact that supplies were provided to both sides revealed the true humanitarian nature of the work being undertaken; it also demonstrated the level of religious tolerance that was present. That the Order of St. John, which was founded to treat the wounded and defend the Holy Land from Muslim invaders, was now providing relief to Muslim Turks was a remarkable development. This would lead directly to the establishment of the St. John Ambulance Association the following year.

The first aid education activities of St. John were expanded in the wake of these conflicts. Duncan worked closely with Surgeon Major Peter Shepherd of the Royal Herbert Military Hospital at Woolwich. Commencing training in a bustling military community, in which ongoing education was an every day part of life, especially for members of the Army, was particularly fortuitous and lead to the rapid spread of St. John first aid courses throughout Britain, and eventually overseas.[49] Sir Edward Sieveking, a noted surgeon, Physician Extraordinary to Queen Victoria, physician to the Prince of Wales, and inventor of the aesthesiometer who had been involved with the Order since the early 1870s, founded the St. John Ambulance Association in 1877. This marked the establishment of the first modern foundation of the Order. The purpose of the association was to "train men and women for the benefit of the sick and wounded."[50] The direct involvement of women, from its founding as a first aid training organization would serve as yet another asset to the Order and its work. Overall, the idea of teaching basic first aid to civilians was a "radical new enterprise,"[51] and one that would launch the newly founded St. John Ambulance Association to national notoriety in Britain and the Empire. Associations with teaching hospitals in London were quickly established and first aid classes began to be offered to the general public. These activities were organized through the Ambulance Department. Another innovation was the triangular bandage, invented in Switzerland by Dr. Mayor [first name not recorded],[52] which was a great improvement over the roller bandage.[53] Another development was the modification of what were known as "litters" or "ambulances," and what today we would call a stretcher with wheels. The first two-wheeled litter was brought from France and greatly improved by St. John for use on battlefields or in industrial and urban areas.

The inaugural first aid class was held in January 1878 in a small church hall in south east London. From there "the concept of first aid teaching quickly expanded," and within a week a similar course was held at Chelsea Barracks.[54] By 24 June 1878 "at least 1,100 people had been taught [St. John first aid] to treat the wounded, and in case of war [the St. John Ambulance Association] had registered the names of 192 men and women, all skilled nurses, who were prepared to go abroad at any moment for the purpose of attending injured soldiers."[55] The first ambulance text book, *Aids for the Cases of Injuries and Sudden Illness,* was published in 1878 and met with great success. Written by Surgeon-Major Peter Shepherd,[56] it was used by the London Metropolitan Police and by the Order of St. John throughout the Empire.

The following year brought more advances, by 1879 a formal syllabus had been developed for teaching first aid, this included:

1. Objects of work, especially consequences of mishandling of sick and injured;
2. Position of main arteries and veins, and extemporized methods of controlling bleeding;
3. Recognition of fractures and use of extemporized material as splints and bandages;
4. Transport of patients by stretcher and ambulance wagon, and methods of extemporizing stretchers or adapting country carts;
5. Immediate treatment of suspended animation due to drowning, sewer gas, fainting, collapse, shock from server injuries, burns, and scalds.

A special sixth part was held for ladies on nursing and how to maintain the room of a person under care. Similar educational material sanctioned by St. John had been published in the Woolwich newspaper the *Kentish Independent* in March 1878,[57] and this had a salutary effect in fostering public interest. With the expansion of training came the introduction of the familiar first aid certificates, which continue to be issued to this day.

The second foundation of the Order was established in 1882 when the Ophthalmic Hospital was opened near Jaffa Gate in Jerusalem. Dr. J.C. Wardell and Lechmere had worked with the British Ambassador to the Ottoman Empire to obtain land for a hospital, "for the alleviation of the terrible sufferings caused by diseases of the eye."[58] The Turkish government was forthcoming with permission and the Ophthalmic Hospital of the Order of St. John was subsequently opened under the name the British Ophthalmic Hospital. The main purpose of the hospital was to provide ophthalmic medical care to the sick in the Holy Land, there being a high prevalence of eye diseases such as, iritis, papilledema, glaucoma, and general infections and nutritional deficiencies that affect the human eye. A small four bed hospital was constructed and within six months more 1,952 patients had been treated.[59] A by-product of establishing the Ophthalmic Hospital in Jerusalem was the prestige that came with it. The Order of St. John, which had been shunned and disowned by the Order of Malta was now present and active in the Holy Land, reviving the hospitaller work of the knights that establish the Order in 1099.

In 1887 the St. John Ambulance Brigade, the third foundation of the Order, was established. In March a conference of physicians and surgeons was held at St. John's Gate by the St. John Ambulance Association. The principal purpose of the conference was to "consider what measures may be adopted to interest the public, and to promote the branch of the work of the St. John Ambulance Association which is connected with the conveyance of the sick of all classes."[60] This meeting set the groundwork for the establishment of the "Ambulance Brigade." It was unanimously agreed first, that a proper system of transport of invalids in London and throughout the country is very desirable and second, that this meeting has confidence in the organization initiated by the association and will use every endeavour to develop and extend this useful work, which has now been underway for nearly four years. Thus the brigade was a child of the association. In June 1887 the brigade was established "as a civilian organization for civilian needs and as army and navy reserves."[61] The brigade in part constituted an amalgamation of the various Ambulance Corps of the association that had been set up since the establishment of the "Ambulance Association" in 1877.

The newly formed St. John Ambulance Brigade would play an important role in Queen Victoria's Golden Jubilee celebrations in London. Fifty members of the brigade, along with horse-ambulances, provided important first aid services during the massive celebrations held in London. During the Jubilee parade more than 200 people were treated by the brigade,[62] and thus the role of St. John at major national, cultural, and sporting events, not to mention in time of conflict, was brought fully onto the national stage in Britain. The purpose of the brigade was different from that of the association in that the brigade was to serve as a pool of trained personnel who could provide first aid treatment during emergencies and public events.

Historic Clerkenwell was purchased by the Order of St. John in 1874. Cardinal Wiseman of the Order of Malta also bid on the building but was unsuccessful in his attempt to buy the property which he intended to give to the English association of the Order of Malta, which was created in 1875. Clerkenwell would become the world headquarters of the Order of St. John. In a period in which the Order of Malta and authorities in Rome regularly questioned the legitimacy of the Order, the re-acquisition of Clerkenwell was a significant symbolic victory in the period before friendly relations were established between the two orders.

Growth Beyond the Seas

Following the revival of the English tongue of the Order, the Priory of Scotland was re-established. As the first aid training direction of the Order expanded, so did its operations throughout the British Empire. Given the fluid nature of the Empire and the relative ease with which government officials moved from territory to territory, it was only natural that the Order and its work was to spread to every corner of the globe. This proliferation was primarily on account of the valuable first aid training, not out of a desire to recreate the ideal of ancient chivalry that was the main attraction to many of those involved in the English tongue immediately after its revival in 1831. The attraction of education and civic betterment was far more enticing, and part of what has been described as the broader "humanitarian impulse of [the British] empire,"[63] as it expanded in influence.

By 1882, the year before the inaugural first aid class was delivered in Canada, St. John had established 130 centres in Britain and throughout the Empire. This included not only the provision of first aid training, but also handbooks and supplies. The Order was forging lasting links with army and police services as well, while bringing home nursing and hygiene courses to the public. Lechmere's vision of the Order of St. John; bringing hospitaller aid to the sick and wounded in the modern era, was being realized.

In 1881 the St. John Ambulance course in first aid was being taught in England, Wales, Scotland, Ireland, the United States, Russia, Germany, and Australia. The first separate overseas centres of the St. John Ambulance Association were set up in Malta and on the French Riviera — where many Britons holidayed — in 1883. Centres were also established in Bermuda, the Bahamas, Gibraltar, and most significantly India, where much suffering was relieved. Hong Kong followed in 1884, while New Zealand, Singapore, South Africa, and Jerusalem were established as centres in 1885. Although St. John first aid had been taught in Canada as early as 1882, it would not be until 1897 that Canada was established as a centre. Throughout the empire the Order was spreading, with its message of self improvement through first aid training. This is the principal reason that it continues to perform first aid training and provide ambulance services in many parts of the modern Commonwealth.

The Order of St. John has spread the hospitaller work — in the form of first aid training and emergency services — in a way never imagined by the original Knights Hospitaller in 1099, to parts of the globe that were not even known to exist at the time. The Order spread throughout the Commonwealth and has become the largest Order of St. John in the world. The Christian characteristics of faith, hope, and charity remain, though the Order has adapted to welcome people of all faiths and backgrounds working together to relieve the suffering of humankind wherever it may occur.

The Sovereign Head

Before the Royal Charter of Incorporation of 1888, the Order of St. John had no official status in Britain or throughout the British Empire as an honour. This situation was not unlike that now experienced by bodies using the name designation The Order of St. Lazarus. The Order of St. John was simply a charitable organization that involved itself in the teaching of first aid ambulance duties that happened to have attached to it an order of chivalry; one that was unrecognized by all relevant authorities — the Order of Malta, Papal officials, and, most important, the government of the United Kingdom. As we have seen, in the early days following the revival most members of the Order were romantics who were more concerned with recreating the ancient concept of chivalry than performing hospitaller work of any description. The involvement of the Prince of Wales was central in affording legitimacy to the Order as it evolved from what was little more than a private club to an official British order of chivalry engaged in important charitable works.

The first formal involvement of the royal family with the Order of St. John came in May 1879 when the Duke of Edinburgh and Prince Leopold became presidents of the Ashford and Oxford Centres of the association respectively.[64]

The Duke of Manchester and Lechmere were well aware of the symbolic power of forging a strong association with the royal family. Members of the royal family undertook various first aid courses and the Duke of Connaught even received donations to the Order from his mother Queen Victoria. Prince Albert, Queen Victoria's consort was made a Bailiff Grand Cross of the Order of Malta in 1839.

The Prince of Wales was greatly interested in the Sovereign Military Order of Malta, having been made a Bailiff Grand Cross of that Order in 1881, one of the few non-Roman Catholics to hold the distinction. The Prince of Wales was fascinated by matters related to honour, honours, and the concept of chivalry. He was after all the heir apparent to the most powerful empire in the world, one consumed with the mythology and history of knights in shining armour, devotion to God and the King, and an ancient code of conduct; that was in the popular mindset seen as being responsible for the success of Britain at home and across the seas.[65] It would not be an unfair assessment to say that the Prince of Wales became involved in the Order of Malta in part because of the robes and decorations associated with the Order.[66] He also shared the Order's love of ceremony and although not a Roman Catholic, was devoted to its broader Christian ideals. Members of the royal family refused to allow their connection to the Order of St. John to be purely nominal, and even continued "to evidence a lively interest in its humanitarian objects."[67]

Another key promoter of the Order was the seventh Duke of Manchester, who was elected as grand prior of England in 1861. Manchester was a close friend of the Prince of Wales[68] and this friendship played an important role in enlisting the support and patronage of the future King Edward VII. The royal family would take a keen interest in the work of the Order of St. John; most specifically first aid training. In 1876, Alexandra, Princess of Wales was made a Lady of Justice of the Order.[69] In 1882 seven female members of the royal family underwent first aid training and received their certificates: The Princess of Wales, Alexandra; the Princess Royal; Queen Maud of Norway; Princess Victoria; Princess Beatrice; the Duchess of Connaught; and the Duchess of Albany.[70] This was evidence of more than a passing interest in gilt baubles and medieval clothing. Princess Louise, Duchess of Argyle and daughter of Queen Victoria became involved in the Order following her husband's retirement as governor general of Canada and was made a Lady of Justice in 1883.[71]

During the 1887 Golden Jubilee of Queen Victoria's accession to the throne, the newly founded St. John Ambulance Brigade played an important role in lining the parade route and providing first aid and medical treatment to members of the military and general public during the massive celebrations that took place in London. The public respect accorded to the St. John first aid training, certificates, and the ambulance brigade had grown significantly since the revival of the Order and inauguration of the earliest-first aid training centre founded at Woolwich in 1877 by Colonel Duncan.

With the profile of the Order firmly fixed in the minds of many in the United Kingdom, the Prince of Wales petitioned his mother, Queen Victoria, on behalf of the prior and members of the Order for a royal charter of incorporation.[72] This charter was to have the effect of officially recognizing the Order as a British order of chivalry and offering royal patronage. The Order was given the style and title: "The Grand Priory of the Order of the Hospital of St. John of Jerusalem in England." It was a unique form of recognition — and remains such — in that while many national organizations in Britain and throughout the Commonwealth possess a royal charter and or royal patronage, only the Order of St. John is also recognized as comprising part of the honours system.[73]

On 14 May 1888, Queen Victoria signed the Royal Charter and it came into force. With this the Order received in essence a new constitution. In August of that same year the Prince of Wales was invested as grand prior of the Order, while his eldest son the Duke of Clarence, was made sub prior. After the Royal Charter of 1888 was granted, Victoria wrote to her eldest son the Prince of Wales from Osborne House:

> Dearest Bertie, — ... I want to ask you now to give me the Order of St. John and to make me a Dame Chevalier or "Lady of Justice," if it can be, as I take so much interest in it all and should like to have it.[74]

As sovereign head of the Order, Victoria was entitled to wear an insignia denoting her office and this was subsequently provided. This is believed to be the only occasion when a reigning sovereign has asked to be appointed to an order.[75]

The Royal Charter had the effect of embedding the Order of St. John into the honours system in the United Kingdom and later throughout the Commonwealth. It also made official and inseparable the connection between the Order and its sovereign head. With this, the Order became totally separate from the Order of Malta and Rome, being subject only to the authority of the sovereign and officials of the Order in the United Kingdom. Unlike members of the Order of Malta, members of the Order of St. John were, and continue to be, permitted to wear their insignia as they are official honours of the Crown. Not surprisingly, the Order of Malta refused to acknowledge the reconstituted Order, even with the Royal Charter. It would not be until 26 November 1963 that a declaration was made jointly by both the Order of Malta and the Order of St. John professing the mutual respect that both Orders have for each other in seeking "ever more ways in which they can collaborate, to promote God's glory and to alleviate the sufferings and miseries of mankind."[76] It was also acknowledged that further discussions of the legitimacy of the Order of St. John should be "relegated to the realms of academic discussion."[77]

Further agreements followed and in 1987 the Order of Malta recognized the legitimacy of the Order of St. John on the basis of its standing as an order of the Crown. This was further enhanced in 2004 when the Order of Malta recognized that the The Alliance Orders of St. John of Jerusalem — Die Balley Brandenburg des Ritterlichen Ordens Sankt Johannis vom Spital zu Jerusalem, The Most Venerable Order of the Hospital of St. John of Jerusalem, Johanniter Orde in Nederland, and Johanniterorden I Sverige — "share a common commitment to the traditions established by The Order of the Hospital of St. John of Jerusalem in the middle ages," and that the "four orders in the Alliance, stemming from the same root, are orders of chivalry as well as being Christian confraternities."[78] This marked an extremely important step for the five orders, where there was once religious animosity and suspicion, a strong and mutually beneficial relationship has been formalized.[79]

THREE

RETURNED TO CANADIAN SHORES

An increased number of classes
have been held in Canada and New Zealand.
Annual Report of the St. John Ambulance Association, 1884.

Although the inaugural St. John first aid training classes were not held in Canada until the winter of 1882–1883, the work of the Knights Hospitaller has a much more ancient connection to Canada, through the governors of New France and Acadia respectively. Until 1759 the French kings had dominion over much of what is modern day Quebec, Ontario, Nova Scotia, New Brunswick, and Prince Edward Island. Some of the governors who administered these territories on behalf of the French crown were themselves Knights of Malta. More than just nominal wearers of the white cross, a number of governors and their subordinates served the Order in a variety of capacities. There was even an attempt to establish a priory of the Knights of Malta in France's North American colonies; alas these efforts came to naught. The "only archaeological memento of the stay of the Knights of Malta on the rock of Quebec,"[1] was uncovered in 1784 in the ruins of the Château Saint-Louis, the official residence of the French governors of New France. A simple stone tablet carved with the white cross of the Knights of Malta remains and now rests on the same spot in the modern day Château Frontenac Hotel.

Although the Canadian connection to the Knights of Malta is firmly rooted in the English tongue of the Order, the presence of Knights of Malta in highly influential positions early in Canada's colonial history provides yet another link between the modern day Order of St. John in Canada and the original Knights Hospitallers who became the Knights of Malta. Indeed, while the Order was being suppressed in England by Henry VIII and Elizabeth I following the Reformation, its members were in charge of New France and Acadia. The Order was flourishing in France and to a small degree among the ruling order of New France and Acadia, the Order found a place. This was natural as "New France was never more than an extensions of France,"[2] thus French institutions and customs were transplanted to North America. This included the Order of Malta.

Charles Huault de Montmagny, the first governor of New France to hold the style and title of governor general, was himself a knight of the Order.[3] This inaugurated a long tradition of governors general having a close association with the white cross in Canada. One of the youngest members of the Order was Jean-Baptiste de la Croix de Chevrières de Saint-Vallier, who had been admitted to the Order at the age of ten as a knight of minority in 1663. He became Bishop of Quebec in 1688. This required a special dispensation from Pope Alexander VII.[4] As in New France, senior French officials in Acadia were similarly involved in the Order. As governor of Acadia from 1632–35 Isaac de Razilly who "lived in as grand a style in the Acadian wilderness as possible," and his brother Gabriel were both members of the Order. Among the possessions left behind by Isaac were his Order insignia and several cloaks bearing the eight-pointed white cross.[5] As well, three knights served in what is modern day Newfoundland. The most notable of these was the Marquis André de Nesmond who had become a member of the Order in 1659, later rising to the rank of naval lieutenant-general in the French Navy, and becoming a Knight Grand Cross of the Order of Saint-Louis and a Knight of the Order of the Golden Fleece in recognition of his distinguished service.[6]

The Sovereign Military Order of Malta, while active among the senior echelons of society in New France and Acadia, was limited primarily to officials from France. There is little evidence to suggest that colonists were involved in a meaningful way. This is not entirely surprising given that French North America was principally administered by officials sent from France, who remained in the colonies for a set period of time, returning to the mother-country upon the expiration of their appointment or upon recall. Colonists failed to achieved high office until the final years of French dominion,[7] thus becoming a member of the Order was socially-unattainable. There was also the fact that the population of New France and Acadia was small, and did not include a considerable middle or upper class from which prospective members of the Order could be drawn, other than transient officials who invariably returned to Europe.

In the Canadian context the cross-pollination of the Order's English and French tongues is particularly fitting. The presence of the Order in Canada before the fall of New France, the revival of the English tongue of the Order by the French tongues and the eventual flourishing of the Order throughout the Commonwealth in Canada can in many ways be traced back to the French connection, like so much of Canadian history.

Canada in the Age of Confederation

Canada was a young country in the period when the inaugural first aid courses were offered to its citizens. With a population of 4.25 million, one third French speakers whose ancestors immigrated from France, and the rest overwhelmingly composed of immigrants from the British Isles,[8] it was not surprising that the culture and public affairs of the country were intensely focused on Britain. The economy of the country was primarily oriented towards agriculture, and there was a small industrial base.

The young Dominion was protected by the Royal Navy, various British regiments, and the Canadian militia. Although internal affairs were governed from Ottawa and the provincial capitals, international matters were still dealt with by the imperial government in London. The British character of the country at this point in history, and the reliance on immigration from

England, Scotland, Ireland, and Wales, played an important role in the development of St. John Ambulance in Canada, as it was British immigrants to Canada who were the people who inaugurated the initial first aid classes.

The 1880s were paradoxically a period of substantial growth,[9] as some historians have noted that it can more accurately be described as steady growth in an economic depression.[10] Growth was considered to be a combination of economic prosperity coupled with growth in population. Over the period 1873 to 1896 Canada's population grew by a mere 40 percent. Over the same period, the population of the United States grew by 100 percent.[11] Thus, St. John first aid was not introduced to Canada in a period of prosperity, as it was in both Australia and Britain.

One reason why the Order of St. John would eventually take root in Canada was closely related to the global nature of the British Empire. Covering a quarter of the surface of the earth and encompassing a fifth of its population one of the by-products of this enterprise was a cross pollination of people from the British Isles to all parts of the world. This meant simply that the Order — the work of the St. John Ambulance Association was transplanted around the globe. The association came into being just as the British Empire was reaching its zenith. The combination of a powerful Empire, administered by military and civil servants around the globe, coupled with immigration and the establishment of first aid as the driving force behind the Order helped to form a potent organization that became empire-wide — and thus global — within two decades.

Attempted Beginnings

While the modern day Order of St. John traces its beginnings in Canada to first aid courses offered in the winter of 1882–1883 in Quebec City and Kingston, there were earlier attempts to establish the Order in Canada, even before first aid — modern day hospitaller work — became the central focus of the organization. The Order in these early days was primarily a group of gentlemen of some influence who were interested in the concept of knighthood and chivalry. In many ways the Order in Canada started off much as it did in England; as a club of men of senior social rank who were keen on reviving and maintaining the ideals of honour, chivalry, and knighthood.

The 1849 *Statutes of the Illustrious and Sovereign Order of the Knights Hospitallers of Saint John of Jerusalem, Venerable Langue of England, Comprehending The Grand Priories, Bailiwicks, and commanderies in England, Scotland, Ireland, Wales* made it clear that one of the purposes of the Order was not only to be active in England, but to spread out around the world, this included the wilderness of Canada. Special dignitaries were appointed and held the title of Preceptors "in India, America [U.S.A.], Canada, Australia and the Mediterranean, with such Delegates as may be deputed."[12] Even before this the Order had been spreading outside England: Given the strong English presence in Canada it should be no surprise that it would return to Canadian shores for the first time since the fall of New France, even though it had only recently been revived in England.

The first permanent resident of Canada to be appointed to the revived English tongue of the Order was Sir Allan Napier MacNab. Son of a Loyalist army officer, MacNab would become an influential pre-Confederation politician. Serving as premier of the Province of Canada from 1854–56, aide-de-camp to Queen Victoria and as a long serving member of the pre-Confederation legislature, serving as Speaker of both the legislative assembly and later the legislative council, he was no stranger to honours, having been made a Knight Bachelor and later a Baronet of the United Kingdom; the first Canadian to hold both of these distinctions. MacNab was first appointed as Knight of Justice of the Order of St. John in 1842 during a trip to England and subsequently appointed as a Bailiff Grand Cross on 20 August 1855.[13] The 1849 statutes of the Order list MacNab as serving as preceptor of the Order in Canada, holding this most senior position in the then colony. MacNab is in many ways Canada's forgotten Bailiff, being not only the first person appointed to the Order but the first Canadian to attain its highest rank.

Although not a great deal of documentation about MacNab's role has survived, he appears to have held this position from 1849 until his death in 1862. MacNab's appointment was followed by that of another premier of the Province of Canada, the Honourable Sir Étienne-Pascal Taché, who was made a Knight of Justice on 18 January 1858.[14] Three other Canadians, Hamnett Pinhey, Warren Hastings Ryland, and Alexander Bell were appointed Knights of Grace.[15] Pinhey was a wealthy land owner, business man, and politician who spent his later years engaged in philanthropic endeavours, even attempting to establish a school open to "all denominations of Christians,"[16] a highly controversial idea at the time. If Pinhey embodied the pluralistic and philanthropic element of the Order in Canada, then Ryland represented the office-seeking, honour-craving side. Like his father, Herman Ryland, Warren had an "insatiable hunger for posts."[17] This was not uncommon, especially in Upper Canada where "people strove to gain appointments by personal connections or by citing long and loyal service."[18] Such attainments were an important part to upward social mobility. In this context it may seem surprising that the Order was not more prolific in pre-Confederation Canada, this can be attributed to two factors. The English tongue of the Order was still young and small, with less than two hundred members. The focus on the organization in the period between the 1830s and 1850s was on developing in England, not on spreading around the globe. It was not until the late 1840s that any designs were placed on spreading the organization beyond England's shores to parts of the Empire. The other reason is again related to who populated the Order in these early days. Until the 1880s the Order was dominated by the social elite of England, and colonial elites, by and large, occupied a lower social strata. Thus, only the most prominent Canadians were able to move between the ruling classes of both Britain and Canada. MacNab was a prime example of someone able to move with ease between elites of both; his daughter married a peer, and he was himself a baronet, knight of the realm, and leading political figure with access to royal and vice-regal courts. In this sense, MacNab and Taché epitomized the class of people who revived the English tongue of the Order in its nascent developmental stage. Pre-Confederation Canada simply did not contain a social elite that was on par with that of England.

Despite the involvement of these high ranking and public figures the Order did not grow in Canada, and there were few subsequent Canadian appointments until after 1888 and the Royal Charter. Given that the St. John Ambulance Brigade work of the Order did not fully get underway until the last decade of the nineteenth century, this is not surprising. Without a cause — beyond the honour side of the Order — the organization had no popular purpose that could draw members from either the top of the social ladder or from the pool of average citizens keen to become involved in civic projects. It was in essence limited to retired military men and politicians, and took root only among a "nascent aristocratic class,"[19] First aid, the work of the association and subsequently the work of the brigade, would give the Order this purpose, much in the same way that it did in England.

Inaugurating of First Aid Training

The earliest recorded first aid training course in Canada was offered in Quebec City during the winter of 1882–1883.[20] A close examination of all the pre-1883 annual reports for the St. John Ambulance Association (England) fail to reveal any mention of first aid training taking place in Canada before this date. The first course was given under the direction of Brigade Surgeon Campbell Mellis Douglas, one of the first Canadian recipients of the Victoria Cross, which he was awarded for conspicuous gallantry and devotion to duty while serving in the Andaman Islands off the coast of India in 1867. The class is described in records of the period as "1 preliminary Female Class 'Detached.'"[21] In accordance with St. John Ambulance Association policy, prescribed by St. John's Gate the examination was carried out by a person other than the instructor. In the case of this inaugural class the test was conducted on 7 April 1883 by Dr. Robert Bruce, a highly respected physician and leading member of the fledgling Canadian medical establishment. With this the fundraising efforts of St. John Ambulance in Canada also commenced, and Brigade Surgeon Douglas's class raised £3.3s.0d.

The same year as the examination was held in Quebec City, first aid instructional classes were commenced for cadets at the Royal Military College in Kingston Ontario. This warranted a "special mention" in the annual report.[22] Thus was signalled the beginning of an almost unbroken connection with Canada's military that continues to this day. There are some accounts that earlier classes were held in Halifax by medical officers in the British Army resident in the garrison;[23] however there is no concrete documentation to support this claim, and no first aid qualification certificates are on record as having been issued to Canadians before 1883. We know that many British Army surgeons were trained and were familiar with St. John first aid education,[24] and that it would seem only logical that they would train others, both personnel stationed in Halifax and members of the local community in the various techniques of first aid.

That 1883 saw the holding of the inaugural first aid examinations, granting of the first certificates and the commencement of first aid training at RMC are the reasons why 1883 has historically been chosen as the benchmark date for when St. John Ambulance was established in Canada. From the events of 1883 flowed the establishment of the St. John Ambulance Association and the introduction of first aid training in Canada. Then came the creation of the first division of the St. John Ambulance Brigade in the first decade of the twentieth century. These comprised the real work of the Order in Canada. Although some could point to 1842 and the appointment of the first Canadian to the Order as the founding date, the only result of this was MacNab becoming a Knight of Justice; it did not signal the founding of an organization. While MacNab's appointment and position as preceptor are interesting events in the broader history of the Order, the fact remains that they were events almost unrelated to the 1882–83 first aid courses and the firm establishment of the Order in Canada. Having classes beginning in 1882 and carrying on into 1885 helped bring the Order in Canada purpose and meaning beyond being an honour, first aid, and civic duty fit well into the Victorian values of self help and social responsibility.

As first aid was taking root in the young Dominion, an unusual, almost made for Canada, first aid device was unveiled in 1883, one that would have particular use in Canada. Herr Dr. Rüdel of Kent, developed a pamphlet entitled "Ice Accidents" along with a floatation and rescue device. "It consists of a wooden ball to which a metal ball and a few yards of rope are attached ... it may be bowled ... and the rope then drawn across the surface [ice] and put within reach of the person in peril."[25]

The period of 1883–84 saw additional classes being held in Kingston, serving either males or females. Montreal held a similar class from which 15 certificates were issued, unfortunately there is no record of how many ladies sat for the Montreal examination.[26] These classes were important in instituting the St. John Ambulance Association as the premier and most significant provider of first aid training in Canada.

The 1884 annual report was written in a hopeful tone, stating that "an increased number of classes has been held in Canada and New Zealand."[27] No doubt officials at St. John's Gate in London assumed that the St. John Ambulance Association was going to immediately flourish in Canada, much as it was in Australia; the early 1880s having been a period of raid growth for St. John in the various Australian colonies.[28] One of the key differences between Canada and Australia in this respect was the presence in Australia of a number of individuals all keen to found an Australian branch of the St. John Ambulance Association. In Canada the focus was primarily of a few individuals who had received St. John training in England who wanted to transplant similar training to Canada. In these early years the Australians and New Zealanders were far more effective at carrying out both first aid training classes and establishing branches to propagate the knowledge further.

The redoubtable Sir Thomas and Lady Annie Brassey undertook a Caribbean tour with their yacht, *Sunbeam*. Aside from their involvement with the Order, the Brassey's were an active couple, Sir Thomas having served as a Liberal member of Parliament at Westminster, holding a variety of posts including civil lord of the Admiralty and later being elevated to the peerage as Baron Brassey. Lady Brassey was much more than just a dutiful politician's wife, and was constantly busy fundraising for the association. Lady Brassey was an accomplished author in her own right and was a noted collector of "natural and ethnological curiosities,"[29] she was a strong willed and independent woman well ahead of her time. Tireless promoters of the work of St. John Ambulance they called at Halifax in 1883.[30] The Brassey's had been engaged in a "vigorous Ambulance Crusade on behalf of the St. John Ambulance Association."[31] The purpose of such crusades was to interest local leaders in various parts of the Empire about founding a branch of the association to bring first aid training to the inhabitants. One historian has noted that "Lady Brassey came ashore and made a serious effort to establish the association on Canadian soil."[32] This however did not have an immediate effect. Brassey would have much better success in Australia where she and her husband played an important role in the growth of the association following her 1887 visit.[33]

Despite these early successes and continuing classes at RMC in Kingston between 1886 and 1895, there is no mention of activity in Canada contained within the annual reports of this period. The first centre in Canada was established in Halifax on 24 June 1892 at Government House in the presence of Sir Malachy Bowes Daly, lieutenant-governor of the province.[34] This meeting included members of the army and navy medical staff — as there was still no separate medical unit for either service — local clergy, and members of the local elite.

Surgeon Captain Lees-Hall, commandant of Cogswell Station Military Hospital in Halifax had recently returned from leave in England and was anxious to promote first aid training in Canada. He was the keynote speaker at the meeting and recited statistics of fatal accidents in Britain and recalled incidents where similar events had occurred in Canada, both in rural and urban settings, noting that many lives could be preserved through basic first aid training. The Anglican bishop of Nova Scotia, the Right Reverend Frederick Courtney moved a resolution to establish Halifax as a centre of the association under the leadership of Sir John Ross as president. Some forty persons present signed the membership roll and that summer first aid classes commenced in the Church of England Institute building.[35] Some of those who took these classes were members of the Halifax Volunteer Fire Brigade and students at the Dalhousie Medical College.[36]

It has been noted that in 1895 a Halifax branch of the St. John Ambulance Brigade was established by the same members of the Voluntary Fire Brigade and Dalhousie Medical College. There is, however, no mention of this in the records of St. John's Gate or in the annual report of the ambulance brigade. It is most likely that an unofficial brigade, consisting of active members of the association, was set up to act in a dual capacity as both persons who offered first aid treatment and first aid training. Although the Halifax Centre had been authorized by St. John's Gate in London, a brigade would not be formally created in Canada until 1909 when the Forest City Division of the St. John Ambulance Brigade was founded in London Ontario. Halifax newspaper articles of the period make reference to "the Brigade" taking part in the celebrations surrounding Queen Victoria's Diamond Jubilee in Halifax as their first public duty.

Members of the Halifax "Brigade" attended military training camp at Aldershot and acted as a supplemental Army medical service unit, on voluntary service. They were designated the

Halifax Bearer Company, which later changed to the No. 1 Bearer Company. Unlike members of the brigade in England and New Zealand, members were supplied with military uniforms, black fatigue dress by the Department of Militia and Defence. In officially recognized brigades the uniforms were supplied at brigade expense by St. John's Gate according to a standardized pattern. The reason for this may have been the interest shown by the Minister of Militia and Defence, Sir Frederick Borden, the man largely responsible for Canada's entry into the Anglo-Boer War, himself a medical doctor and Knight of Grace of the Order.

During the Anglo-Boer War a number of members of the company, including Major Guy Carleton Jones, a noted first aid instructor, served with the No. 10 Canadian Field Hospital in South Africa. In 1906 the No. 1 Bearer Company became the First Field Ambulance of the Canadian militia. Jones would continue to play an important part in the growth of the association and brigade in Canada throughout his lifetime, rising to the rank of surgeon-general by the end of his career.

The 1895 annual report erroneously makes references to centres being founded in Halifax in 1889, Vancouver in 1890, and Toronto in 1895. References exist to 45 certificates being issued in Vancouver in 1892,[37] but the centre became dormant after that year. There is no evidence that first aid courses were held in Halifax until after 1892.[38] None of these centres submitted reports until Toronto in 1896 following the establishment of the Council of the St. John Ambulance Association for the Dominion of Canada. The presence of members of the Royal Navy in the various military establishments more than affords the possibility that St. John first aid training was being given to members of the garrisons and local communities, but again there is a gap in documentation. In his memoirs George Sterling Ryerson, founder of the Canadian branch of the St. John Ambulance Association makes references to classes being held in Halifax and Victoria under the "auspices of the medical officers of the Royal Navy and the Army."[39] Once again no dates are attached to when these classes took place. Before 1896 there are records indicating that 296 people took first aid instruction in Halifax, while 45 persons attended St. John first aid courses in Vancouver.[40]

Although the first Canadian centre was established at Halifax in 1892, it was from central Canada that the great push to spread the work of the association across the country came, from that hub of activity that is Toronto.

George Sterling Ryerson

It will be recalled that the Order's first aid work in England flowed directly out of a series of conflicts that gripped mainland Europe during the middle years of the nineteenth century; from the Danish-Prussian War of 1864 to the Franco-Prussian War, these conflagrations illustrated the immediate need for first aid training not only targeted to military personnel, but also civilian populations. Canada too was not immune from conflict. There were the Fenian Raids of 1866 and 1870, along with the Red River Rebellion of 1870 and the North-West Rebellion of 1885. It was this later conflict that helped to firmly establish the Order's first aid training in Canada, and that helped to spur on one of its great supporters to coordinate and energize the nascent organization.

The Order's institution in Canada as a first aid training organization was in large part attributable to the work of George Ansel Sterling Ryerson. If Furley, Lechmere, and Duncan were the founders of the Order's work in England then it would be fair to say that Ryerson was the Order's Canadian founder. He was one of those eminent Victorians who was not confined to a single profession, equally at home in the university lecture theatre, operating theatre, provincial legislature, drill hall, and battlefield, Ryerson was a polymath of the first order. Ryerson was born on 21 January 1855, and is a direct descendent of the eminent United Empire Loyalist and Methodist minister Egerton Ryerson who was largely responsible for the establishment of standardized schooling in what was then Canada West (Ontario). The Ryerson family had a history of civic involvement and of establishing institutions; this would be impressed upon George at a young age. Socially, Ryerson was of the same class as Furley, Lechmere, and Duncan, all relatively wealthy and talented men looking to make a contribution that would not only better their position in society, but improve the lives of those less fortunate.

At the age of 15, Ryerson served in the Canadian militia during the Fenian Raids of 1870. Following this adventure, Ryerson began his training as a medical doctor in Toronto, eventually undertaking additional medical studies in Edinburgh, Paris, London, Vienna, and Heidelberg. Here he learned not only the intricacies of general surgery but also took an interest in ocular surgery and became one of Canada's first ophthalmologists and otolaryngologists (ear, nose, and throat specialists).

As a young army surgeon serving in the North-West Rebellion, Ryerson saw first hand the savagery of armed conflict. The bitter battle of Batoche gave Ryerson experience in dealing with battlefield injuries and made him witness to the violent deaths of a number of colleagues.[41] One of Ryerson's non-commissioned officers (NCOs), Staff Sergeant Curzon, of the Royal Grenadiers who was also at the battle on 12 May 1885 saw a sergeant in the Midland battalion wounded in the upper arm:

> Sergeant Curzon had fortunately attended the regimental ambulance class, and had learned the simple art of applying the improvised tourniquet. He made out with his hand-kerchief and tightened it with a stick, thereby saving his comrade from a severe hæmorrhage, if not his life.[42]

During the Rebellion, Ryerson was responsible for the presence of a horse drawn ambulance, which was used during the battle of Batoche. The ambulance displayed the flag of another organization that he would be instrumental in establishing, the Canadian branch of the British Red Cross Society.

It was Ryerson who gave the infant Canadian branch of the association purpose, as he was so effective at articulating the need for first aid training and conveying a vision of just how important first aid could be in times of crisis — whether it be an accident or during a battle. As in England, the Order in Canada had gone through a period of slow growth; a period when it was dominated by an inactive group of gentlemen more concerned with fancy dinners and chats about chivalry, than participating in the modern day hospitaller work of the Order — the administration and teaching of first aid. In this context Ryerson noted "the members began to look for a means and methods to put to practice the motto of the Order, *pro utilitate hommium*."[43] Ryerson served as the catalyst for the expansion of the association, not only in Ontario but throughout Canada.

As a militia officer he initiated the Association of Medical Officers of the Canadian Militia in 1892, which lobbied for the establishment of the Canadian Army Medical Corps:

> It became apparent to those medical officers who took part in the North-West Rebellion of 1885, that something must be done to ensure a supply of trained men for the ranks of the medical service.[44]

Until 1904 there was no permanent or militia medical corps in Canada, medical officers were simply attached to individual battalions and regiments along with individual stretcher bearers.[45] This was modelled on the British Army, which also lacked a specific Army Medical Corps until 1898. Ryerson's contributions were to military medicine in Canada on the widest scale. He later rose to become deputy surgeon-general in 1895. Throughout his life he maintained an inexhaustible interest in "military medical affairs."[46] Beyond the medical field, Ryerson served as a member of the Ontario provincial legislature from 1893–1989, sitting as a Conservative. He devoted this period of his life to founding and maintaining the St. John Ambulance Association in Canada and the Canadian branch of the British Red Cross Society.[47] Proud of his achievements, in later life, when asked what his involvement with the Order was, he simply said "I organized the St. John Ambulance Association in Canada."[48]

In 1894 Ryerson wrote to St. John's Gate in London requesting permission to establish a Canadian branch of the St. John Ambulance Association, as up to this point Canada only possessed a centre in Halifax, which had by this point fallen dormant. Encouraged by his friend Sir George Airey Kirkpatrick,[49] lieutenant-governor of Ontario, on 8 March 1895 Ryerson was granted permission to establish a branch called the "Dominion Council." In November 1895 at the Royal Canadian Military Institute in Toronto the Ontario centre of the association was established, which marked the formal establishment of the Dominion Council of the St. John Ambulance Association. With a organizational structure now in place for not only Ontario but also — theoretically — for the entire Dominion, the work of St. John Ambulance could finally be taken to all parts of the country. That there was a pre-existing, yet dormant, centre at Halifax helped to ensure that the organization was not going to be entirely dominated by central Canada. The fact that a Halifax centre had been established in 1892 helped to ensure that the association in Canada would adopt a federal structure, whereby each province would establish its own centre. These would later grow into what are today known as provincial and territorial councils.

In recognition of medical services rendered during the North-West Rebellion, Ryerson was made an Honorary Associate of the Order,[50] in 1892, the first Canadian to be appointed to this grade. For Queen Victoria's Diamond Jubilee, 1897, he was made an Esquire of the Order, and was made a Knight of Grace following the Anglo-Boer War. At the time of his death in 1925, he was the most senior ranking Canadian member of the Order. Until the replacement of the Dominion Council with the Canadian branch in 1910, Ryerson served as the general secretary. This made him responsible for the day to day operations and administration of the Dominion Council. Upon his retirement from this post, there being no other accolades or honours to offer, Ryerson was presented with an illuminated scroll that states "in appreciation of the unselfish and gratuitous labors and valuable services rendered by Colonel G.S. Ryerson to the people of Canada in the cause of humanity."[51]

Growth and Stagnation

In November 1895 the Ontario Centre was organized in Toronto, this was followed by the establishment of the Toronto Centre on 5 February 1896. This centre would be the one constant in the early history of the association in Canada. Being the industrial engine of the country it was not surprising that first aid training would take root so quickly in late Victorian Toronto. As early as 1889 the chief of police of Toronto requested that all constables "be instructed in how to render first aid in cases of accident or illness in the streets."[52] Police, factory workers, women seeking basic nursing skills, and labourers all saw the value in first aid training, and St. John was there to offer it.

Following the establishment of the Toronto centre first aid classes began being offered. In 1896 alone 238 pupils attended seven courses: four first aid for women, one first aid for working men, and two first aid for men. Lieutenant-Governor Sir George Kirkpatrick presented the first certificates on 8 October 1896 at St. Georges Hall in Toronto. This same year saw centres established in London, Halifax, Fredericton, Westmount, Guelph, Orillia, and Brockville. Officials at St. John's Gate in London seemed pleased with the way things were developing in Canada, noting "the prospect of work by these several centres is encouraging."[53] On paper it looked impressive, but the truth of the matter was that some centres were inactive, aside from the holding of a founding meeting. There was however a tinge of disappointment that Canada had taken so long to establish a branch of the association and begin the first aid work of the Order. In India, Australia, and New Zealand there had been great progress over the preceding decade.

No doubt officials at St. John's Gate looked at a giant map of Canada, tinged pink and dotted with towns and cities and viewed it as having great potential, but they must have also been daunted by the sheer size of the place. Not wanting to "blame" Canadian officials for not being more proactive, officials in London simply noted that while pleased with the development of the Canadian branch, "results up to the present … would have been still better, had it not been for the commercial depression which has prevailed on the country for several years."[54] Indeed the economic situation in Canada was not as strong as it was in the United States or Britain at this point in history.

The earliest first aid medallions were awarded to sixteen women in Toronto in 1896.[55] Toronto was the largest centre, holding a wide variety of courses for men, women, and children. Aside from appealing to women interested in nursing and first aid, it was the working class for which first aid courses were the most attractive; they were the people most at risk from injury or death while on the job. Ryerson noted that the association's "work is appreciated by those whom it is chiefly intended to benefit, the industrial classes, as witness a resolution recently passed by the Toronto Trades and Labour Council."[56] The association was seeking to help train and protect the most vulnerable in society.

Table 1

Toronto Centre, Courses, and Certificates

Course	1895	1896
First Aid Men	53	634
Men who earned certificate	48	33
First Aid Women	196	88
Women who earned certificate	141	72
Women nursing	144	73
Women who earned nursing certificate	97	49

The first junior first aid course was held in Toronto in 1896, with forty-nine attendees, twenty-six of whom received their certificates. The best evidence of the success of the association in these early years can be found in the record of instances of first aid being administered. During Queen Victoria's Diamond Jubilee celebrations in Toronto, St. John first aid certificate holders came to the rescue on many occasions:

At Exhibition Park on Jubilee day two cases of fainting; three similar cases in Queen's Park at the reception to the Jubilee contingent. First aid was rendered to a young lady at Hanlan's Island, who fainted in the crush, and to whom two policemen were endeavouring to administer an emetic of salt and water. Among accidents treated were the following: injury of right hand, with partial severance of the ends of two of the fingers; a punctured wound of the head; a severe cut in the thigh with many smaller cuts and abrasions, the result of a bicycle accident whilst racing; scalp wound caused by a heavy maple plank; a cut on the sole of the foot by a piece of glass.

The North End Class reports as follows: at Niagara Falls, on the opening of the New Grand Trunk Railway Bridge, promote aid was rendered to the aeronaut who fell with his balloon some 50 feet and received severe injuries; a case of epilepsy occurring on the public street; also several minor cases such as sunstroke, incised wounds.[57]

The Queen's Diamond Jubilee year brought an expansion of the administrative structure of the association in Canada. With the establishment of so many branches and centres and not wanting to lose momentum in the movement, officials at St. John's Gate suggested that the activities of the association in Canada be coordinated. With this, the Ontario Provincial Centre was enlarged to a Dominion Council. Sir George Kirkpatrick was elected president along with fourteen vice-presidents, and ten members.[58] This was the first time that leaders from all the various branches and centres were brought together to discuss the development of the association on a national scale. In some ways the federal nature of the country was manifesting itself in the Dominion Council set up for the association in Canada. Despite the desire for some degree of central coordination, there was a realization early on in the association's history that it would be impossible for the organization to be centralized and run from one part of the country. If branches and centres were set up properly the decentralized nature of the association could become one of its great strengths in a country as big as Canada. The absence of representatives from Alberta and Saskatchewan is not surprising as the two provinces did not yet exist, still being part of the North-West Territories, which was the most rural part of the country, not yet containing sufficient populations to found centres.

Ryerson was instrumental in enlarging the provincial centre for Ontario into the Dominion Council. "I hope this will give wider interest, stability, and permanency to the Association in Canada."[59]

Throughout the late 1890s growth would continue throughout Ontario and eventually spread outside the province. The Orillia centre was established in 1897 and promptly elected Elizabeth Greene as its president, the first woman to hold such a post within the association in Canada. Brantford would follow this pattern, being established in 1898, the entire executive of the centre was composed of women.[60] During 1898 the Montreal centre met with some success training seventeen men and eighteen women in first aid, the previous year the chief of the Westmount Police began requiring his constables to take St. John first aid training. A centre was established in Fredericton on 1 October 1896, noting that some training had occurred in previous years. Toronto remained the largest centre, with 31 medical staff. In 1899 the Toronto centre began offering an important new course known as the "Railway Men's Class."[61] This course was designed for tramway drivers, railway workers, and anyone involved with the movement of railway cars. The various railway companies in Britain, and their workers, quickly saw the value in first aid training and it was thus natural that a similar relationship be established in Canada between railway workers, companies, and St. John Ambulance.

In 1899 war broke out between Britain and the Boer Republics in what is today the Republic of South Africa. As part of the British Empire, Canada sent a contingent to help fight the Boers. Over the course of the conflict more than 7,000 members of the Canadian militia would serve. The Toronto centre provided each Canadian officer who was going overseas with a copy of *Shepherd's First Aid Text Book and Illustrated Triangular Bandages*, "which were much appreciated by these men."[62] The conflict had erupted quickly and there was no time to offer first aid courses to the men going overseas. This might have been possible had centres in other parts of the country not been dormant.

The period leading up to and following the Anglo-Boer war saw the Canadian Dominion Council come near to extinction. From 1899 to 1901 only the Toronto centre of the Canadian association submitted an annual report to London. By 1901 even the Toronto centre had fallen largely dormant and it is noted "there is a marked revival of interest in this centre this autumn."[63] From 1902 until 1906 neither the Canadian branch nor any Canadian centre submitted an annual report to St. John's Gate. Other dominions and colonies were making great progress, especially India, South Africa, Australia, and New Zealand. It is worth noting that other colonial centres, such as Hong Kong, did not report during this period either. By 1905 the annual reports ceased listing Canada as having a branch of the association, this was repeated in 1906. The following year 1907 saw the revitalization of the Toronto centre, and seven first aid classes were held, three of which were given to members of the Toronto Police Force.[64] Despite the existence of the Dominion Council, which was supposed to oversee the creation and development of new centres the organization became stagnant. The lack of regulations and oversight of the centres meant that it was relatively easy to set up a centre, all that was required was a group of well-meaning citizens of middle-class background who had a vague interest in first aid. As anyone who has been involved in a volunteer organization knows, it is easy to become immersed in administration and holding meetings and not actually get any real work done.

Another reason for the sudden decline of the association in the last part of the Victorian era is related to the activities of one of its principal promoters, George Ryerson. Although still general secretary of the association, Ryerson was increasingly focused on matters related to the Department of Militia and Defence and was also serving in the Anglo-Boer War as a Red Cross commissioner. Upon his return to Canada he was again focused on his own medical practice and re-entering politics. The Canadian economy was experiencing a significant downturn during this period. Given that the association was a volunteer organization largely administered by members of Canada's middle and upper classes, this does not seem to be a sufficient reason to explain the decline it suffered during the first few years of the twentieth century. This accounts for a decline in the number of first aid courses being taken by railwaymen and labourers, but given that all centres ceased offering first aid courses one must attribute the decline more to administrative and internal difficulties within the organization than to the economic situation. The Toronto Trades and Labour Council was "eulogistic of its [the

Association's] work and [there were] favourable comments from the Ontario Inspector of Factories,"[65] about the value of St. John Ambulance Association first aid training. A group that exists solely to protect the rights of workers would not be likely to abandon first aid training even in times of economic depression. During this same period the Canadian branch of the British Red Cross Society did not experience a similar decline, indeed during the Anglo-Boer War the Canadian branch of the British Red Cross Society established 63 local branches across Canada, "the support which these received in their work undoubtedly affected adversely public interest in the St. John Ambulance Association."[66] For all his administrative skills, Ryerson had not done any succession planning and often found himself overcommitted, having responsiblities to his medical practice, work with the association, the Red Cross, Canadian military, and politics.

By 1907 the association was in desperate need of revitalization, the only centre that had met with any consistent success was Toronto, and even it seemed to be on the verge of collapse.

So perplexed by the decline of the Canadian association were officials at St. John's Gate that they sent Colonel C.W. Bowdler on a fact finding mission, known as the "Crusade to Canada." In the fall of 1904 Bowdler travelled across Canada by train visiting Quebec, Montreal, Ottawa, Toronto, and Winnipeg. In each city he met with military and civil officials to discuss the potential for the work of the association to be revived. Where possible, Bowdler also met with members of the various centres. While visiting Montreal he found a first aid class being taught at the local YMCA. The instruction was being given from the St. John First Aid Manual, accompanied by the St. John Ambulance Association First Aid syllabus. Bowdler advised the instructor how he could contact St. John's Gate and get the proper authorization to teach the class. The instructor, Charles Copp became an instant supporter and promoter of St. John Ambulance. Also while in Montreal, he met with workers and managers at the Canadian Pacific Railway (CPR) Angus Shops, the largest railway yard in the country. This would directly lead to the creation of a CPR Angus Shops centre of the association. While Bowdler's Crusade to Canada had helped inform St. John's Gate about the decline of the Canadian centres, it did not result in an immediate revival of any centre, it did however play a role in the ongoing project of rewriting the Royal Charter and the sections that related to overseas branches and centres.

1907 Royal Charter

The circumstances affecting the Canadian branch of the association did not go unnoticed in London at St. John's Gate. Canada was seen as having great potential, especially in light of the success the association had achieved in Australia, India, and New Zealand. There was a general realization that although the Order would continue to be administered from London, a greater deal of autonomy needed to be given to the various dominion and colonial branches of the association and brigade. "The time was fast approaching when it would be necessary for the Order to consider the question of decentralization."[67] Much as the dominions — Canada, Australia, New Zealand, and Newfoundland — were gaining more control over their own affairs, the overseas branches of the association and brigade were in need of more dominion autonomy.

In 1907 King Edward VII, sovereign head of the Order assented to a new Royal Charter. The new charter allowed for the establishment of priories outside the United Kingdom. The realization that if St. John was to flourish beyond the shores of Britain, it could no longer be tightly controlled from London, was implemented. This was seen as the most effective way to allow overseas branches to autonomy. The fact remained that all parts of the Order, no matter what part of the Empire they were located in, were united through the Crown in the person of the sovereign head. In the case of Australia and New Zealand there was a desire to be elevated to priories much sooner than in Canada. Again, Canada was not quick to avail itself of greater independence, the simple reason for this was that the association in Canada was almost defunct aside from the much reduced Toronto centre. The new charter would allow overseas branches to become truly national in scope, in many ways foreshadowing the independence that would be achieved by the dominions in the decades following the First World War. Standards and records would still all be regulated by St. John's Gate.

The year following 1907 was a momentous one for St. John in Canada. It would see steps towards the establishment of the first brigade and the revitalization of the association. The period between the adoption of the new Royal Charter and the beginning of the First World War, although not even a decade in length was remarkable for both organizations.

FOUR

RENEWED PROGRESS

Before the First World War

*The promotion of instruction and carrying out of works for the
relief of suffering of the sick and injured in peace and war,
independently of class, nationality or denomination.*
Act Incorporating the Canadian Branch of the St. John Ambulance Association

The period immediately preceding the outbreak of the First World War was one of increased economic prosperity for Canada, coupled with an upswing in immigration. A confluence of factors helped the Canadian branch of the St. John Ambulance Association and the St. John Ambulance Brigade to become firmly ensconced in the country. Increasing interest from employers such as the CPR and Grand Trunk Railway (GTR) helped to bring St. John Ambulance first aid training to more Canadians than ever before. The same training was also rapidly expanded among police and fire departments, miners, and those working in industry. The arrival of the grand prior, HRH Prince Arthur Duke of Connaught as governor general of Canada in 1911 also helped to encourage the growth and spread of the organizations throughout the Dominion. The renewed work was also in part a result of the dynamic leadership of Dr. Frederick Montizambert and Dr. Guy Carleton Jones, a Colonel in the Canadian Army. Montizambert served as president of the newly formed Canadian branch of the St. John Ambulance Association from 1910 to 1914, while Jones, "slight and formal ... open minded and without predications,"[1] served on the executive committee of the association and was one of the most persistent promoters of first aid within the Canadian militia. Under the leadership of Montizambert and Jones, the Canadian branch was established, incorporated by an act of Parliament, and new centres were opened in every province. The growth of the association in Canada after the establishment of the branch was much more systematic than it had been before 1910 under the Dominion Council. Both St. John's Gate and supporters of the association in Canada had learned that simply allowing centres and branches to be established across the country with little oversight was not a viable plan. A new national management structure, based on federal, provincial, and local cooperation was put in place; one which focused on region wide development on a province by province basis. Previously there had only been the Dominion Council of the association, which was a loose confederation of centre presidents, lacking a national vision. The newly formed Canadian branch, which included provincial councils and local centres and branches was far more suited for expansion and long term success. However this did not preclude certain growing pains that would be felt in Alberta, Saskatchewan, and New Brunswick to a much greater degree than in other parts of the Dominion.

Following the Anglo-Boer War the association went through a period of stagnation in Canada. Only Toronto and to a lesser degree Montreal continued to operate centres, and even in these locations the number of first aid certificates issued was not changing. There were entire years where annual reports were not submitted, and thus it is difficult to paint any picture of the events, although anecdotal evidence suggests that little work was done. One of the main supporters of the association in Toronto remained the Toronto Police Force. In 1908 a total of 368 members of the force had trained in St. John's first aid and by 1912 this had grown to 621 members.[2] The Toronto Force was also one of the earliest to order stretchers and to have its members trained in their use.

Given that there was no central coordinating body, other than St. John's Gate in London, it was not surprising that the only centres to continue in operation were those located in Canada's two largest and most industrialized cities. These centres were overwhelmingly focused on local matters and first aid training, with little emphasis on growth beyond their particular region. There was no province-wide or national conception of the association. The attitude was typically provincial in nature, and like other events in Canadian history it took external involvement to spur growth and development.

Establishment of the Canadian Branch

The impetus to establish a Canadian branch of the association did not come from Canada. The process was set in motion by a recommendation of the Chapter-General at St. John's Gate dating from 1909, which dispatched a second Canadian crusade. A previous crusade had been carried out in 1904 by Colonel C.W. Bowdler on behalf of officials at St. John's Gate, but this had been met by mediocre progress at best. St. John's Gate was impressed with the way in which the brigade had been established in London, Ontario, and felt that given the presence of a somewhat moribund association in Canada, most notably in Toronto, the time was now ideal to restart the group of centres on a national scale. Harold Boulton, MVO, was appointed as honorary organizing commissioner for Canada, and it was up to Boulton to invigorate and organize the Canadians who were interested in establishing a branch. By the end of 1909 he had "engaged in the organization of work all through the provinces and is receiving great assistance and encouragement from H.E. the Governor-General and Countess Grey."[3] It was noted that "Ambulance classes were started in the Dominion many years ago, and a certain limited number of centres have been in existence which have been worked with more or less efficiency, but thanks to the official encouragement now given to the movement the Canadian branch has been properly organized."[4]

On 24 February 1910 at the Parliament Buildings in Ottawa the Canadian branch of the

St. John Ambulance Association was organized. The meeting was directed by Harold Boulton[5] and His Excellency the Governor General, Lord Grey presided. Among the attendees were many senators and members of Parliament. It was a high profile beginning to the Canadian branch of the association. "At this meeting it was resolved that it was advisable to establish a Canadian Branch to carry on the work of the St. John Ambulance Association in Canada, and a provisional Committee was appointed to perfect the organization, with His Excellency the Governor General of Canada as [interim] President."[6] For the first time the association in Canada had high-profile support from the governor general and federal politicians, not to mention the general membership. The governor general was chosen as patron of the Canadian branch, his wife Lady Grey was named patroness, while it was also agreed that the lieutenant-governors and territorial commissioners should be invited to become patrons of their particular jurisdictions. In Ontario, Alberta, Nova Scotia, and Saskatchewan the various lieutenant-governors would become key participants offering logistical support along with organizational expertise.

Dr. Frederick Montizambert was elected as the Canadian branch's first President. Montizambert was the father of the effective quarantine in Canada, and for many years served as the Superintendent of Grosse Île. Born into a well established Quebec family, Montizambert would become one of Canada's leading public health advocates. He believed strongly in the value of public health and was an early "advocate of compulsory vaccination."[7] Apart from his role as president of the Canadian branch of the St. John Ambulance Association, Montizambert had served a wide variety of other national and international organizations. He was president of the Canadian Medical Association, Canada's first director general of Public Health (1899–1920), president of the American Public Health Association, and one of the members of the founding council of the Canadian branch of the National Society for Aid to Sick and Wounded in War (the Red Cross). It is not surprising then, that a man with such a keen interest in the health of his fellow citizens was a great promoter of St. John first aid. A critical assessment of his career could discern an eager office-seeker who jumped from cause to cause, yet Montizambert's long service as director general of Public Health, more than fifty years as a Canadian public servant and four full, and highly productive years, as president of the Canadian branch reveal a man who was committed to a host of endeavours, all aimed at decreasing mortality and improving quality of life.

Other leading members of the newly formed Canadian branch of the association were R.J. Birdwhistle, who was appointed general secretary of the branch, and provided all of the administrative work and advice of the branch as it sought to form not only local centres, but provincial councils. Two members of the executive committee were particularly active and instrumental in the work of the association in the period immediately preceding the First World War, Dr. Jones, who was the director general of Medical Services for the Canadian militia and Dr. Charles Hodgetts.

A special committee was formed to draft a constitution, petition the Dominion government for funds, and plan towards incorporation of the branch, although this later detail did not occur until 1914.[8] By April 1910 the constitution of the Canadian branch was completed and a request for funds from the Dominion government was sent forward to assist the work of the branch. A onetime grant of $5,000 was given to the association over 1911–1912.

With the formation of the Canadian branch it was decided that the national headquarters of the association should be formed in Ottawa, the capital. This was not the obvious choice for some, as the Toronto centre had been particularly strong and had the largest membership, while Ottawa did not have an established branch until November 1910, this would later become the Federal District Centre. Given that the federal apparatus of government, both civil and military, were centred in the Canada's capital city, it was a necessity, especially with the newfound patronage of the governor general, director general of public health, and surgeon general. There was the additional fact that placing the headquarters in Toronto, home to an existing branch and future home of the Ontario provincial council would have given Ontario much more influence, which had hitherto not advanced the national interests of the association. Nevertheless, association officials in Toronto remained critical of the decision to move the headquarters to Ottawa right into the 1930s.

Contained within a number of St. John Ambulance Association publications were leaflets that outline how to form a local centre. These were included with annual reports and periodic mailings done within Canada shortly after the establishment of the Canadian branch. These were usually accompanied by information about first aid kits and equipment, and provided basic instruction on founding a centre, the equipment that was required, and the cost of the kits.

One influential St. John Ambulance publication, which was not a first aid text, was a leaflet included with the bylaws, entitled *How to Form a Local Centre*. It included advice about "interesting citizens of your locality in the work of instruction in First Aid." Along with the usual details related to governance of the centre, it included information on holding a public meeting "to which you should invite … the most prominent men and women in your locality." The intent of the meeting is to explain the work of the St. John Ambulance Association and to elect the executive officers to plan out the future work. Emphasis was placed on involving trade and commerce, clubs, and women's organizations.[9]

At this early stage in the development of the association in Canada, the provision and sale of first aid kits, as today, was one of the most outreach oriented services that St. John offered. While the price for first aid equipment has increased the contents of these early first aid kits has remained fairly constant. A First Aid Box, for use with the Rea-Edwards Litter (ambulance) contained splints, 12 triangular bandages, 12 roller bandages, 2 1/4 pounds of cotton wool, boric lint, adhesive plaster, a pair of scissors, a knife, 2 ounces of olive oil, eucalyptus BPC, sal volatile, and ether, graduated measuring glass, kidney-shaped dressing basin, 7 tampons for washing wounds, tourniquet pins, safety pins, needles, thread, and tape for a cost of $15.

The St. John Ambulance Association First Aid Box "Compressed" was available for $5, and contained 2 packages of absorbent gauze, 1 bandage, 1 absorbent cotton between gauze, 4 ounces of absorbent cotton, 1 pleated boric lint, 6 packages bandages, 3 yards of bandage, 4 packages of bandage, 1 bottle of sal volatile, 1 pair of scissors, 1 paper safety pins, 1 bottle of boric acid, 1 camel hair brush, 1 package of aromatic ammonia, 1 tincture iodine, and booklet *What to do in Case of Accident*. "The best value ever offered in a First Aid box."[10] For centres and brigades looking to purchase more substantial equipment there was always the 1899 Model Furley Stretcher for $14.00. It could be ordered with options such as an awning, chest strap, and legs for additional costs.

Building a National Organization

The intense interest of the CPR and the GTR helped to rapidly spread first aid training to all parts of the country. The railways did after all link the nation together, and the training of its workers had a cascading effect that brought first aid into communities across the country. The renewed St. John Ambulance Association in Canada grew out of two centres, one in Montreal and the other in Toronto.

After six years of failing to submit an annual report the Dominion Council of the association had become defunct, it was no longer reporting to St. John's Gate, and it had been reduced to a centre in Toronto, with centres in other parts of the country operating sporadically at best. In 1907 the Toronto centre resumed submitting its annual report, however the contents were far from enthralling. Under the presidency of Lieutenant-Colonel James Mason seven first aid classes were held, three of which were taken by the Toronto Police Department, which maintained a desire to take St. John's first aid courses even when the branch was not fully operating.[11] Some credit is due to the forethought of the chief of police who encouraged constables to take first aid training. The interest of the Toronto police helped keep the Toronto centre afloat in a time of little activity and financial difficulty. At this time, Toronto was the only functioning centre that was carrying out first aid training.

The most significant step forward in revitalizing the association in Canada was the relationship founded between it and the Canadian Pacific Railway, specifically at the CPR's Angus Workshops in Montreal. This was the hub of the CPR's operations and the rail centre for all of Canada. During Colonel Bowdler's 1904 "Crusade to Canada" he had occasion to meet with CPR officials to encourage them to engage association to teach first aid to their workers.[12] Classes were inaugurated in July 1908, and a centre was established in that same year at the Angus Shops, with 61 first aid certificates being issued.[13] The value of first aid training was realized in the prevention of blood poisoning "by the application of antiseptic dressings." There were also great plans for expansion of association first aid training, "it is the intention of the Company [CPR] to organize ambulance classes throughout their entire system."[14] Not coincidentally the introduction of first aid training spread quickly and in October 1907 a centre was established in Vancouver, where it was strongly supported by the British Columbia Electric Railway (BCER), which subsidized the cost of classes for its employees and their families. The Vancouver City Police and Fire Department were similarly drawn to association first aid classes, with the city council voting a grant of $100 to promote the work. The managing director of the BCER was an enthusiastic promoter, commenting "it is almost incredible that of the work so well known in England, so little should be known here."[15] A number of his employees were immigrants from England and had previously earned association certificates. The BCER went so far as to buy the first Rae-Edwards litter to be imported to Canada's west coast.

By 1909 the CPR centre was reporting that St. John first aid was rendered to 420 persons who were hospitalized and over 15,000 minor accidents.[16] In Toronto a formal relationship had developed between the Toronto centre and the Canadian Army Medical Corps (CAMC), with the association instructing all members of the No. X and XI Field Ambulance Units of the CAMC in first aid. Increasingly other civic organizations such as the Salvation Army, Young Men's Christian Association (YMCA), and the Young Women's Christian Guild (forerunner of the Young Women's Christian Association [YWCA]) were offering first aid classes under the aegis of the association. The Toronto centre finally began to look beyond the city limits and member of the centre were sent to Winnipeg; London; Peterborough; Berlin (Kitchener); and Yarmouth, Nova Scotia to help establish centres.

While the CPR Centre was becoming more firmly established and members of the Toronto centre were seeking to propagate the association in various parts of the province, London, Ontario, would be the site of the first official division of the St. John Ambulance Brigade in Canada. The brigade had been founded in England in 1887 with the purpose of serving as a "civilian organisation for civilian needs and as army and navy reserves."[17]

The first overseas division of the brigade was founded in Dunedin, New Zealand in 1892. In the 1890s Halifax had an unofficial brigade division, consisting of members of the association, but this brigade was never registered with St. John's Gate in London and was thus not part of the St. John Ambulance Brigade Overseas. It did however assist in the 1897 Diamond Jubilee Celebrations held in Halifax for Queen Victoria and trained with local militia units. While the association seeks to impart first aid knowledge the brigade was set up to provide first aid treatment and assist the military, participating in both military and civil events. Beyond the purpose of the brigade, there were other differences between it and the association. The brigade, as its name suggests, was much more structured along military lines. In the early stages each brigade division in Canada reported directly to the chief commissioner of the brigade at St. John's Gate in London, it was a highly centralized governance structure, not ideal for growth or a country the size of Canada. In other parts of the British Empire, the Brigade Overseas operated with ambulance divisions, made up of men, and nursing divisions comprised of women. In cities where there were more than three divisions, a corps was formed, all reporting to a deputy commissioner, although this was not the structure immediately adopted in Canada. Requirements for becoming a member of the brigade were:

> Good character and suitable physique. Age not under seventeen years or over fifty five years. Height not under 5 ft 4 in. Chest not under 32 inches.
>
> The possession of a First Aid Certificate (not a Junior Certificate) of the St. John Ambulance Association. This is absolutely necessary for all members of the Brigade

Overseas with the sole exception of qualified medical men and women. For membership in the Nursing Division, a certificate in Nursing from the St. John Ambulance Association must be obtained in addition to the certificate in First Aid, except in the case of a trained nurse from whom the certificate in First Aid is only required.

The maintenance of efficiency as defined in the Brigade Overseas General Regulations.[18]

The Forest City Ambulance Division of the brigade was established by a British immigrant who had served in the Anglo-Boer War. This was done independently of the association, which at the time was still in flux and trying to arrange its own affairs and take root across Canada. While the executive of the Toronto centre took an active interest in the establishment of the division, they were primarily involved from the standpoint of providing support, not taking the lead in founding the brigade in Canada.

The founding of the division came about as part of a men's Bible class at the Southern Congregational Church in London, Ontario. During a meeting, between resolutions to hold an Old Folks Concert and hold a late summer watermelon social it was decided that "Mr. Loveday and the Secretary make arrangements for Ambulance Drill."[19] The following month, presumably before any ambulance drill could be undertaken, the value of first aid was demonstrated totally by "accident." On 17 September 1908 a group was playing a game of handball, one of them, Byron Simmons suffered a serious injury when the ball struck him in the nose, presumably breaking it, and unleashing a torrent of blood. William Loveday, administered first aid, stopping the bleeding and comforting the man. Loveday had received St. John Ambulance first aid training while in England before moving to Canada as a stonecutter. A local doctor, H.H. Black was called to the scene. Arriving after treatment had been administered, he commented on its high quality.[20] During the following winter, interest grew and a series of first aid classes were held in the church by association certificate holders. That same summer William Pinnock arrived from England. Pinnock had served with the brigade in South Africa during the Anglo-Boer war and in October of 1908 he proposed a motion "would a Division of the St. John Ambulance Brigade be of benefit to London."[21] At this time in Canada few municipalities had an ambulance service of any sort.[22] The usual reaction in a medical emergency was to call the fire department or the police. Pinnock received a positive response, so he and Loveday set about finding all the men in London who held St. John first aid certificates, as being a qualified first aider was a prerequisite for joining the brigade. On 30 November 1908 a meeting was held under the chairmanship of Dr. J.S. Niven, vice-president of the association's Canadian Central Committee, which was headquartered in Toronto at that time. The project had the support of the general secretary of the association, George Sterling Ryerson. With this support and the enthusiasm of those present it was agreed to establish a division of the Brigade Overseas in London, Ontario.

On 13 May 1909 the names of nineteen men were entered on the brigade registration form; five policemen, three carpenters, three shoemakers, two machinists, a granite-cutter, a stone mason, a printer, a gardener, a florist, and a crater. This was representative of the labouring class, there were no bankers, doctors, or lawyers involved at this stage. More than half were born in Britain and this demographic would come to be ingrained in the brigade until after the Second World War. This would cause friction between the brigade and association in coming years. Loveday and Pinnock would continue their involvement in the brigade for more than fifty years, each holding increasingly senior positions and continuing to make a significant contribution to its growth and welfare in Canada. The Forest City No. 1 Ambulance Division went into action for the first time during the Western Ontario Fair in the summer of 1909 where it set up a first aid tent. Three charter members of the Forest City Division lived to celebrate the brigade's golden anniversary in 1959; William Loveday, W.H. Pinnock, and F.H. Morton. All three men provided entertaining reminiscences of their service over the previous half century. It was a remarkable achievement, in that within five years of the London Division being founded, the brigades were being established in communities all across Canada.

By 1912 the Brigade Overseas had established eight new divisions[23] in Canada and was optimistic about the development of brigade and nursing divisions all across Canada, "special attention is being paid to those large cities where the work has not yet been started and arrangements have already been made for several visits and others are being arranged."[24] As with the association, women were encouraged to participate, although within the standard gender-specific roles of the time. Thus women could not become member of brigade divisions, however, they could found or join a nursing division. The first Canadian nursing division, the Toronto (Central) No. 1 Nursing Division, was organized on 6 August 1912. There had been earlier attempts to create a brigade division in Toronto, both in 1904, after Colonel Bowdler's visit and again in 1908, however both failed to gain sufficient membership and were never registered with St. John's Gate. A Toronto brigade division was finally founded in 1911, following a series of meetings that were held in the YMCA Central building in downtown Toronto. Captain G.R.N. Collins, with strong support from the newly formed Ontario Provincial Council of the association was responsible for the successful inauguration of the No. 2 Toronto Central Division, and within half a year three more divisions were established in Toronto and one in Winnipeg, Manitoba.

As the number of brigade and nursing divisions grew the organizational structure of the Brigade Overseas in Canada became cumbersome, and in late 1911 the chief commissioner of the St. John Ambulance Brigade Overseas at St. John's Gate in London gave Sir Henry Pellatt permission to establish a Canadian district of the Brigade Overseas.[25] With the establishment of the Canadian district a new governance structure came into being, the Brigade Overseas, Canadian District was placed under the control of a deputy commissioner who reported directly to the chief commissioner of the Brigade Overseas at St. John's Gate in London. Pellatt, the Toronto stockbroker and financier responsible for building *Casa Loma*, and a prominent supporter of the work of the association, was appointed deputy commissioner of the brigade in Canada. He was assisted by two assistant commissioners. Dr. Charles Copp became assistant commissioner for Ontario, while Major F.L. Vaux was appointed assistant commissioner for Manitoba. Copp had joined the association and later the brigade following Bowdler's Crusade to Canada in 1904. At that time Copp was not a member of the association yet he was giving instruction in first aid at the Toronto YMCA using St. John Ambulance first aid teaching materials.[26]

The headquarters of the brigade in Canada was therefore established in Toronto, in part because Pellatt was resident there and also because the majority of brigade divisions were located in that city. A small office was provided at 554 1/2 Young Street. Pellatt's generosity, both through his philanthropy and organizational skills, was a driving force behind the success of the Canadian District. Brigade and nursing divisions in Canada tended to be established from the grassroots level, as evidenced by Pinnock and Loveday's founding of the No. 1 Forest City Division, and William A.R. Daniels's and Charles E. Arlidge's organization of a unit of the brigade at Elmwood, just outside Winnipeg.[27] Most of the founding members were immigrants from the British Isles who had taken association training before moving to Canada.

In 1912 King George V held a royal review at Windsor Castle. Pellatt not only equipped fifty members of the various Toronto divisions with uniforms, he covered the cost of transportation for the brigade members to Britain. On 22 June the sovereign head of the Order reviewed the Canadian contingent of the brigade along with members of the brigade from all over the Empire: New Zealand, South Africa, Australia, India, and Newfoundland.

There was an expectation that the CPR and GTR would take a direct interest in establishing divisions of the brigade but this did not occur, the railways were more concerned with having all of their employees trained and putting the effort into reaching a high level of training, than establishing company-wide ambulance divisions. This was unlike the various railways companies in England which actively set up ambulance divisions. Although enlisting the support of the railways for establishing ambulance divisions was not successful, the brigade was cooperating with the Mines Ambulance Rescue Corps (MARC), which operated in many of Canada's larger mines. The MARC would eventually be absorbed into the brigade, a process which began in 1912.[28]

The second Canadian nursing division was founded on 19 May 1913 as No. 2 Fort Gary Nursing Division, with Lady Divisional Superintendent Edith Hudson as its head. Hudson was a registered nurse, as were a number of other members of the newly-minted division, including Alfreda Jean Attrill, who would become one of the first women to enter the Canadian Army Medical Corps after the beginning of the First World War.[29] By the beginning of 1913 Canada had 24 ambulance divisions and three nursing divisions, with approximately 700 officers and men along with 54 nursing officers and sisters. With five ambulance divisions, Toronto had the largest establishment, followed by Winnipeg with five, London with three, Hamilton with two (one at the Westinghouse factory), and one each at Brampton, Brandon, Muskoka, North Bay, Oshawa, Owen Sound, Saskatoon, Sutherland (SK), and Welland. The three nursing divisions were located in Toronto, Winnipeg, and Owen Sound. In less than five years the brigade had grown greatly and although the early focus was overwhelmingly on Ontario, the events of the First World War would help to spread it from sea to sea. The number of nursing and ambulance brigade divisions in Toronto and Winnipeg warranted the creation of a Toronto Corps, No. 1 and the Winnipeg Corps No. 2. Winnipeg was especially interesting as it included a fire brigade division, CPR division, and trades and labour division, demonstrating the high value that workers and employers, whether it be transportation, manufacturing, or public safety, placed on the work of the brigade and St. John Ambulance first aid training in general.

Despite the success of the first brigade divisions, the association continued to experience difficulty finding enough funds to maintain solvency, and it was the railways that helped to prop up its finances in the first two years of operation, which preceded the patriotic call of the First World War that caused donations to rise substantially. Officials at St. John's Gate were impressed with the progress of the new Canadian branch, and although concerned about the financial situation, they noted "remarkable progress [has been] made in the face of financial difficulties."[30] This was no understatement given that a firm donation/subscription base had not yet been built up. Sir Thomas Shaughnessy, president of the CPR, John Manuel, a prominent Ottawa lumber merchant, Sir Edward Clouston, vice-president of the Bank of Montreal, and George Drummond, a Montreal businessman, donated a combined total of $3,000 in 1910.[31] In monetary terms, these four men donated three quarters of all the funds for the 1910–1911 year in which the work of the Canadian branch got underway.[32] While the general membership of the association was high on enthusiasm and organizational skills, until the beginning of the First World War they would largely rely on the generosity of a few influential men. It is interesting to note that of these four benefactors, three, Shaughnessy, Clouston, and Manuel came from humble backgrounds, starting their working lives in hazardous environments where first aid skills were invaluable. We can only speculate that the interest of these gentlemen was in part on account of their own experiences, this would have been especially true for Shaughnessy who worked on American and Canadian railways and Clouston who worked in the lumber and sawmill trade.[33] Without this seed money and early support the work of the new branch in Canada "would have [had] to be suspended."[34]

Although the brigade and association cooperated, and there was a great deal of crossover between their members at the senior levels of the organizations, they operated as separate entities. Provincial councils for the association had been inaugurated in 1910 following the establishment of the Canadian branch. It helped that Dr. Montizambert, Colonel Jones, and Dr. Hodgetts, all held positions in the federal government that allowed them to travel across Canada in their official capacities and concurrently carry out association work, attending meetings or helping to set up local centres. In September 1910 the Canadian branch began organizing in the maritime provinces. As a result the first provincial councils were founded in St. John, New Brunswick; Halifax, Nova Scotia; and Charlottetown, Prince Edward Island. New Brunswick was the first province to be organized. The lieutenant-governors of each of these provinces were enlisted as patrons, forming a long and profitable relationship between the provincial representatives of the Crown and the association that continues to this day. In Prince Edward Island even the elected government wanted to be involved, supporting the training of the Intercolonial and Prince Edward Island Railroad workers.

The Ontario Provincial Council was formed on 21 December 1910 in Toronto at the

Normal School Assembly Hall. Governor General Lord Grey was present to offer the keynote address on the importance of the association and first aid training. Although "the work of the Association has been more active in the province of Ontario during the past few years than in any other part of Canada,"[35] the fact remained that outside of Toronto, Ontario's was developing slowly in this period. In part this was because the various Toronto centres tended to dominate the affairs of the association.

Growth in Quebec was slow as well, although this was more on account of the absence of two leading members of the executive, George R. Drummond and William Molson Macpherson. It was not until 8 November 1911 that the Quebec Provincial Council was established following a meeting at the Windsor Hotel. The lieutenant-governor replaced Lord Strathcona and Sir Thomas Shaughnessy as patron of that council, but the two railway barons would remain engaged in the work of the association becoming patrons of the CPR centre. One of the early successes of the Quebec council was a grant given by Montreal's city council of $250 towards the training of members of the municipal police force and fire department in first aid. Within a year of being established the Quebec Provincial Council set about having St. John Ambulance first aid training materials translated into French, an important step in opening up association to francophones. It had been noted that "the absence of a text book on first aid in the French language has been felt for a long time and it is expected that the distribution of this book [*Cantlie's First Aid*] will mean an advance among our French speaking citizens in the provinces of Quebec and New Brunswick."[36] There was a nearly immediate increase in classes being taken by French Canadians.[37]

The first western province to be organized was Manitoba. The inaugural meeting was held on 6 January 1911 at the Oddfellows Hall in Winnipeg and was presided over by the Lieutenant-Governor Sir Daniel MacMillan. The city controller made a presentation on the importance of first aid and suggested that all police, fire, and civic employees should undertake training. From Winnipeg the general secretary travelled to Alberta to help establish yet another provincial council. He was slowed by a snowstorm and the Edmonton meeting was delayed, but finally held on 11 January at the Edmonton YMCA, presided over by Lieutenant-Governor George H.V. Bulyea. The chief of police, fire chief, and other civic officials attended the meeting, and, as in Winnipeg, agreed to undertake a vigorous training program. In September of 1910 a preliminary meeting of what would become the British Columbia Provincial Council as held in Victoria at the Canadian Club. At that meeting the provincial health officer, Dr. C.J. Fagan proposed its creation. On 24 June the council was created. One of the more interesting developments out of the meeting was a promise made by the police chief to have every member of his force trained in first aid. Victoria was unusual in that the police department operated the city ambulance, and thus first aid training was all the more necessary.

Saskatchewan was the last western province to be organized as a provincial council. A public meeting was held on 27 January in the presence of Lieutenant-Governor George Brown. The president of the Saskatchewan Medical Association strongly supported the work of the St. John Ambulance Association and encouraged the creation of a council.

General Secretary Birdwhistle put considerable effort into organizing his cross-country tour, managing to involve all the lieutenant-governors, senior medical officers, the press, and persons holding St. John first aid certificates, "speakers at the meetings in all the provinces were impressed with the possibilities of the work."[38] Aside from problems caused by inclement weather in a few of the western provinces, each meeting was well attended by members of the general public. Birdwhistle's whirlwind tour was perhaps too focused on soliciting high profile support for provincial councils in the form of judges, lieutenant-governors, and other high ranking officials.[39] It is difficult not to think that the general secretary was more concerned with holding impressive social gatherings involving the social elite, sprinkled with speeches about first aid training, than getting people at the most general level interested in the work of the association. Not a great deal of effort was put into enticing more average citizens to partic- ipate in the organization and permutation of provincial councils, or, more importantly, local centres. The provinces that suffered most as a result of this top down approach were Saskatchewan, Prince Edward Island, and New Brunswick. The latter province failed to even submit a report in 1914, while the PEI Provincial Council noted that "activities of our branch had been more limited than desirable,"[40] Saskatchewan was more blunt in assessing their work, "little progress [has been] made by the St. John Ambulance Association in this Province."[41] Alberta had made a solid recovery after a rough start in 1911 and 1912, but it was the First World War that would vitalize theses provincial councils and their community work.

With the development of the councils the association in Canada now consisted of many layers, which offered the young organization structure that it did not have under the old Dominion Council, which was essentially composed of local branches with no broader regional structure. It was a period of optimism for the association, even King George V was pleased to note "with satisfaction that the organization of the St. John Ambulance work in Canada is proceeding so well."[42] During their cross country travels, Montizambert, Jones, and Hodgetts were assiduous in making use of the local media. Newspapers in each town and city were visited and presented with information of the value of first aid training and the work of the association in other communities. It was a clever way to spark local interest and ensure large turn outs for inaugural meetings.

The Canadian branch acquired a new headquarters in Ottawa, the Castle Building on Queen Street. This would provide a suitable location for the association until the conclusion of the First World War when the headquarters was moved to the Banque Nationale Building. Two staff were employed, the general secretary and a stenographer. It was a remarkably small staff for an expanding organization, one which relied more than ever on volunteers and donations.

The Grand Trunk Railway followed the example set by its leading competitor, the CPR, by covering the cost of association first aid courses. Under the chairmanship of William Molson Macpherson, the company's chief medical officer, Dr. Alex Huchinson, had commenced first aid classes in early 1909, and would go on to teach association first aid by 1910. In 1910 the course was offered to a small class of 15 men, and an ambulance room, outfitted to association standards, was set up at Pointe St-Charles Shops in Montreal. The Winnipeg centre held classes at the College of Pharmacy and members of the local Boy Scouts unit and the ladies belonging to the Lord Selkirk Chapter of the Imperial Order of Daughters of the Empire were among the first to take courses.

Involvement of government agencies was not uncommon. By the beginning of the First World War many municipal police and fire departments encouraged or required their members to take association first aid training. At the 1913 convention of chiefs of police, held in Halifax, Assistant General Secretary S.A. Gidlow made a presentation about the value of first aid training, and "the convention endorsed the work, and a motion was unanimously carried, recommending that first Aid instruction should be given to Police Forces."[43] The Dominion Police, who guarded the Parliament Buildings in Ottawa and served as Canada's first secret service, were also required to hold association first aid certificates.[44] When suggestions or regulations were not enough legislation was enacted to ensure that certain employees were trained in first aid. The first example of this was the Department of Education in British Columbia which required every teacher employed by the provincial Normal Schools to possess a certificate. Shiftbosses, firebosses, and shotlighters were also required to hold a first aid certificate. This was not always at St. Johns Ambulance Association certificate, as other organizations such as the Mines Ambulance Rescue Corps also issued certificates. It is notable that that organization was eventually absorbed into the association. Indeed, British Columbia's provincial government was the most proactive in requiring first aid training for workers who worked in injury prone occupations. The 1912 annual report of the province's chief inspector of mines made special mention of the work undertaken:

> the St. John Ambulance Association has established centres in most of the coal-mining communities, and from now on there will be a fixed standard of examination and uniform training throughout the Province.[45]

In 1914 British Columbia's premier, Sir Richard McBride, who was also the minister of mines, appointed a royal commission to investigate a number of labour problems. This resulted in the appointment of a permanent first aid instructor by the Ministry of Labour, after consultation with the association. McBride had spent much of his youth working in a salmon cannery,[46] another environment where first aid was regularly required.

In other provinces, association first-aid courses were being taken up by miners and labourers alike. Operations such as the Copper Cliff Copper Company in Northern Ontario quickly adopted association first aid courses. Mine operators had been training their employees in general first aid, one of the first was the Dominion Coal Company in Nova Scotia, which began doing so in 1908. With the growth of association first aid the responsibility quickly fell to it. In British Columbia and Alberta miners had been required to take first aid courses from the colliery doctor. For British Columbia this became a legal requirement in 1912, with the Coal Miners Regulation Act. Such articles of legislation greatly assisted the association's work. The military also began taking an increased interest in St. John Ambulance first aid courses, especially as so many militia doctors and surgeons were involved in the organization. Many units began liaising with the association, often through their commanding officers, to offer first aid training. The 3rd Regiment of the Victoria Rifles had their stretcher sections trained by association; all members of the No. XXI Cavalry Field Ambulance and the No. XVI Cavalry Field Ambulance units in Winnipeg took association first aid courses in 1912.

Outside of the railways, association first aid training became a staple of employee training. A number of industrial companies inaugurated ambulance divisions of the brigade. The first among these was the Canadian Westinghouse Company located in Hamilton, Ontario. The division was founded by Samuel Holland, who had worked for the British Westinghouse Company until his immigration to Canada in 1905. At the Hamilton plant he was responsible for plant safety and was in charge of the fire watch and ambulance department. He enlisted seventeen other plant employees to undertake association first aid training to earn their certificates and by 1912 the No. 7 Canadian Westinghouse Ambulance Division was registered. Holland had the assistance of Dr. J.A. Simpson who taught the first aid courses, and who periodically acted as the plant physician.

With provincial councils in every province by the end of 1911, "at the present time there is no portion of the Dominion, outside of the Yukon Territory, that is not properly and efficiently equipped for spreading a knowledge of first aid, nursing, sanitation etc."[47] Centres of the association were now present in Toronto, Montreal, Ottawa, Hamilton, London, Quebec City, Vancouver, Victoria, Winnipeg, Halifax, St. John, Galt, West Toronto, Michel, Bowmanville, Eholt, North Bay, Port Burwell, Cranbrook, MacLeod, Calgary, Coleman, Bankhead, Jaw, Belleville, Brandon, Goderich, Swift Current, Woodstock, Kenora, Glace Bay, Fort William, Paris, Berlin, Farnham, Windsor, Carlton Place, Smith's Falls, Revelstoke, and "many others" as the 1911 annual report noted. There were still weak areas, such as Saskatchewan, Prince Edward Island, and New Brunswick.

Given the success that the association was continuing to experience with the CPR and GTR, a directive went out from headquarters in Ottawa that each centre should "encourage employees of all public utilities to take up first aid work, largely because of these men and women so frequently coming into contact with the general public,"[48] and because of the hazardous nature of their work. Other organizations such as the Boy Scouts, Girl Guides, Police, Fire Departments, YMCA, YWCA, and the Women's Christian Temperance Union (WCTU) were also approached with a good deal of success.

The CPR provides the most tangible example of why association first aid training was so popular and so highly valued by worker and employer alike. It also helps that the CPR centre kept fairly detailed statistics on the number of accidents and deaths experienced by their employees. By 1911 more than 2,000 CPR employees had been trained in association first aid. Over this same period 6,722 accidents were treated of which 964 were classified as "serious," which meant they required the injured party to spend time in hospital.[49] As compared with 1909 this was a decrease of 3,426 cases. The CPR hired two permanent association instructors to travel across the country training CPR employees and fitted out two railway car classrooms for teaching.[50] Each car provided a lecture theatre that seated up to 30 students, although much of the instruction was given to smaller groups, given the unusual teaching hours of 8 a.m. to 10 p.m. The CPR and the association set up a flexible system for employees to take training when they had time, and not during specific set class hours. A system of attendance forms was set up for travelling railway workers who would take classes in various towns and cities they were travelling through. Major CPR railway stations were kitted with a large association first aid box "throughout the CPR system," along with Furley pattern stretchers.

During an address to the annual general meeting of the Canadian branch of the association, Lieutenant-Colonel Lacey R. Johnson, chair of the CPR referred to the average railway man as a "happy go lucky" sort of fellow, who is regularly exposed to danger, yet takes it as part of his job:

You will see him jumping on to the footboard of an approaching switch engine, and on to moving cars, without the slightest hesitation or apparent thought of risk to life and limb in every case of a mis-step. In fact he will be witness to the mis-step with its horrible consequences, and immediately turn around and do it again, notwithstanding the rules and warnings laid down by the Railway Companies to prevent it.[51]

In the same address Johnson recalled an incident where the provision of aid by a trained association first aider saved the life of a CPR employee:

A section man had one of his feet badly torn and left leg broken through his hand car being struck by a train on a sharp curve. The conductor of the train took charge of the case and rendered First Aid. The doctor who was called was so pleased with the work done by Conductor Leach that he wrote the Local secretary in Ottawa as follows: — "having learned that you are interested in First aid to the Injured, I desire to let you know of the excellent services rendered ... I have not the least doubt but that Sectionman Courchaine would have bled to death had it not been for the timely and efficient assistance of Mr. Leach, who not only stopped the hemmorage [sic] by his proper application of the tourniquet, but in several other ways shewed the advantage of his training in this direction. I cannot speak too highly of Mr. Leach, and his work on this occasion goes to show that all railroad men should be so trained."

Even office work could be dangerous:

A lady stenographer, engaged in a railway office, severed an artery in her hand by a piece of glass, another young lady, who possessed a St. John Certificate, arrested the hemmorage [sic] until the arrival of a doctor.

Such testimonials from employers, medical doctors, and onlookers often appeared in the press and helped to bolster interest in first aid training and the association.

The CPR and GTR were not alone in vigorously supporting first aid training. By 1913 all of Canada's major railways were involved, as the Intercolonial and Canadian Northern had each commenced training their employees through association courses. One reason that industry and various levels of government were supportive of the work of the association was because of the number of people it saved, and thus improved productivity. Between 1904 and 1910 there were on average 1,300 deaths of working men per year, and another 10,000 were seriously injured. The view of many government officials was that "we permanently impair the nation"[52] through these sorts of injuries and deaths. Association first aid training saved lives and treated injury in an expeditious fashion, speeding recovery and reducing days off.

The Grand Prior Moves to Canada

The installation of governors general has been a regular event in Canada since the late years of the French regime. Yet the arrival of the Duke and Duchess of Connaught along with their youngest daughter Princess Patricia, on 13 October 1911 in Quebec City was met with great enthusiasm. The Duke was after all the youngest son of Queen Victoria and a member of the royal family. Members of the Canadian branch of the association also had reason to rejoice with the arrival of the new governor general, as he was also grand prior of the Venerable Order of St. John and an enthusiastic promoter of the association and brigade.[53] Early on during their tenure at Rideau Hall it was noted that "both Their Royal Highnesses have shown much interest in the work of the Association in Canada, and have by their encouragement assisted in speaking a knowledge of the work."[54] Even Princess Patricia, whose name is born by one of Canada's most famed regiments, Princess Patricia's Canadian Light Infantry, became involved; first aid training was not limited to working men alone. An association first aid course was held at Government House where Princess Patricia along with a number of staff earned their certificates.[55]

Connaught's enthusiasm, peerless social status, and prestige all helped the work of the association in Canada. One cannot underestimate the symbolic power of having such an individual involved in the work of the Canadian branch, especially in a period when so much of the Canadian identity was focused on the British connection. It also helped that Connaught was a popular governor general who travelled extensively throughout the Dominion.[56] He was present at many of the annual meetings of the Canadian branch and allowed Government House to be used regularly for special meetings. Connaught's support had a salutary effect, as the lieutenant-governors, who had been made patrons of the various provincial councils were keen to emulate his example; they were after all tantamount to provincial viceroys much as the governor general was the viceroy of Canada.[57]

The value of association first aid training and organizational skills were proven following the Regina Cyclone of 1912. Ironically the Saskatchewan Provincial Council had experienced some difficulty in commencing operation — "work in this province has been at a standstill"[58] — and it was the most underdeveloped in Canada. Nevertheless small classes had been held in Moose Jaw and Regina during the previous year resulting in 32 first aid certificates being issued. The cyclone (actually a tornado) was the first natural disaster that the association would involve itself in. At 5:00 p.m. on 30 June as residents began preparations for Dominion Day celebrations, 400 km/hr winds hit Regina. It still stands as one of the most deadly natural disasters in Canadian history, killing 28 people and leaving 2,500 homeless.[59]

As soon as news was telegraphed across the country an emergency meeting of the executive committee of the Canadian branch was held in Ottawa. It was decided to send the general secretary, Major Birdwhistle, to Regina immediately to work with the newly formed Saskatchewan Provincial Council on the relief effort. Simultaneously the Ottawa Board of Control voted a grant of $2,000 to the association to assist with the relief effort in Regina. The reaction from Regina was almost instant, on 3 July Saskatchewan Premier Walter Scott telegrammed, "Please accept thanks of people of Saskatchewan, as well as those of Regina, for the steps taken by your Executive to aid those stricken in Sunday's calamity."[60] Major Birdwhistle played an important role in the relief work undertaken in Regina as part of the Relief Committee, he also provided the cabinet, through Acting Prime Minister Sir George Perley, with reports on the devastation. Subsequent telegrams of thanks and appreciation were received in the weeks and months following the disaster.

The Regina Cyclone proved to members of the Canadian branch of the association and the deputy commissioner of the brigade that further expansion was necessary, the lethargic pace of development in Saskatchewan and Alberta was unacceptable, and the disaster provided an excellent example of why immediate progress was necessary. Even with increased interest from headquarters in Ottawa and a diligent effort to improve the situation in these provinces, it would take the First World War to fully activate the work. The rural nature of Canada's west and its poor economic health at this time were key factors behind the situation.

St. John in Parliament

With the development of provincial councils and expansion of the work of the association, it became necessary to take legal steps to incorporate the Canadian branch, so it could function as a truly national organization. This would allow it to purchase assets such as buildings and to legally hold large donations. Under the leadership of Dr. Frederick Montizambert the Canadian Branch of the St. John Ambulance Association was formally incorporated by act of Parliament.[61] This occurred scarcely two months before the outbreak of the First World War. The *Act to incorporate The General Council of the Canadian Branch of the St. John Ambulance Association* was typical of such acts of incorporation passed by the Senate in this period.[62] Other organizations that incorporated around this period were the Canadian branch of the British Red Cross Society (1909) and the Canadian General Council of Boy Scouts (1914).

The Bill was drafted by the association's honorary solicitor Mr. J.F. Ordre who would later serve as president of the Canadian branch from 1920–21. Colonel James Mason, senator for Toronto introduced the bill for first reading on 30 April 1914.[63] Second reading occurred soon there after, and the third and final reading occurred on 15 May 1914. Senator Hewitt Bostock reported on behalf of Senate Miscellaneous and Private Bills Committee noting that the committee "have in obedience of the reference …. examined the said Bill and now beg leave to report the same without any amendment."[64] There was no great debate or controversy surrounding the incorporation of the Canadian branch of the association. The Senate was all the more gripped by inquiries related to salaries and retiring allowances for judges and proposed amendments to the Juvenile Delinquents Act. The committee report tabled, third reading was discharged by Senator Bostock and the bill was transmitted to HRH The Duke of Connaught for royal assent, which was given on 12 June. Bostock would go on to become president of the St. John Ambulance Association in Canada from 1928 to 1929. It did not hurt that both Mason and Bostock were deeply involved in the affairs of the association, as was the governor general, and Sir Louis Davies, a judge of the Supreme Court of Canada.[65] Others listed in the articles of incorporation included gentlemen from every province and the Yukon — demonstrating the pan-Canadian nature of the organization, though with notable absences, French Canadians in particular. The Quebec Provincial Council was almost entirely dominated by the English Montreal elite, and it would be some years before the organization became more open to francophones. Effort had, however, been put into having association teaching materials translated into French, and while not involved in the senior ranks of the association, French Canadians were eligible for first aid certificates. This situation was indicative of the period.

The act set out the purpose of the Canadian branch of the association:

To promote and carry out in Canada the objects of the said Canadian Branch, namely:
- The instruction of persons in rendering first aid in cases of accidents or sudden illness, and in the transport of the sick and injured;
- The instruction of persons in the elementary principles and practices of nursing, and also of hygiene and sanitation;
- The manufacture and distribution by sale or presentation of ambulance material, and the formation of ambulance depots in mines, factories, and other centres of industry and traffic;
- The organization of ambulance corps, invalid transport corps and nursing corps (provided that any scheme for the formation of organization of such corps be first approved by the Chapter General) … and the assistance of the St. John Ambulance Brigade Overseas within the Dominion of Canada;
- And generally the promotion of instruction and carrying out of works for the relief of suffering of the suck and injured in peace and war, independently of class, nationality or denomination.

The act was surreptitiously passed in the period leading up to the First World War, and from a legal standpoint would be crucial to the association playing a key role on the national stage, both in Canada and overseas.

The bylaws of the Canadian branch of the association set out that it was a foundation of the Grand Priory in the British Realm.[66] The administrative structure of the association was also delineated, with the General Council being the governing body, with subordinate provincial councils, special company councils, and special centres under it. At the top of the organization was the Executive Committee, which was elected by the General Council, this was, as its name suggests, the main decision making body, and consisted of the president, vice-presidents, two honorary treasurers, and the deputy commissioner for the St. John Ambulance Brigade Overseas in Canada. Previously the association and brigade operated as separate entities, despite a high degree of cooperation. The inclusion of the deputy commissioner signalled that there was to be a continuing close relationship between the organizations. Indeed, the brigade was in practice, subordinate to the Canadian branch of the association, although it remained under the command of the commissioner for the St. John Ambulance Brigade Overseas, who was an official based out of St. John's Gate in London. The Executive Committee had control over the approval of and withdrawal of approval for provincial councils and local centres.

The required structure for provincial councils and local centres was also set out in the bylaws with the desire to have uniformity in governance structures across the country. Given the difficulties experienced in the first five years of the twentieth century in keeping local centres viable and functioning, it is not surprising that so much effort was put into outlining their structure and role within the broader Canadian branch of the association. The local centres were subordinate to the provincial councils, while they in turn reported to the General Council, thus much like the federal structure of Canada there were three levels with varying degrees of responsibility and authority.

Passage of the act was a fitting event to precede the outbreak of war. The Dominion government recognized the national character of the Canadian branch of the association and the fortunes of both the brigade and the association were positive. In 1911 a total of 3,179 people took an association first aid course, and 2,138 received a first aid certificate. By the beginning of 1914 this had increased to 6,364 people taking classes and 3,588 earning their certificates. The Ontario Provincial Council and CPR centre had the highest overall enrollment, but with the beginning of the war the number of Canadians trained, both civilians and military would balloon.

The Forgotten Colony

Given that until 1949 Newfoundland was not part of Canada, it would be incorrect to simply combine events in that colony in with the rest of Canada. Newfoundland was at one time a dominion, equal in status to Canada and, although possessing a small population, rendered extraordinary services during the First and Second World Wars, both at sea and on land.

The development of the association and brigade in Newfoundland mirrors that of many Canadian provinces in the same time period, with the establishment of the association and first aid training preceding the creation of a brigade unit. There is no evidence to suggest that the establishment of a branch of the association in Canada played a role in the creation of the Newfoundland centre of the association and division of the brigade. St. John Ambulance first aid training had been given in Newfoundland as early as 1905 under the supervision of Dr. Cluny Macpherson, at a time when the association in Canada was almost dormant. Macpherson had returned to Newfoundland in 1902 upon completion of his medical training at the Royal Infirmary in Edinburgh. He spent a great deal of time working in costal Labrador and helped to successfully control a smallpox epidemic. He would found a medical practice in St. John's in 1904 and shortly thereafter he began teaching first aid using St. John Ambulance Association materials. His experience in remote communities in both Newfoundland and Labrador gave him a strong appreciation for the value of basic first aid training, especially in communities where there was no resident doctor or surgeon.[67] Macpherson took a keen interest in all matters that touched upon public health, along with helping to found the Newfoundland centre of the St. John Ambulance Association and a division of the brigade, he was one of the founders of the Newfoundland Medical Association and the Newfoundland Outport Nursing and Industrial Association. The early courses held by Macpherson were given before the formal establishment of the Newfoundland centre of the association, but there is ample evidence from the annual reports of the association that theses were undertaken with the knowledge and consent of St. John's Gate.

Almost simultaneous with the establishment of the Canadian branch of the association, Newfoundland established its first centre. On 11 April 1910, under the patronage of Governor Sir Ralph Williams, the Newfoundland centre was brought into being. From 1905 to 1909 the previous governor, Sir William MacGregor, who was himself a medical doctor and keen exponent of St. John Ambulance first aid training, worked to ensure that skippers and seamen were given basic training in first aid. During the first year of operation, the centre in St. John's gave instruction to more than 400 people, since the population of St. John's was only 32,242,[68] this was an impressive achievement.[69]

Given the rural nature of the population and the high proportion who engaged in either the fishery or merchant navy, Newfoundland was a natural place for the first aid work of the association and brigade to take hold. The high degree of self sufficiency and ingenuity required to survive in the adverse conditions faced by those working by the sea made first aid training popular. Dr. Macpherson was instrumental in ensuring the initial success of the branch, and Chief Justice Sir William Horwood, was appointed president. This followed the standard St. John Association pattern of enlisting the support of prominent citizens in the organization of branches and centres.

Following the founding meeting the Newfoundland centre of the association petitioned the colonial government for a grant of $500 to help underwrite the costs of setting up a fully functioning centre. Such petitions by the association in other colonies and dominions were not uncommon. The association was awarded a grant of $100, certainly the patronage of the governor and chief justice, among many other prominent local citizens, helped the application. By the summer of 1910 first aid and home nursing classes were being held in St. John's. In the first year, six classes were held with 138 attendees, 107 exams were given, and 71 passed. Special classes were held for members of the Newfoundland Constabulary and members of the St. John's Fire Brigade.[70] It was a solid beginning.

Following the success experienced by the association in 1910 and 1911, it was speculated that "a branch of the St. John Ambulance brigade will be formed within the next two months,"[71] an optimistic prediction, that was not far off the mark. There was a general trend in other dominions and colonies that once the association had been established for a few years and as the pool of first aid certificate holders grew, that the establishment of a brigade was almost inevitable. On 7 May 1912, two years after the establishment of the Newfoundland centre of the association, and the holding of many classes, the No. 1 Church Lad's Brigade Division of the St. John Ambulance Brigade was established. Under the direction of Dr. Macpherson, an active member of the association, the brigade came into existence with seventeen members.[72] As the name suggests, all the founding members of the brigade were members of the Church Lad's Brigade.[73] During the First World War, most of the medical staff attached to the Newfoundland Regiment was trained by the association and many were members of the No. 1 Division of the brigade. It was a exemplary start to both the association and brigade in Newfoundland, setting the foundation of two organizations that would cooperate during the First World War to render highly notable service to King and Country.

FIVE

CALL TO SERVICE

The First World War

We are all cooperating on the same level, in a good, patriotic service.
Annual Report of the Canadian Branch Association, 1916

The First World War provided both the St. John Ambulance Association and the St. John Ambulance Brigade with an opportunity to serve King and Country. This service was rendered with distinction in Canada, Newfoundland, and abroad. Perhaps the greatest contribution made by the association and brigade was the training of approximately 200,000 members of the Canadian Expeditionary Force (CEF), not to mention the training given to every medic and stretcher bearer in the famed Newfoundland Regiment, most of whom were members of the brigade before the outbreak of war. Other significant contributions included Newfoundlander, Dr. Cluny Macpherson's invention of the first gas mask to be widely used by British and Empire troops. The war allowed the St. John Ambulance to offer training to an ever-expanding number of people, bringing relief to the sick and injured on the battlefield and on the home front. The war and the demand for the skills offered by St. John Ambulance helped the organization grow into a modern entity, truly national in scope, focused on serving humanity in its hour of greatest need. The war also brought about a change throughout Canadian society in the position held by women. Although they already held a prominent place within the Order, the nursing services rendered between 1914 and 1918 were among the most significant contributions of St. John Ambulance in Canada. Twenty-two members of the St. John Ambulance Brigade, who enlisted or became VADs (members of a Volunteer Aid Detachment, see next section), died while serving during the war; five women and seventeen men in total.[1]

An important internal change also developed during this period, the emergence of St. John Ambulance, as a term used to identify both the association and the brigade. Although the two organizations were linked together as two of the three foundations of the Order, they had hitherto been considered separate in terms of administration and structure. However, in Canada at least, the two were increasingly referred to as "St. John Ambulance" despite retaining separate command structures. This was in part because of the significant degree of cross-over between members of the two organizations. There are indications that this increased sense of cooperation was brought about by the War, the focus being overwhelmingly on winning and not on squabbling over jurisdictional issues between the association and brigade. Another area, in which jurisdictional issues would cease to be a significant problem for the duration, was in the relationship between St. John Ambulance and the Canadian branch of the British Red Cross Society, commonly known as the Canadian Red Cross. The Duke of Connaught's patronage of the Order of St. John, as grand prior and patron of the Canadian branch, and as patron of the Red Cross Society in Canada eased the pre-existing tensions; few would be bold enough to question the Duke's loyalty to the Order or his desire to see victory achieved.

From its founding in Canada, the Canadian branch of the association had a strong link to the Canadian militia and these links were strengthened in the period leading up to the outbreak of war. Through this connection St. John Ambulance was able to make a direct contribution to the welfare of CEF members serving at home and overseas. Cooperation between the association and militia was not surprising given that so many members of the association were members of what would become the Canadian Army Medical Corps, and in the case of the brigade there was similar cross-pollination between the organization and military. In Britain during the last quarter of the nineteenth century a plan was arranged for the "deployment from civil sources of voluntary aid to the Militia and medical services."[2] As we have seen, this resulted in the offering of courses for men and women in general first aid. This would be duplicated in Canada. Most of these first aid courses were offered by the St. John Ambulance Association, while a smaller number were given by the Red Cross Society. From this a medical reserve was amassed for use in hospitals and in mobile field units.

A leading figure in the success of the association, brigade, and fledgling Canadian Army Medical Corps was Colonel, later Major-General, Guy Carleton Jones. A native of Halifax, Jones was educated at the Halifax Medical College and later King's College London. In the early 1890s he became involved with the association in Halifax, long before the Canadian branch was established. In 1898 he became the first commanding officer of a bearer company attached to a militia unit in Canada. Along with Ryerson, Jones helped to create the Canadian Army Medical Corps. This was a process that was started following Ryerson's and Jones's return from service in the Anglo-Boer War. The two men were also founding members of the Association of Medical Officers of the Militia of Canada,[3] leaders in the field of military medicine.

The Militia Council, the body responsible for advising the minister of militia and defence, approved a plan for the organization of "Voluntary Medical Aid" in Canada on 29 November 1911, this plan would subsequently be augmented and approved by the Milita Council on 3 March 1914, well before the outbreak of war. The scheme provided for the creation of voluntary aid committees (VACs) in each of Canada's nine military districts. Members of each VAC were appointed by the minister on the recommendation of the association and Red Cross. Each VAC was made responsible for organizing voluntary aid detachments in its district. Naturally this required a good deal of cooperation between St. John Ambulance and the Red Cross. A similar scheme had been developed in England in 1877 "as part of the country's Voluntary Aid

Movement."[4] In the United Kingdom, the first full test came in the Anglo-Boer War when 1,871 men trained by the association were seconded to British medical units.

On 14 August 1914, shortly after the outbreak of war a special meeting was held at Rideau Hall between senior officials of the Department of Militia and Defence, the association, brigade, and the Canadian branch of the British Red Cross Society. This was done under the direction of HRH the Duke of Connaught, who was governor general and patron of both organizations. It was "decided that in order that there should be no overlapping of work or energies that the obligations be coordinated, and that a general plan … [be] administered by an executive body of the whole."[5] This body was given the title "The National Relief Committee [Joint Committee]." It was at this meeting that an agreement was developed between St. John Ambulance and the Red Cross under the designation "the Joint Committee."

The entire association and brigade in Canada rallied behind the training of CEF members. Sir Louis Davies, president of the association made it his primary objective. "It was thought desirable that the force [CEF] should be so far as possible instructed, in First Aid … we are sending a quarter of a million of the best blood of Canada, across the seas to defend our liberties and our country, and we ought to see to it that every man, as far as possible is instructed in First Aid."[6]

It was realized how important first aid training was to those who would be serving at the front. One officer in the Canadian Field Artillery commented to the *British Daily Whig*, "Men of this kind could save dozens of lives per day. Men who are wounded and can walk go straggling back to the dressing stations. Sometimes they have some one to accompany them and sometimes not. In any case they often get lost when it is dark, and that is the last of them. I took probably a dozen such men into my dug-out and tied up their wounds; then sent them to the dressing station. This was in our last position on the Somme, where we were about 2,500 yards from the front line."[7]

Another innovation introduced under the plan devised with the militia department was the appointment of association and brigade first aid instructors with the rank and pay of a senior non-commissioned officer in each unit for a sufficient time to enable him to take up the work, so that each officer, NCO and man would have a general knowledge of First Aid to "enable him to be of service in case of accident, sudden illness."[8] These instructors were also attached to divisional staff headquarters and seconded to other units from time to time as necessary. The association selected suitable first aid instructors from each military district and also developed a short pamphlet on first aid "so that study could be taken up in private, and which could also be used as a reference book as required."[9] St. John Ambulance instructors were appointed with the rank and pay of quartermaster sergeants in the Canadian Army Medical Corps. One unintended problem with this scheme was that as the war dragged on many of the instructors enlisted or took commissions in the CEF, thus depriving St. John of its cadre of trained instructors.

It was not until late 1915 that first aid training of CEF members got fully underway. In November, "the General Executive Committee prepared a memorandum for the Minister of Militia and Defence on the subject of First Aid instruction for members of the CEF. The course proposed included instruction under the following headings, "a) fractures, dislocations and sprains; b) Haemorrhage or bleeding; c) artificial respiration and insensibility; d) bandaging; e) methods of carrying."[10] This proposal was accepted by the militia minister, Sir Sam Hughes. One of the key promoters of this project was the Duke of Connaught who would continue to play an important role in the work of St. John Ambulance. His campaign to ensure that all members of the CEF receive first aid training.[11] Given that Connaught was not on good terms with Hughes — whom he considered "a lunatic"[12] — it is testament to the Duke's devotion to and belief in the value of first aid training. As a result of this and the work of Jones, 150,000 copies of *Cantlie's First Aid* were printed by the King's Printer on behalf of the department, and more than 130,000 members of the CEF were trained in first aid by the association and members of the brigade in 1916.[13]

The Joint Committee: St. John Ambulance and the Red Cross

Commensurate with the outbreak of war St. John Ambulance and the Canadian branch of the British Red Cross Society (Red Cross Society of Canada) entered into an agreement to ensure that there was minimal overlap in the war-work of the organizations. Cooperation was encouraged by the governor general and senior members of the brigade who were similarly involved in the Red Cross. This agreement set up the Joint Committee, sometimes referred to as the Executive Committee, of the Red Cross and the association. Members of the Canadian militia and Dominion government were also involved in an *ex-officio* manner to provide a maximum level of coordination.

The Canadian agreement was worked out by the end of August 1914, and the parent bodies of both St. John Ambulance and the Red Cross in Britain would arrive at a similar agreement in October 1914, nearly two months after Canada. One reason an agreement was so rapidly developed in Canada was the hands on approach of the Duke of Connaught. There was also a high degree of overlap between the Red Cross and St. John Ambulance. Perhaps the best example of this was Ryerson, who it will be remembered was the founder of the association and of the Red Cross in Canada. Ryerson remained involved in both organizations, thus participation was not viewed as being disloyal to either the Red Cross or St. John Ambulance, but rather was seen as natural. Members of the association and brigade also become involved in the Canadian Patriotic Fund, Canadian Club, and other philanthropic organizations that sought to make a contribution — there was no mutual exclusivity.

As the Red Cross had international treaty recognition through the various Geneva Conventions, it was designated the umbrella organization under which the association and brigade operated for the duration of the war; thus both the organizations in Canada were made subordinate to the Red Cross. The principal goal of the agreement was to prevent duplication and competition for funds, while maximizing the efforts of volunteers working for each organization. The Red Cross had a history of working primarily in war zones, hence their inclusion in various treaties, being focused on providing relief during conflict, while St. John Ambulance worked to provide relief and training in times of war and peace. It was the training aspect that gave St. John a multifaceted purpose. Many Red Cross VADs and orderlies were trained by St. John Ambulance instructors. For the duration of the war the association included the sub-heading "A part of the Red Cross Organization of the British Empire" on all publications and letterhead. All VADs wore a Red Cross on their nurses uniform, usually accompanied by a St. John first aid medallion. All this was undertaken in an effort to emphasise the level of cooperation.

The relationship with the Red Cross was cordial, each organization not wanting to either duplicate the work of the other or impede the war effort by causing administrative or logistical difficulties. From an administrative standpoint it helped that one organization was placed over the other, the Red Cross had a larger membership and was serving throughout the British Empire alongside the association and brigade. There was nevertheless some discontent with St. John Ambulance's position as junior to that of the Red Cross. Perhaps Connaught explained the situation most succinctly on 24 February 1916 in the City Council Chamber of Ottawa City Hall. St. John Ambulance "is relatively in the same position as the Red Cross, except that we work in time of peace, whereas the Red Cross only works in time of war. Ladies and gentleman, what did we do when war broke out? We felt that during the war the Red Cross had the right to step forward, and we took second place. We have loyally supported the Red Cross and I am happy to say that there has never been any real friction."[14] This was a slightly glossy view of the relationship, as at least one aspect would become detrimental to the association in the immediate post-war period. Some were nevertheless uncomfortable with the degree of integration and cooperation. Dr. J.W. Robertson was incensed that the association was to be subordinate to the Red Cross "we are all cooperating on the same level, in a good, patriotic service."[15] Indeed Connaught's comments were directed at those who shared Robertson's view.

As part of the St. John Ambulance-Red Cross agreement in Canada the association agreed to cease actively petitioning for monetary donations, there being a desire not to confuse the general public or start a competition with the Red Cross. Along with this through 1916–1918 the association curtailed its solicitation of new membership — other than VADs and first aid instructors, "no special effort has been made to secure a large membership in the Association, as it was not desired to compete for subscriptions during war-time with the Red-Cross."[16] The association ceased to grow in membership, indeed one of the only reasons it remained stable was because of the number of VADs recruited, when set against the loss of membership to enlistment in the CEF the organization was stagnant in terms of expansion.

Agreeing to become subordinate to the Red Cross for the duration of the war made sense on paper and in the wartime context of the organization, "all Red Cross work in the Dominion has been done in the name of the Canadian Red Cross Society and our own workers in many instances constituted themselves into the Red Cross organizations where such did not previously exist."[17] The focus was overwhelmingly on war-work and cooperation, not taking advantage of the crisis at hand. The funding channelled through the Red Cross was sufficient and that the Red Cross took the lead in fundraising allowed the association and brigade to focus on their traditional activities of first aid instruction and treatment. With hindsight it is easy to second guess the decisions made, however in spite of all this St. John Ambulance was still able to make a significant contribution and work more closely with the Red Cross than any other organization in Canada.

An example of how donations were channelled through the Red Cross to St. John Ambulance is best illustrated by a $10,000 donation made by A.D. Miles, president of the Canadian Copper Company[18] in 1915. Miles requested that the money be directed to defraying the expense of sending twenty graduate nurses overseas and equipping them. The Joint Committee agreed on the details of the donation and how the money was to be disbursed. The graduate nurses were supplied with equipment purchased jointly by the Red Cross and St. John Ambulance — thus accruing a significant discount on account of the quantity — and transport was arranged through the Red Cross, the balance of the funds being put aside in a VAD current account. It not only saved money from an administrative and resource consumption standpoint, but it provided for coordinated purchasing of medical supplies and other necessities, which became increasingly important as the war dragged on into 1917 and 1918 with rationing of many goods being imposed by the Dominion government. The overall fundraising efforts of the Joint Committee were impressive. Special "Our Day" collections were held each year from 1915 to 1918. In 1915 the collections raised $2,340,982, while raising $1,897,000 the following year, both immense amounts of money in an era when a loaf of bread cost 10 cents.[19]

The president of the association, J.M. Courtney was aware of the post-war disadvantage that such close cooperation with the Red Cross was placing St. John Ambulance at, and he attempted to explain his reasoning, "the more we can extend this cooperation with great municipalities and similar institutions throughout the length and breadth of the country the greater will be the benefit which will accrue to the community as a whole."[20] This was tempered with the statement that "it is not only to its war organization but to its peace organization as well that we must keep our thoughts directed."[21] Part of this plan included a vigorous campaign to increase first aid training in the provinces. By the end of the war the numbers of civilians trained had doubled with a tripling in the number of first aid certificates awarded.

By the end of 1915 in England there were 970 hospitals being run by the British Red Cross Society and 150 hospitals being operated by St. John Ambulance. The St. John Hospitals were staffed entirely with St. John Ambulance personnel, while the Red Cross hospitals had a mix of Red Cross and St. John Ambulance personnel. In France there were nine Red Cross Hospitals, with 1,040 beds and these were staffed by both Red Cross and St. John Ambulance personnel, primarily VADs. There was also the St. John Ambulance Brigade Hospital at Étaples in France, which had 520 beds.[22] The St. John Ambulance organization as a whole proved itself to be both an effective cooperator with the Red Cross and remained capable of fielding stand-alone St. John hospitals and convalescent establishments.

The $10,000 donation made by the Canadian Copper Company was used to send the first group of Canadian graduate nurses to serve overseas. As graduate nurses were unable to serve as VADs the association and brigade looked for ways to utilize their training and skills. The initial contingent was made up of 20 nurses who had all worked in hospitals with more than 100 beds and had been involved with the association or the brigade. Along with 10 Red Cross nurses they sailed from Montreal on 20 May 1915 aboard the S.S. *Missanabie*. An additional 15 graduate nurses sailed for England in July. Many of these nurses would see service at the large St. John Ambulance Brigade Hospital at Étaples in France.

The First Voluntary Aid Detachments: The VADs

One of the most visible and remembered contributions made by St. John Ambulance during the First World War was the provision of Voluntary Aid Detachment personnel (VADs) to work in hospitals treating and ministering to wounded soldiers. Canadian VADs served in Britain, France, Egypt, and Salonika, not to mention on the home front. They tended wounded soldiers, sailors, airmen, and civilians at home in Canada during the Influenza Epidemic of 1918–1919. "The spirit of V.A.D.'s is the same the world over. The one desire is to be of service."[23]

Most VADs acted as what today we would call nursing assistants, as trained nurses were ineligible to serve as VADs. Most trained nurses involved in St. John were part of the brigade or took commissions in the Canadian Army Medical Corps. VADs in the First World War were typically Anglo-Protestant, middle class, unmarried women, ranging in age from mid-twenties to early thirties. Many of them held university degrees and left paid employment for the chance to undertake unpaid VAD service abroad.[24]

There were different VAD classifications: Nursing Members, Functional Trainers, Special Service, and General Service. Nursing members had to be between the ages of 21 and 48 and hold a St. John Ambulance first aid certificate and nursing certificate. Functional trainers had to be between 21 and 50, hold a St. John first aid and nursing certificate, and undertake a three month course at the military School of Orthopedic Surgery and Physiotherapy at Hart House in Toronto. These VADs were also called functional trainers, and were the VADs who would go overseas to serve in Britain and France. Then there was the Special Service Section, which took women aged 22 to 38. They underwent a six-month masseur training program at Hart House and were deployed to military hospitals throughout Canada to undertake physiotherapy services. Lastly there was the General Service Section, which was made up of women between the ages of 18 and 50. These VADs were not required to hold a St. John first aid certificate as they undertook non-medical logistical tasks, holding positions as stenographers, secretaries, clerks, telephone switchboard operators, cooks, housemaids, sewing women, orderlies, cleaners, drivers, and stock clerks.

What exactly was the work of a VAD functional probationer? Their principal role was to apply their training in home nursing and first aid to help the wounded; this included such things as making beds, applying and changing bandages/dressings, applying compresses, preparing invalid diets, and ensuring a clean environment for every patient. VADs were also trained to assist graduate nurses in the care of the sick and wounded in hospital, and to serve as probationers under trained nurses in military convalescent homes. As a group, VADs were trained to transform any building into an emergency or makeshift hospital. This latter task was of particular importance during the Influenza Epidemic when VADs became the sole staff operating a number of hospitals in remote areas throughout Canada.

The first VAD detachments were set up in mid 1915 at the ports of re-entry for members of the CEF (Halifax and Quebec City) where wounded soldiers returning from Europe would transit home. VADs would meet the returning soldiers at the docks and travel with them to a convalescent home, train station, or awaiting family. In serious cases VADs would travel the entire journey home with the wounded. This was in addition to the general nurse assistant duties that VADs were entrusted with.

In July 1916 the first Canadian VADs sailed for England to undertake similar duties closer to the conflict. In total sixty were sent as a trial, "all of these members have proved entirely satisfactory to the authorities."[25] They sailed on the S.S. *Grampian* wearing the white cross and burgeoning with supplies. Of these sixty women, fifty would initially be posted to military hospitals in England, while ten were immediately sent to military hospitals in France. "Many of them have had rough work and long hours, but their principal duties have been to assist the nurses with dressings, taking temperatures etc."[26] By 1917 a total of 318 Canadians (plus twenty-three from Newfoundland) were serving overseas.[27] By the end of the war 432 had served overseas. Canada provided the largest overseas contingent of VADs to serve, as might be expected the overwhelming majority of non-overseas VADs were from Britain.

St. John Ambulance VADs from throughout the British Empire made a significant contribution. By the end of the war more than 45,000 had served as VADs, with 8,707 serving in military hospitals during the war.[28]

Table 1

Strength of the St. John Ambulance Brigade in the British Realm

	Strength	Detachments
Men	271	15,016
Women	719	30,073
TOTAL	990	45,089

The administration of VADs was originally assigned to the association in conjunction with the Red Cross as part of the Joint Committee. The Red Cross like St. John Ambulance was training VADs who undertook very similar tasks. In 1917 the administrative responsibilities for the VADs was transferred to the brigade; given their structure, the VADs were ideal for becoming a part of the brigade as nursing divisions. The VADs were originally part of the association because they were small in number and only located in a few centres, but as the number of members and detachments grew it became more and more difficult to coordinate the efforts of the VADs with the brigade and the Red Cross VADs.

VADs in Canada were formally recognized as care providers by the Department of Militia and Defence and operated a number of convalescent homes. Their skills and efforts not being limited to ministering to the injured alone, they also assisted in furnishing homes and providing comforts to both returned solders and those going overseas. In conjunction with the Red Cross they helped in the making and packaging of medical supplies for use in Canada and overseas.

Six VAD detachments were established in Canada by wars end: Ottawa, Montreal, Quebec City, Victoria, St. John and Halifax.[29] In New Brunswick, the VADs worked with the Canadian Club to establish a convalescent home. As a result of the war-work of the association and the need for more women to become VADs, the association began coordinating first aid training classes with women's institutes, home economics societies, and home makers clubs. Perhaps the Duchess of Devonshire, patroness of the Canadian branch of the association and strong supporter of the Order, summed up best the services rendered by the VADs, "I feel that the call which you have all answered is one which requires considerable self sacrifice. May I say how much I admire the spirit in which you and the members have undertaken this work which takes you so far from home."[30] Service overseas would claim the lives of six VADs, who succumbed to illness or infection. Their selfless devotion to the service to humanity was in the highest tradition of St. John Ambulance.

Comfort, Explosions, and Epidemics: St. John Ambulance on the Home Front

The work of the association and brigade on the home-front was not limited solely to first aid training and traditional brigade work. There was the "comfort" dimension aimed at providing members of the CEF with various amenities and St. John Ambulance also provided important relief services during various crises that occurred away from the battlefield. All this was carried out alongside the important war work, such as fund raising and training of CEF members and VADs. Never had the association and brigade been so multifaceted in their provision of training and relief to so many different elements of Canadian society.

We tend to think of the CEF as an organization of 650,000 men and women, yet before the First World War the Canadian regular Army was small, numbering just over 3,000 officers and men. The Royal Canadian Navy had a similarly minute establishment of 350 officers and ratings. Not since the Fenian raids of 1866 and 1870 had the country mobilized all of its military forces, and even then the crisis was nothing of the magnitude brought about by the World War. The Department of Militia and Defence had a difficult time equipping all members of the CEF with the appropriate kit, thus local and national civic organizations joined in the effort to provide certain supplies. Key among these groups was the Order of St. John, which worked in conjunction with the Red Cross, indeed it was the two organizations that developed some of the first care packages for prisoners of war, which were initially part of the "Prisoners' War Parcels and Bread Fund." These parcels later gained the moniker "Red Cross Parcels," as their distribution was coordinated by the International Committee of the Red Cross, even if the production of the parcels was a joint effort of St. John and the Canadian branch of the Red Cross. Along with the Red Cross, Canadian Patriotic Fund, and Canadian Club, the association also helped put together Christmas gift parcels and Christmas cards for those serving at the front.

That the association was divided into provincial councils with local branches throughout the Dominion was ideal for the type of grassroots-based collections undertaken. Each provincial council coordinated with the local general officer commanding the particular military district in which the province was located to determine what supplies were needed. Often over-enthusiastic St. John Ambulance officials would even collect items not required as it was seen as helping the overall war effort. Every provincial council participated in the gathering of goods, some such as Manitoba were highly successful in putting together large quantities of goods that they felt would be useful to members of the CEF in France.[31] In September 1916 the Manitoba Council sent one of the largest care parcels, in what was almost certainly amounted to a boatload of goods, both medical and non-medical:

Manitoba Provincial Council donation to the CEF, September 1916:
- 280,128 pairs of socks;[32]
- 2,139 scarves;
- 866 helmets;
- 432 woolen caps;
- 4,416 pairs wristlets and mitts;
- 1,726 service shirts;
- 126 suits of underwear;
- 1,165 cholera belts (flannel cumber band);
- 47 sweater coats;
- 4,747 surgical gowns;
- 324 helpless case shirts;
- 1,229 pairs of pyjamas;
- 2,316 night shirts;
- 482 dressing gowns;
- 566 night gales;
- 508 pairs of bed socks;
- 108 hospital convalescent suits;
- 645 sheets;
- 3,572 pillow slips;
- 1,746 towels;
- 1,250 pairs blankets;

- 1,490 pillows;
- 919 hot water bottle covers;
- 443 housewives (sewing kits);
- 412 pneumonia jackets;
- 102 hospital kit bags;
- 6,786 packages surgical dressings;
- 12,664 assorted bandages;
- 2 artificial legs;
- 6,465 respirators[33]

Beyond providing comfort and supplies for those serving overseas, St. John Ambulance developed a reintegration program for returned members of the CEF who were usually invalidated home on account of physical or mental injury. There was the "Outing in the Country for Returned Soldiers Free of Cost Programme," which was inaugurated in Manitoba early in 1916 and which spread across the country. This had the dual purpose of not only re-integrating returned soldiers into civil society and getting the injured out of hospital, but in helping "advertising the cause."[34] Long before the Department of Militia and Defence began considering reintegration programs and orientation regiments for the injured who were returned to Canada, the association and VADs were working to help with resettlement.

Other services provided to returned soldiers came in the form of transportation from the rail station home. Those who were injured, mainly those with fractures and flesh wounds that were partially healed, were driven home in brigade ambulances. The "comfort" dimension included the delivery of refreshments and meals to CEF troop trains passing through communities. This was usually done in concert with other local civic organizations, although the association and brigade, along with the Red Cross, played the leading role.

After the departure of the Duke of Connaught from vice regal office, the office of governor general retained a strong connection with the Order and the work of both the brigade and the association. The Duke of Devonshire was installed as governor general in 1916 and on 16 November 1917 he was made a Knight of Justice in recognition of his war work and work with the association in Canada and the Red Cross.

Beyond the war front, St. John first aid training remained popular and was increasingly seen as a necessary part of educational training, both in schools and in the workplace. First aid regulations were adopted by the Workers' Compensation Board (WCB) in Ontario, "making it compulsory for all establishments having fifteen or more employees to supply suitable first aid equipment." This lead was later followed by Workers' Compensation Boards in Manitoba, Saskatchewan, and Alberta. Normal schools in Alberta, British Columbia, and Manitoba began offering summer St. John Ambulance first aid teaching programs for teachers.

The Canadian Pacific Railway continued to have large numbers of its employees trained by the association, and began to include its hotel and steamship employees in receiving first aid training. A testament to the ubiquity of St. John Ambulance first aid training within the

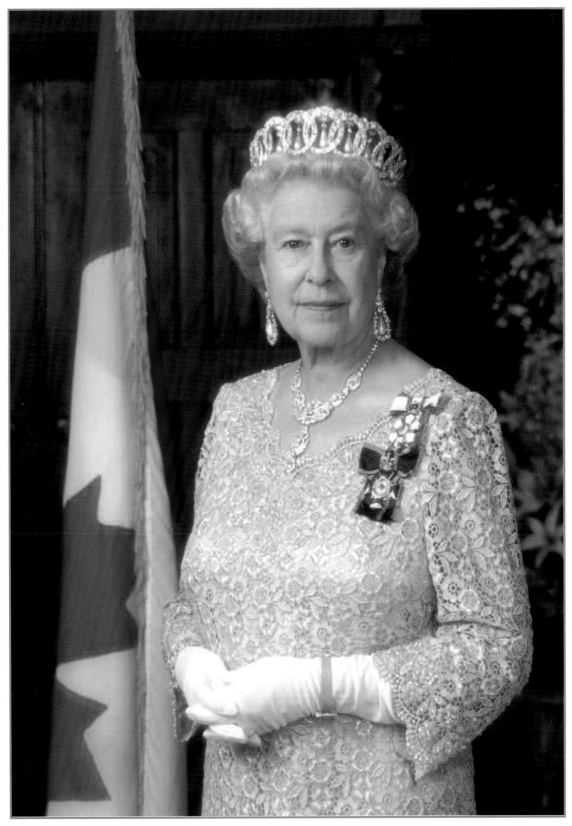

Her Majesty Queen Elizabeth II
Sovereign Head of the Most Venerable Order of the Hospital of St. John of Jerusalem.

Plate 2   The Grand Prior of the Order of St. John

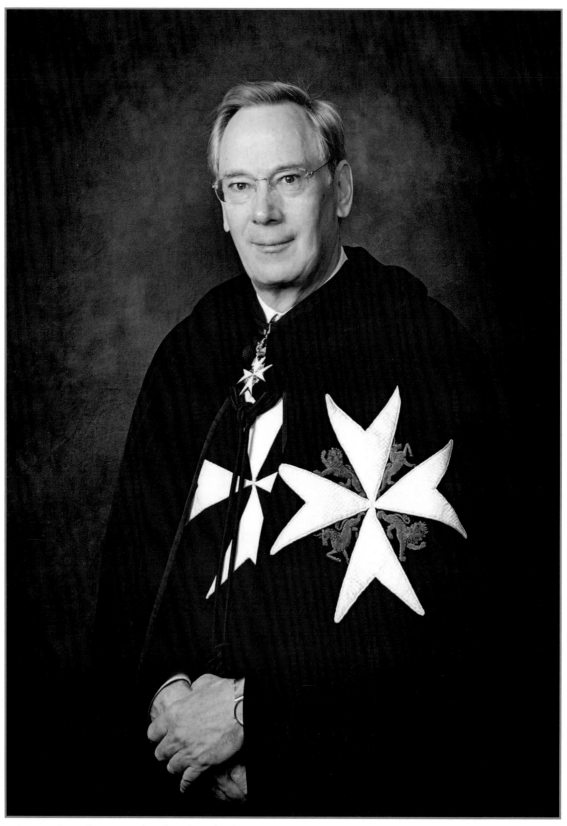

His Royal Highness, Richard Duke of Gloucester, KG, GCVO, GCStJ
Grand Prior of the Most Venerable Order of the Hospital of St. John of Jerusalem.

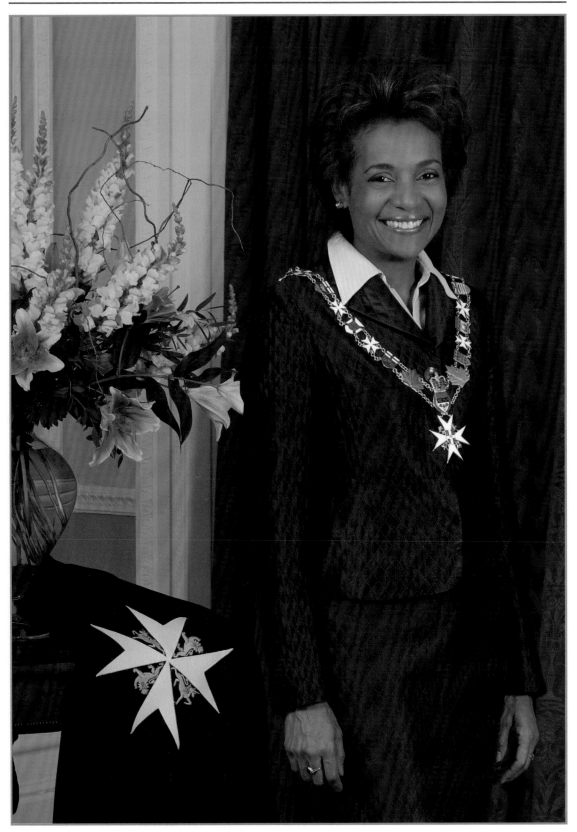

Her Excellency the Right Honourable Michaëlle Jean, CC, CMM, COM, DStJ, CD
Prior of the Priory of Canada.

Plate 4   The Order of St. John in Canada Prior to the First World War

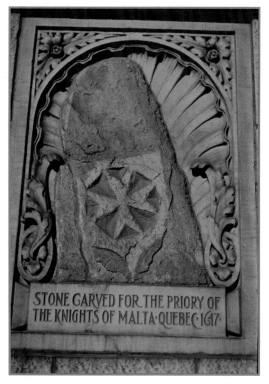

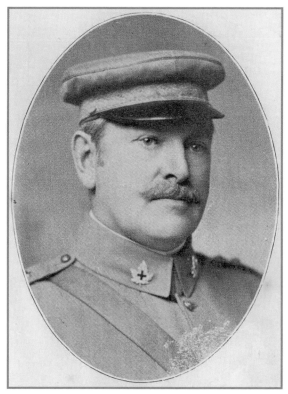

Stone bearing the arms of the Order of Malta, found in the ruins of the courtyard of the Chateau St. Louis in Quebec City, 1784. The stone has been on display in the Chateau Frontenac since 1893.

George Sterling Ryerson, KStJ, VD, founder of the Canadian Branch of the St. John Ambulance Association, wearing his Red Cross uniform, taken during the Anglo-Boer War.

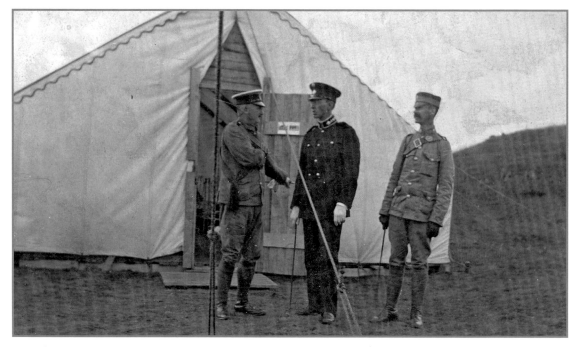

Dr. Cluny Macpherson (centre), CMG, OBE, KStJ, a leading figure in the establishment and operation of both the Association and Brigade in Newfoundland.

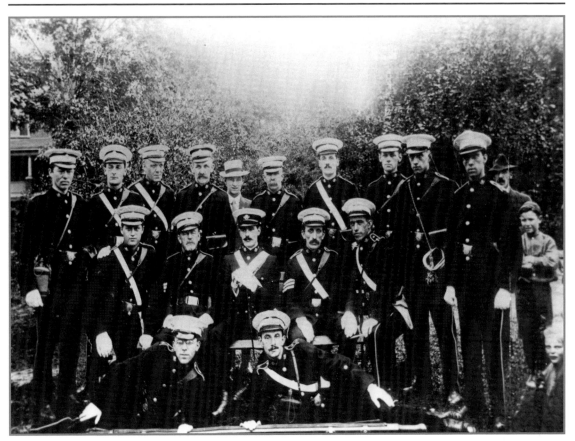

The second Brigade Division founded in Canada. Members of the No. 2 Toronto Central Ambulance Division on duty at Dovercourt Park in Toronto on 1 July 1914. More than three quarters of these men would join the Canadian Expeditionary Force.

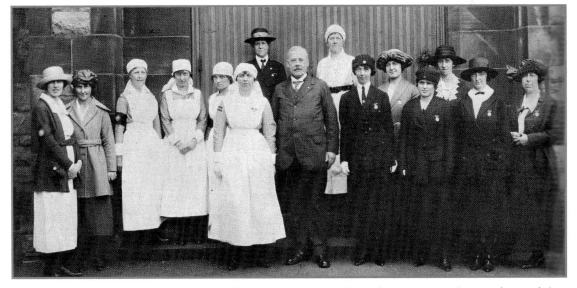

A group photograph taken in the fall of 1914 shows a number of nursing members in front of the old St. John's (Stone) Church Hall, Saint John, New Brunswick.

Plate 6

St. John Ambulance in the First World War

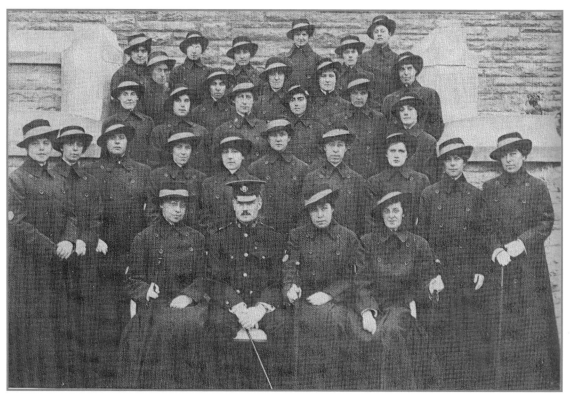

Canadian St. John VADs shortly before departing for England in 1916.

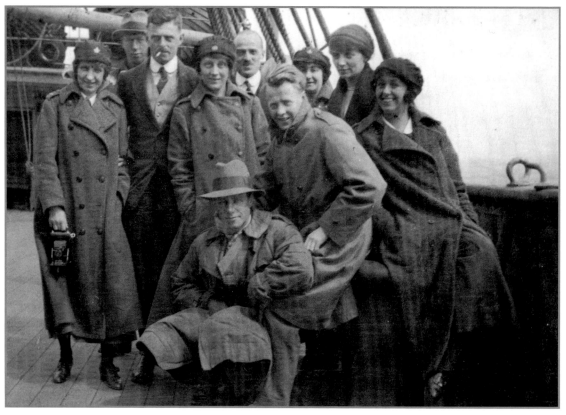

Group of Canadian VADs in a lighter moment aboard the S.S. *Missanabe* sailing to England, 1917.

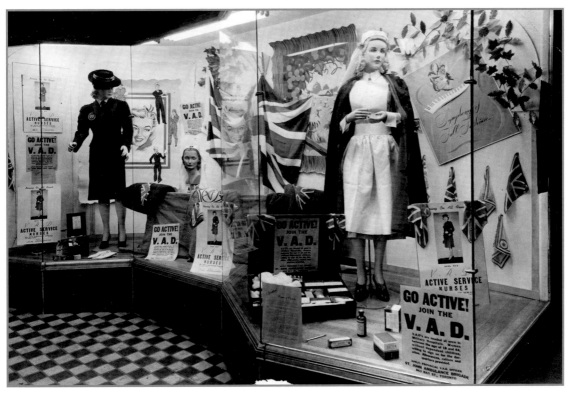

A Second World War VAD recruiting display from 1943.

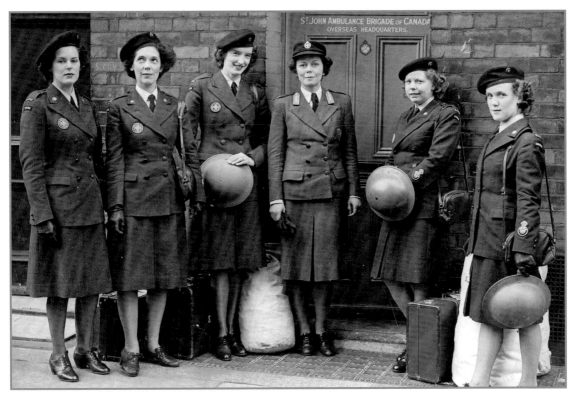

St. John VADs in London at Headquarters on 42 South Audley Street. Kay Gilmour bids farewell
to Janet Whitten, Violet Kemp, Margaret Hicks, Frances Stubbs, and Jean Nixon, who were
departing for the Far East in May 1945 shortly after VE Day.

Plate 8   St. John Ambulance in the Second World War

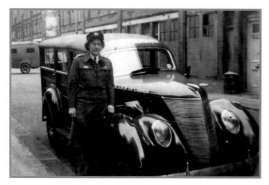

Con Hutcheon with the 1937 Ford Woody Wagon in London, 1945.

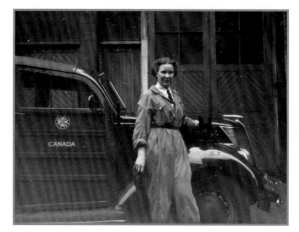

Peggy Horner with the Ford Woody Wagon in London at VAD HQ.

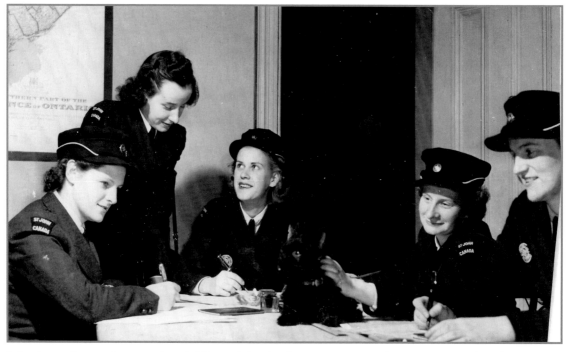

Members of a contingent of 37 VADs arriving in the UK on September 17, 1945. This photo was taken at Headquarters on Audley Street, London. Eilain McMullen, Jean MacLennan, Hilda Gilchrist, Dorien Freeman, and Betty Gray. Also present is Baron "Jock" Mackenzie, the VAD HQ Mascot.

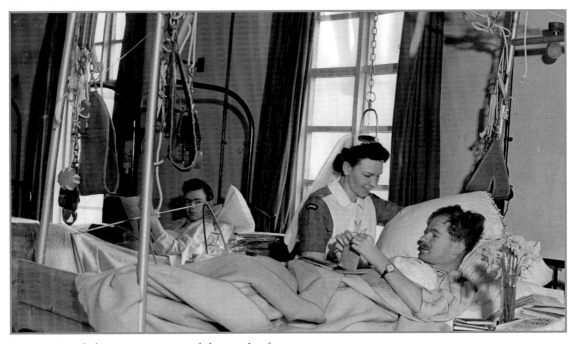

Occupational therapy was part of the work of members of the St. John Ambulance Brigade who served in both the First and Second world wars. Here Elizabeth Lothian helps a convalescent soldier to regain the use of his hands while recovering in an Emergency Medical Services Hospital in the United Kingdom.

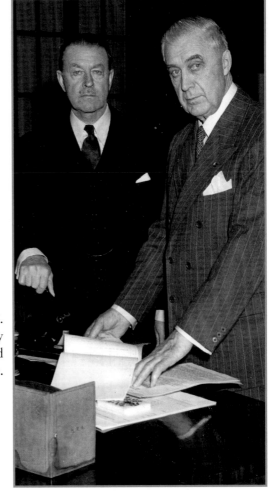

Establishment of the Priory of Canada, 1946. Lord Alexander (Prior) and Charles Gray (Chancellor) surveying a variety of related documents at St. John House.

Plate 10   St. John Ambulance in the Post-War Period

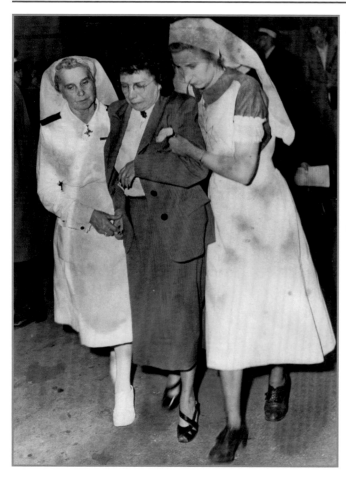

Two St. John Ambulance
Nursing Division members
assist a survivor of the
S.S. *Noronic* Disaster on
14 September 1949 in
Toronto.

HRH Prince Philip
speaking with George
Hayden, a survivor of the
23 October 1958
Springhill Mine Disaster.
Hayden's wife and
daughter look on with St.
John Ambulance Brigade
Divisional Superintendant
Mrs. E.M. Fife supervising
the care. In a lighter
moment Prince Philip
signed Mr. Hayden's
plaster leg cast.

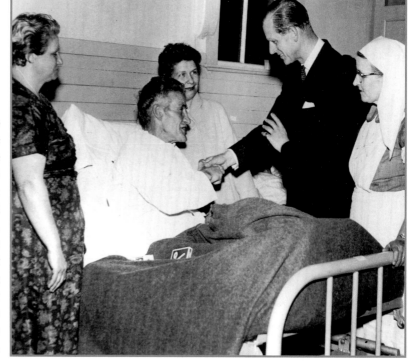

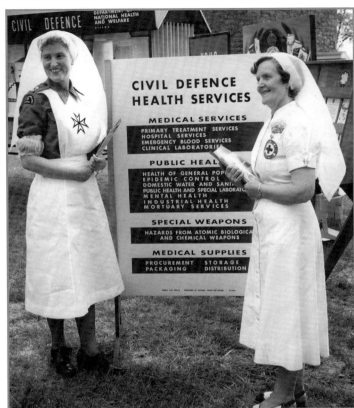

Civil Defence Preparations. St. John Ambulance and Red Cross volunteers participate in a Civil Defence drill, 1957.

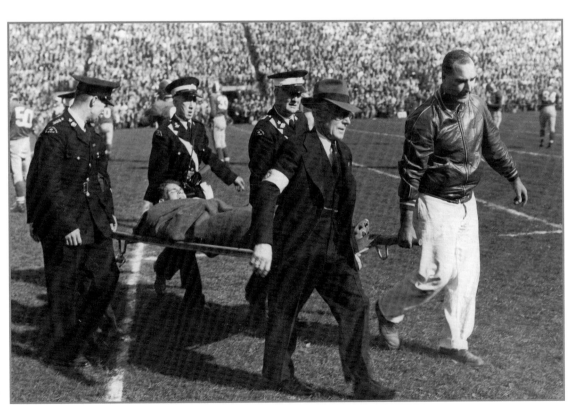

Brigade volunteers on duty at a CFL game during the 1957 Canadian National Exhibition.

Plate 12

St. John Ambulance in the Post-War Period

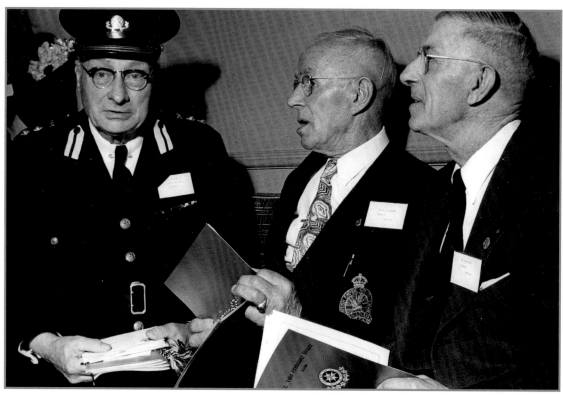

Three charter members of the Brigade, honoured at the Golden Jubilee Banquet in London, Ontario, June 1959. William Loveday, W.H. Pinnock, and F.H. Morton.

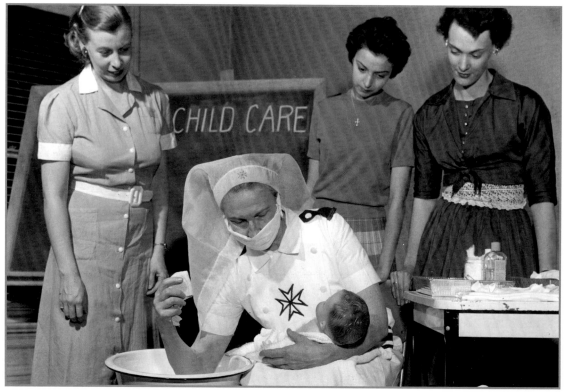

Throughout the 1950s and 1960s St. John Ambulance retooled its Home Nursing Courses.

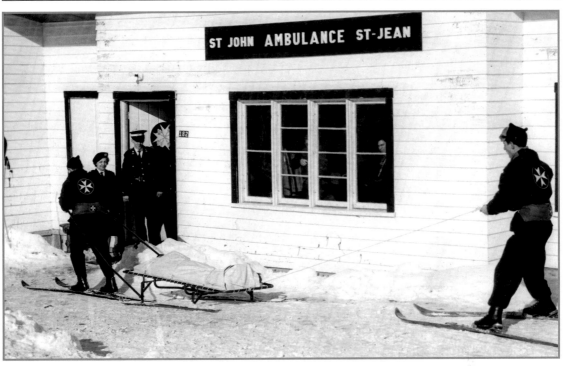

One of the familiar St. John Ambulance Ski Patrol stations that were first instituted in Quebec and would later spread to Ontario and Canada's west.

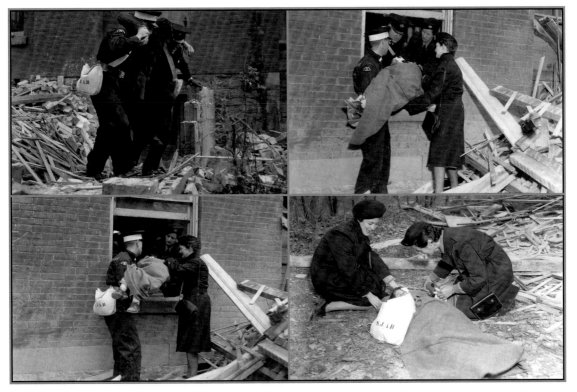

A Civil Defence disaster drill. Throughout the 1950s and 1960s St. John Ambulance provided training to Civil Defence authorities and members of the general public.

Plate 14   St. John Ambulance in the Post-War Period

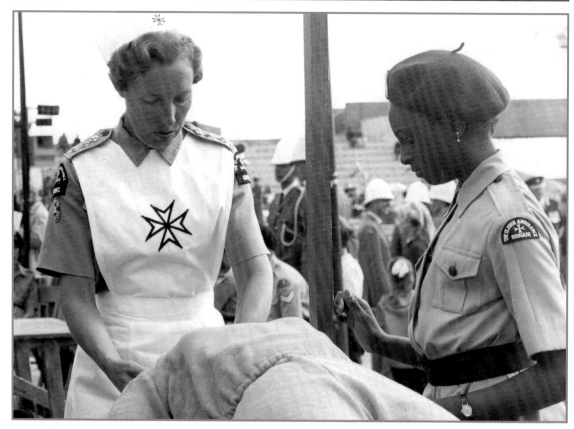

One of the many demonstrations put on by St. John Ambulance during EXPO 67. Here a young girl learns about how to bandage a head wound.

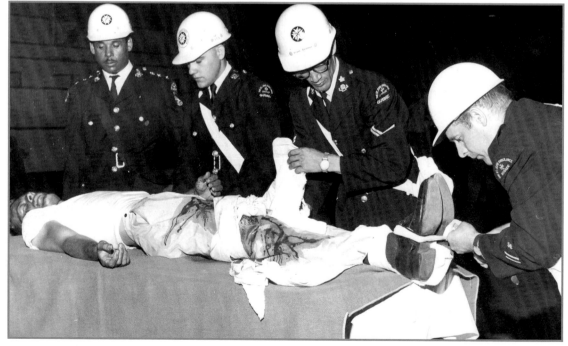

Another St. John Ambulance first aid demonstration. EXPO 67 brought together members of the Brigade from all across Canada for the Centennial Year.

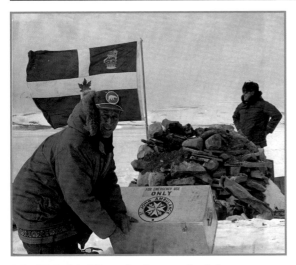

Mr. N.C. McClintock places a St. John
Ambulance survival kit in Canada's north.
John Scullion looks on in the background,
June 1974.

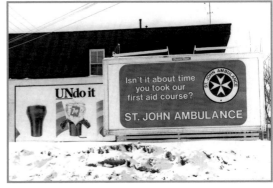

One of the many billboards rented by St. John
Ambulance to increase awareness of the need
for first aid training. This was part of the outreach campaign that commenced in the 1970s.

A group of Inuit youth receive
their first aid pins after having
successfully completed training
in Emergency and Standard
First Aid. Don Johnston
presents an Instructors pin to
Peter Buggins. Looking on are
Mr. J.J. Ootes, Lloyd Dahl,
Alexis Pameok, Joachim
Bonnetrouge, Betty Brewster,
Susan Husky, David Audlakiak,
and Peter Liske.

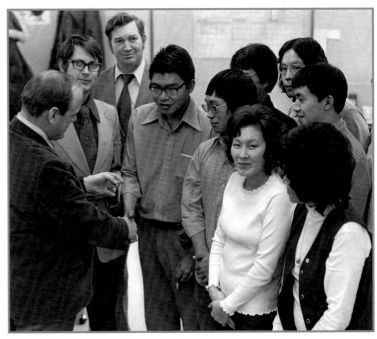

Plate 16   St. John Ambulance Today

Ann Midgley and her dog Jamie
visit a senior citizen as part of the
Therapy Dog Visitation Program.

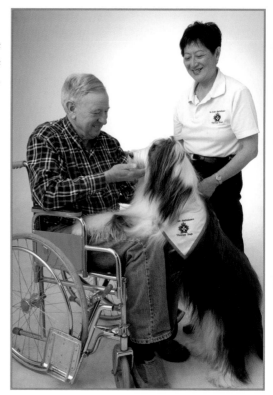

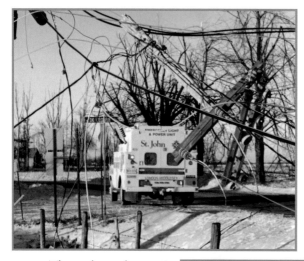

Throughout the 1998
Ice Storm, which left much
of Ontario and Quebec
without electricity, St. John
Ambulance provided a wide
variety of services, from
emergency power
generation and first aid to
the provision of emergency
shelter and food services.

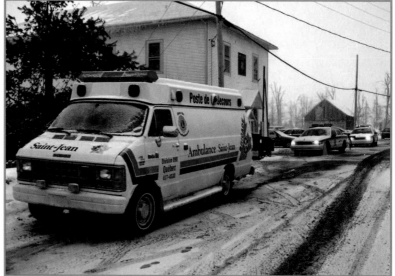

CPR system, in 1917, of the 7,502 employees who had enlisted in the CEF for service all had been trained in St. John first aid, thus providing a "splendid auxiliary to the Army Medical and Ambulance Services."[35] Understandably the number of CPR and GTR (which would become the majority part of the CNR) employees who were taking St. John first aid courses began to drop, not because of lack of interest but "by reason of our instructors going abroad."[36] In many jurisdictions remaining members of the brigade were trained to act as instructors so that first aid education could continue. Other Canadian industrial concerns maintained their connection to the association and brigade. The Canadian Westinghouse factory in Hamilton, which had its own ambulance brigade division sent twenty members overseas to serve in the Canadian Army Medical Corps. [37]

By 1918 first aid training continued to increase in every Province and Territory, except Nova Scotia, where there was an acute shortage of qualified instructors. Nova Scotia, like Newfoundland had one of the highest enlistment rates in the British Empire and given that members of the association and brigade were among the first to respond to the call the situation was not entirely unexpected. British Columbia had experienced significant growth between 1915 and 1918, holding the record for relative expansion in 1915 when the number of persons instructed rose from 667 in 1914 to 2,117 the following year. The Quebec Provincial Council continued to experience difficulties. In the early days of the association in Canada the great potential of this province was never realized, this was in partly a result of internal difficulties experienced within the provincial organization, and partly because association headquarters in Ottawa found it easier to deal with the large and instantly successful CPR centre than with the provincial council. No doubt there were also language difficulties, given that most members of the association were anglophone Montrealers. A revealing comment was included in the 1916 annual report of the Canadian branch, "it is sincerely hoped that 1917 will usher in a live executive who will make themselves properly acquainted with the details of our work."[38] The Quebec Provincial Council had just over $744 in the bank, while their counterparts in the much more rural and agrarian province of Manitoba had just under $5,000. The lack of documentation and impossibility of gauging the personality conflicts that undoubtedly existed prevents us from fully understanding the dynamic that resulted in such a poor showing on the part of the Quebec council; however, the simple financial fact that the council based out of the richest and largest city in the country could only muster one-fifteenth of the funds raised by a significantly less affluent province tells its own story. The Canadian branch of the Red Cross was successful in Montreal, enlisting help and funds from many members of high society, but in other large centres such as Toronto the presence of the Red Cross did not impede the work of the Order. Lady Julia Drummond, wife of Senator Sir George Alexander Drummond a leading member of the Conservative Party and one of Canada's wealthiest men, was appointed a Lady of Justice of the Order in 1916 in recognition of the "keen interest shown at all times by Lady Drummond, in all branches of humanitarian endeavours in the Dominion, and her splendid work with the Canadian Red Cross."[39] Lady Drummond became the first Canadian woman to be appointed a Lady of Justice. Although her work was primarily with the Canadian branch of the

Red Cross, it was not uncommon for members of the Red Cross to be recognized with the Order because of the high degree of cooperation between both organizations. Drummond would continue to be a supporter of the work of St. John throughout her life. As prophesized in 1917, the new executive of the Quebec Provincial Council did usher in a period of modest expansion and growth, beyond the CPR centre, and by the end of 1918 there was a substantial increase in the number of first aid classes being taken "our prospects for 1919 are exceptionally good and our financial position is sound."[40]

Summer first aid programs were inaugurated in 1917 for normal school (public school) teachers in Edmonton, Victoria, Winnipeg, and Saskatoon. The following year the program was expanded to operate throughout Saskatchewan and Manitoba.

The retaking of Jerusalem by General Sir Edmund Allenby[41] and the Egyptian Expeditionary Force (EEF)[42] on 9 December 1917 was cause for celebration for the Order. Jerusalem was part of the Ottoman Empire, and the Ophthalmic hospital had operated without serious difficulties in the period leading up to the outbreak of war. In August 1914, however, shortly after the outbreak of the European part of the First World War, the Ottoman-German Alliance was signed, bringing the Ottoman Empire into the war on the side of the Central Powers, against Britain. In December 1914 the Ottoman-Turks pillaged the ophthalmic hospital of all its supplies and by January 1915 the Order had been expelled, the hospital having been converted into an ammunition depot.[43] On 11 December 1917 General Allenby and the EEF entered Jerusalem on foot. This was wonderful news for the Order, which had essentially lost one of its three foundations for the three years between December 1914 and December 1917. The Canadian branch of the association was greatly heartened by the news and at the annual general meeting the Canadian branch "takes this opportunity of expressing its gratitude for this glorious achievement, and further, that a message be sent to the grand prior and Chapter General affirming the sense of gratitude, and the hope that the retaking of the Holy City and the re-establishing of the Order of St. John in its original home will be an incentive to continue its great work of "service in the cause of Humanity."[44] In February 1919 General Allenby reopened the St. John Ophthalmic Hospital in Jerusalem, the building having sustained some damage during its time as an ammunition dump.

Halifax Explosion

During the devastating Halifax Explosion both the brigade and association played a prominent role in the relief effort in the immediate aftermath of the disaster and as the city recovered. On 6 December 1917 the French cargo ship *Mont-Blanc*, heavily laden with explosive materials, collided with the *Imo* a Norwegian cargo ship resulting in the largest artificially created non-nuclear explosion ever to occur. More than 1,500 citizens were killed instantly and another 500 would die as a result of injuries, and 9,000 were wounded. As a city, Halifax was well serviced by four large public hospitals, four military hospitals, and seven smaller public hospitals, nevertheless the total bed count numbered under 1,000, most of which were in use before the explosion.

Halifax was home to No. 17 Nursing Division, with 129 active members under the direction of Lady Divisional Superintendent C.H. (Clara) Macintosh. The explosion injured thirteen members, others lost homes and family members, nevertheless 111 nurses reported for duty and immediately set to work removing glass and arresting bleeding. They were eventually attached to dressing stations and hospitals throughout the city. Eight members were given the tragic task of searching the city for 140 missing children.[45]

The city's military hospitals were immediately opened to receive civilian casualties, and many large public buildings that remained standing were converted into temporary hospitals. Lady Divisional Superintendent Clara MacIntosh opened her damaged house to the injured, and her parlour and entire abode was converted into a make-shift treatment centre within a day. In her 1917 annual report MacIntosh reported "I can never express ... the admiration I have for our girls, who unaccustomed to the horrors of this kind have shown the greatest endurance ... I know of cases where they have stayed on duty twenty hours at a stretch and rendered service which at any other time would have been considered impossible."[46] Members of the brigade from outlying areas also played a role, most notably members from St. John New Brunswick. Many of the injuries were caused by flying debris, most notably glass, "faces torn to tatters as if clawed by a tiger. The wounds were stuffed with plaster and dirt."[47] Depressed cranial fractures and compound fractures were also prevalent among survivors.

St. John first aiders sprung into action throughout the city, aiding the injured, transporting them to what could best be described as makeshift casualty clearing stations and where possible hospitals. Apart from first aid work, members of the brigade handed out clothing and food throughout the city in concert with the Red Cross and Salvation Army.[48]

"Hundreds were grateful for the assistance rendered by our First Aid Members on that occasion, and too much praise cannot be given to such voluntary workers.... The medical profession has been loud in its praise of the work done and the injured have not yet ceased their expressions of gratefulness."[49]

Following the explosion the somewhat lethargic progress of the Nova Scotia Provincial Council was overcome, with more than 700 people attending 27 first aid classes throughout the province — a new record. Interestingly of the 700 who attended classes, only twenty were males; women were quickly taking a leading role in the affairs of the association at home, as they had already been doing overseas at VADs. Also as a result of the explosion a second division of the brigade was established in Halifax, "the young people have dipped deeply into the social and military life of our city, rendering aid in our hospitals, at steamboat piers, on the arrival of our wounded from overseas, travelling with helpless wounded on trains to their destinations."[50]

Influenza Epidemic

It was not only war that would take its toll on Canadians, disease would have an equally debilitating effect. In early 1918 an influenza epidemic broke out in the Canton Province of China, the epidemic, which erroneously gained the name "the Spanish Flu," spread around the globe in less than a year and would claim the lives of 50 to 100 million people over a year-and-a-half. This dwarfed the estimated 20 million people killed during the course of the entire 1914–1918 war. It is estimated that one in six Canadians became ill with the disease, and estimates of the number of Canadian deaths ranges from 30,000 to 50,000.[51] The disease was airborne and had a high morbidity rate, coupled with a high incidence of mortality. The unprecedented amount of travel being undertaken by Canadians during the war increased the transmission of the disease which "spread along the railways and highways into remoter parts of all provinces."[52]

The flu arrived in Canada in late July 1918 and was carried inland from the ports by the returning troops. Its onset was fast and there was no effective treatment. Unable to contain the disease or cure it, "authorities were forced to turn their attention to the immediate problems of caring for the sick."[53] Acting Prime Minister Sir George Foster noted the urgency of the matter as the disease spread across the country, "with increasing cases of illness from influenza in Ottawa there is a very urgent call for women's care."[54] It was women who bore the heaviest burden and who rendered the most outstanding service in the most serious national health crisis in Canadian history.

Throughout major cities and in each province boards of health were set up to manage the sick, arrange for their comfort and attempt to prevent the wanton spread of the disease. One of the first things that provinces such as Ontario and Quebec did was ask the brigade to provide a list of all the trained nurses, this later expanded to all those who were trained in association first aid. Nursing divisions and voluntary aid detachments in particular were thrust to the frontline of patient care. The epidemic had "stretched available [medical] staffs beyond their limits. In addition, morbidity was high among the medical profession."[55]

The association and brigade, primarily through the VADs and members of Canada's nursing and ambulance divisions, and even holders of association first aid certificates were actively engaged in the treatment of those afflicted with the disease. Given the high transmission rate those association and brigade members on the home front faced a far greater risk of death than their St. John counterparts serving near the armed conflict in Europe. The disease, not being limited to urban areas wreaked havoc on rural Canada, and VADs were sent into many rural communities to minister to the sick and dying. The Red Cross and Victorian Order of Nurses also participated in the relief effort.[56] The VADs and VON worked closely, the efforts of the VON were greatly expanded through their cooperation with VADs and members of the brigade. Superintendent Charlotte Hannington of the VON was unequivocal in her praise for the work undertaken by the VADs in cooperation with VON nurses, saying that they were "of invaluable assistance to the trained nurses."[57] It was the skills demonstrated and versatility of the VAD nurse probationers that really impressed Hannington:

> The teaching that these young women get must be remarkable when they are able to go out and do the work they did. In several cases the staffs of small hospitals in Northern Ontario all went down with the Flu during the epidemic of 1919, and we were obliged to staff these hospitals entirely with VADs ... in Alberta a party of VADs were sent ... and

not only did they skilfully nurse these men but they cleaned the bunkhouse, chopped the wood and built fires.[58]

In Ontario, the assistant commissioner of the brigade set up the Emergency Voluntary Health Auxiliary, which helped to coordinate nursing services in Toronto and other communities throughout the province. It served primarily as a supplemental reserve to the brigade and VADs; operating mainly in larger communities such as Toronto, Ottawa, and Hamilton.

Into 1919 the epidemic continued to spread and reappear in areas considered to be safe. The Association and brigade sent out a call across Canada through the newspapers "asking graduates of the association to report to their local or provincial organization" and to cooperate with local Health Boards and other relevant authorities in treating the sick.[59] Some VAD nurses returned from the field hospitals of France simply to be placed in civilian hospitals and make-shift wards where they treated the afflicted. The epidemic actually temporarily increased the number of people taking first aid courses, it convinced "many that the ability to nurse the sick may at any time be made of incalculable benefit."[60] In 1917 a total of 8,935 first aid certificates were issued by the association, this jumped to 10,094 for the following year. The number of pupils who attended first aid classes jumped from 5,075 to 6,952 between 1917 and 1918. As the epidemic passed the numbers dropped significantly, this is best demonstrated by the decline in first aid certificates issued.

Table 2

Total First Aid Certificates Issued, 1917–1919

Year	Total Certificates Issued
1917	8,935
1918	10,094
1919	5,755

Only the railway centres increased the number of courses and certificates issued through the 1918–1919 period. Despite this sharp decline, almost a 50 percent drop in certificates, public officials continued to extol the work of the brigade and the association:

The splendid work of the women and girls of the Association of this city during the influenza epidemic has called for the admiration and praise of all citizens, and the assistance of the Association officers and members both men and women has been unestimable [*sic*][61]

The war in Europe was over and the war against influenza had coming to a close. By 1919 the brigade in Canada consisted of eleven ambulance divisions and forty-eight nursing divisions. More than 200,000 members of the Canadian Expeditionary Force had been trained by the association during the war, not to mention the 61,000 civilians who undertook first aid training between 1914 and 1918.[62]

Honour in Jeopardy, 1918–1919

Towards the end of the First World War debate erupted in Canada around the subject of honours and titles, specifically peerages and baronetcies (hereditary knighthoods). A number of influential, wealthy, and unpopular public figures were recognized, most notably Sir Hugh Graham, who became Lord Atholstan and Sir Sam Hughes the cantankerous minister of militia and defence. There had long been an opposition in Canada to hereditary titles and, to a lesser degree, knighthoods which conferred on the recipient the style "Sir" or "Dame."

The result of this debate was the adoption of the Nickle Resolution, which requested that:

Your Majesty hereafter be graciously pleased to refrain from conferring any titles upon your subjects domiciled or living in Canada.[63]

Although the Resolution only sought to restrict the bestowal of "titular" honours on Canadians — such as peerages and knighthoods — a subsequent report of the House of Commons Special Committee on Honours and Titles expressed a desire to ban *all* honours in Canada, save those being awarded for military service in the First World War.

Prime Minister Sir Robert Borden, decided to cease nominating Canadians for honours from the King, thus all honours came to an end after 1919 in Canada. Borden's immediate successors, Arthur Meighen and William Lyon Mackenzie King followed this policy assiduously, neither man wanting to be drawn into the acrimonious and politically explosive topic of honours in Canada. The Order of St. John was not drawn into the debate in the same way other honours such as the Order of the British Empire were. A detailed examination of this debate is contained in Chapter Eleven, however it is worthy of mention herein, as the way which the Order dealt with it reveals much about the relationship between the association and the brigade.

With passage of the Nickle Resolution and adoption of the report of the committee, the flow of civilian honours in Canada came to an end, with the conclusion of the War the Canadian military was similarly included in this prohibition on honours. Because recipients of the Order of St. John were not nominated by any government department, as was the case with other honours, such as the Order of the Bath, Order of St. Michael and St. George, and Order of the British Empire, it was outside the control of the Canadian government. For the association, the nomination list simply went forward from headquarters in Ottawa to St. John's Gate in London and was then sanctioned by the grand prior on behalf of the King. For the brigade the process was slightly different in that brigade commanders in Canada sent their nominations directly forward to the commissioner for the Brigade Overseas at St. John's Gate where the nominations were vetted and then sent on to the grand prior.

During the First World War few Canadians were appointed to the Order of St. John, the total compliment was below 100 members, so the Order was not known to many Canadians, but it was included in the broader honours system, just as in the United Kingdom. After the House of Commons adopted the Nickle Resolution the association decided not to nominate any members of the association for appointment to or elevation within the Order. Even the list of living members of the Order ceased to be printed in the annual report, in an effort to avoid controversy. It was deemed most prudent by the executive of the Canadian branch of the association to cease nomination so as not to raise the ire of the government or the general public, both of which were groups it relied upon for financial support.

The brigade did not follow the lead of the association, believing itself to be outside the jurisdiction of the resolution because of its direct connection with the Brigade Overseas headquartered at St. John's Gate in London. The command structure was arranged in such a way that individual ambulance and nursing units sent their nominations directly to the commissioner for the Brigade Overseas in London, essentially bypassing Canadian authorities all together. Appointments to the Order and awards of the Service Medal of the Order of St. John continued for Canadian members of the brigade even after the bestowal of other official honours had come to an end in Canada. The small number of annual Canadian appointments to the Order, and similarly small number of Service Medals awarded during this period meant that government authorities were likely unaware of the situation or simply were not concerned by it.

It would not be until 1931 that members of the association resumed being appointed to the Order, following the relaxation of the government's policy towards official honours. The association had taken a definite wait and see attitude and did not want to become part of the honours debate, in part because the main goal of the association was to teach first aid, not to award honours. Also, given the number of senators and members of Parliament involved in the association there was undoubtedly some pressure from them to deal with the issue in a delicate manner. As an important mechanism for recognizing service to the association and brigade, the Order was also a morale tool, and a draw for some people to become involved. However, the removal of this mechanism during the period 1920–1932 seems to have had only a limited effect on the success of the organization.

The work of the association and brigade continued in communities across the Dominion as soldiers, sailors, airmen, and nurses returned to their families. In 1918 the association in Canada had adopted an instructional movie about first aid. This would become one of the first instructional films to be provided with French and English subtitles. "All titles and subtitles now appear in English and in French. This change has greatly appealed to the French speaking students in the province of Quebec and Northern New Brunswick. With French text books in first aid and home nursing also available, considerable progress in instructional work, should be made during the ensuing year among our French speaking compatriots."[64] *Cantlie's First Aid to the Injured* was translated into French in 1916 as *Premiers Secours Aux Blessés*. Both English and French editions of the publication were made available at thirty-five cents per copy, the initial French edition being printed almost at cost. This was a remarkably forward looking move for the association to take at a time when few services from any level of government were available in French outside Quebec, especially when one considers that the association was still largely dominated by anglophones.

• • •

The First World War transformed the Order in Canada from a new and somewhat wobbly organization into a truly national force, which grew to become one of the leading civic organizations that made a significant contribution to Canada's overall war effort. It is impossible to quantify the contribution even on a financial basis given the high degree of integration between St. John Ambulance and the Canadian Red Cross Society, however one fact is easy to quantify: that 200,000 members of the CEF were trained in St. John first aid methods. If each one of those men and women prevented just one infection or tended to one injury for each year of the war the number of people saved from infection and possible death is staggering. That throughout the conflict the association and brigade was able to continue with the provision of first aid classes to an ever increasing number of Canadians, 61,000 over the duration, while simultaneously collecting goods for the CEF, offering comfort to those overseas and the returned injured, not to mention dealing with such home-front crises as the Halifax Explosion and Influenza Epidemic proved the versatility and meaningful nature of the services provided by St. John Ambulance in Canada, even if the branch was scarcely a decade old. The increase in number of courses taken and certificates awarded had never been more substantial. Even with a decline in the number of instructors, caused by enlistments and the pressures of war, the provision of first aid instruction to civilians continued to climb, demonstrating the need and desire for such training.

Table 3

First Aid Courses Offered to Civilians, 1913-1918

Year	Instructed	Certificates
1913	6,364	3,588
1914	10,443	5,887
1915	14,742	10,181
1916	10,024	8,160
1917	13,076	8,935
1918	13,327	10,094

The success of the VADs ensured that women would continue to have a prominent role in the association and brigade, as they had been the primary St. John care givers at home and overseas during the conflict. With the end of the war and Influenza Epidemic the work of the

VADs slowed, with most returning home. In total, 432 Canadian VADs served in England, France, and Egypt, and by the end of 1919 all but twenty-two had returned to Canada; they remained in England, continuing to serve wounded soldiers.

Despite this exemplary and notable service the association was denied, through the Nickle Resolution, the ability to nominate its membership for appointment to the Order of St. John. It was a strange way to offer thanks for services, but this was beyond the control of the Canadian branch as they did not want to arouse controversy, the main focus being on continuing to provide first aid training to people throughout the Dominion. The prohibition on honours was not mirrored by Canadian units of the brigade. With the end of the war every provincial council was on a sound footing, even those that had experienced difficulties in the period immediately preceding the war. The various railway and industrial centres continued to function effectively and the relationship with Canada's military that had been tested under fire was now unbreakable. The Order had given its all during the conflict, as had other civic organizations from the local to the national level. The success of St. John Ambulance was solely the result of the services rendered by the thousands who sought to work in the service of humanity in one of the most tumultuous periods in the young country's history.

Newfoundland at War

Despite its small size and population Newfoundland succeeded in making a most remarkable contribution during the First World War. The contribution was so great that it would paradoxically sap the St. John Ambulance of much of its strength and ability for years to come. This is evidence of the high price paid by Newfoundland's inhabitants for the valour and service they rendered overseas.

Before the outbreak of the war the brigade in Newfoundland consisted of three divisions, the Church Lad's Brigade Ambulance Division, the Dalton Ambulance Brigade Division, and the No. 4 Ambulance Brigade Division.[66] Dr. Macpherson was appointed assistant commissioner in Newfoundland for the Brigade Overseas in 1914 and would play an important role not only in the affairs of the brigade but also in the Newfoundland Regiment.

Newfoundland was beset by disaster in 1914 when in March of that year two calamities at sea resulted in the deaths of 251 Newfoundlanders. In March various fishing vessels headed to the Gulf of St. Lawrence to undertake the annual seal hunt, two of the main ships were the S.S. *Newfoundland* and the S.S. *Southern Cross*. Towards the end of the month the weather worsened and both ships experienced high winds and snow squalls. The S.S. *Southern Cross* was lost in the ensuing storm, last being sighted on 31 March; all 173 members of the crew perished. Although the S.S. *Newfoundland* did not sink in the storm, 89 of its sealers were left in the blizzard for 53 hours.[67] Of these only eleven survived, all with permanent injuries. As the General Hospital in St. John's was full, the survivors were taken to the King George V Seamen's Institute. "The two top floors of the Institute [were opened] as a St. John Ambulance Hospital ... the whole scheme worked beautifully."[68] It was members of the brigade who tended the survivors under the direction of Macpherson.

In September 1914, with the outbreak of war, Newfoundland's first nursing division, the Lady Davidson Nursing Division was established. Lady Davidson was the founder of the Women's Patriotic Association of Newfoundland, and called upon "the women of Newfoundland to assist in aiding the British Empire in the present crisis by providing the necessities needed by our soldiers at the front."[69] Lady Davidson was aided by Eleanor Macpherson, the wife of Dr. Macpherson, who had immigrated to Newfoundland from Britain in 1902. A trained nurse, she, along with her husband, had organized a tuberculosis sanatorium in the colony and carried out other philanthropic works. Following the outbreak of war Macpherson became the honorary secretary (chief organizer) of the Women's Patriotic Association of Newfoundland, which organized women from all over the island to aid the war effort. Throughout the war she was active in both the association and brigade serving as an instructor. Through the work of Mrs. Macpherson the Lady Davidson Nursing Division of the brigade was established scarcely three weeks after her initial call for assistance. Lady Davidson would be made a Dame Commander of the Order of the British Empire (DBE) in 1918 for her work with both the brigade, association, and the Red Cross Societies in Newfoundland and Australia where her husband was posted in 1916. Mrs. Macpherson would be made a Dame of Justice of the Order of St. John and be appointed one of the first Newfoundland female Officers of the Order of the British Empire for her charitable work.

Many members of the brigade joined the Newfoundland Regiment and would see military service overseas, no doubt making good use of their first aid skills. Dr. Macpherson held the dual responsibilities as chief medical officer of the Newfoundland Regiment and assistant commissioner of the Brigade Overseas in Newfoundland. He was noted to alternate between his army tunic and brigade tunic on an almost daily basis.[70] In February of 1915, Macpherson travelled to England for meetings at the War Office in London, and to look into setting up a separate hospital for Newfoundland casualties and make arrangements at St. John's Gate so members of the Lady Davidson Nursing Division could be brought to Europe to serve as VADs. Macpherson was responsible for ensuring that "the Ambulance detachment of the First Newfoundland Regiment is composed entirely of holders of the Associations first aid certificates."[71] It is doubtful that any other regiment in the British Empire could boast such a strong connection to the association or brigade.

While at the War Office, Macpherson was assigned to sit on the Army Medical Advisory Board's Special Committee on Protection Against Poisonous Gasses.[72] In April 1915 the German Army introduced the use of chlorine gas with terrible results. It was feared that the Turks, with German assistance, would use gas at Gallipoli where members of the Newfoundland Regiment would soon see service. As a member of the board, Macpherson helped to develop one of the earliest types of gas masks known as a "smoke helmet."[73]

As in Britain and Canada, the war work of Newfoundland's association and brigade was coordinated with the local branch of the Red Cross Society, so as to reduce duplication of services and make the most of donations and volunteer time. The working arrangement seems to have been a cordial one in which differences were set aside so as to better serve the greater cause.

Aside from military matters the association continued to carry out first aid instruction. Up to this point its efforts had focused on the capital, St. John's, however in 1915 instructors were sent to the outlying communities of Grand Banks and Greenspond. More than $2,500 in donations was raised towards the formation of the St. John Nursing Division Hospital. An additional $11,173.84 was raised and used towards filling a warehouse in St. John's square with supplies for members of the Newfoundland Regiment.[74]

As in Canada, throughout the war the ambulance divisions of the brigade experienced membership retention problems, because many eligible men had enlisted in the Newfoundland Regiment or were involved in other essential services that were not located in St. John's. People focused on winning the war, not the effect that a depleted membership would have on the brigade in Newfoundland. The absence of Dr. Macpherson, who was in England for much of the war, did not help matters.

Despite depletion of its ranks the brigade was successful in sending a nursing division to France, largely through the efforts of the female population of the island and with the support of the Women's Patriotic Association of Newfoundland. On 4 August 1915, one year to the day that Britain declared war on Germany, schoolchildren throughout the island began raising money, which was to be used towards the purchase of hospital beds. The "cot fund" was a stellar success initially raising enough money for thirty beds. By 1918, money would have been raised for 239 beds, which were donated to various military hospitals, including the Naval Convalescent Hospital, Waterford Hall, in St. John's. The first thirty were set up at the Newfoundland Ward of the St. John Ambulance Brigade Hospital in Étaples France in 1915. A wooden sign was erected in the ward stating "Presented by Members and Friends of the St. John Ambulance Association and Brigade Overseas In The Colony of Newfoundland."[75]

The Battle of Beaumont Hamel on 1 July 1916 brought with it one of the most important days in Newfoundland history, one that would have a lasting and profound impact on the people and government of the island. A total of 22 officers and 758 non-commissioner officers were involved in the Battle, of which all of the officers and 658 of the non-commissioned officers became casualties; being either wounded or killed. It is estimated that only 110 survived the battle unscathed. The 1916 annual report makes no mention of the Battle, simply noting that £50 was donated to the association for war work.

One non-St. John VAD came to represent the service of all VADs from the island. In total approximately 60 Newfoundlanders served as VADs, and more than a third were brigade VADs.

VAD Ethel Dickenson, a former schoolteacher, who served as a VAD at Lady Roberts' Convalescent Hospital in Ascot, returned home to St. John's in August 1918 and resumed her teaching duties that September. When the Influenza Epidemic was brought to the island, Dickenson "reverted to her VAD role, to assist in one of the many emergency hospitals."[76] She ultimately succumbed to the disease and died on 26 October 1918. In an extraordinary gesture Dickenson's sacrifice was commemorated in the erection of an eight-metre tall granite Celtic

Cross, which was unveiled in 1920. A historian of the Canadian and Newfoundland VADs has noted that this was recognition "by extension [of] the efforts of all nurses ... who had served Newfoundland in the cause of the war and the epidemic."[77] This remains the largest single memorial to VAD service in Canada.

As the war dragged on the brigade began to lose more members, with twenty-three enlisting to serve as VAD nurses in England. One former member of the Church Lad's Brigade Division, Private Stewart Dewling, had entered the Royal Army Medical Corps and been awarded the Military Medal while attached to the Newfoundland Regiment during the battle of Beaumont Hamel.[78] Two other members of the Church Lad's Brigade Ambulance Division were honoured for valour: Arthur Hammond, was awarded the Military Medal for bravery in the field while acting as a first aid medic, and John Fitzgerald was awarded Mentions in Dispatches for his attempt to save a comrade's life at the Battle of Gallipoli. Like many other young Newfoundlanders, Fitzgerald did not survive the battle.

By the end of the war, Newfoundland was sapped of financial resources and had lost many of its most capable young men on the battlefields of Europe. Despite great hardship at the end of the war Newfoundlanders raised a £1,000 endowment that was given to the St. John Ophthalmic Hospital in Jerusalem. The "Newfoundland Cot" was dedicated to the memory of the sailors and soldiers of Newfoundland who gave their lives for King and Empire in the war. To this day a bed at the St. John Ophthalmic hospital remains dedicated to their memory.

The association and brigade suffered a similar fate as the rest of the island in the period following the end of the First World War: that of decline. Annual reports were only sporadically submitted, and although first aid training would continue under the direction of Dr. Macpherson, it was at a much reduced pace.

S I X

DIFFICULT GROWTH

The Interwar Years

A Delegation is being sent by Chapter General to discuss
the formation of a Commandery in the Dominion.
Beatrice H. Dent to Colonel Sleeman
7 July 1933

The development of the association and brigade following the First World War was uneven,
presenting St. John Ambulance with significant challenges. In the years immediately
following the armistice the number of first aid courses being taken by Canadians dropped
substantially, and the once robust compliment of nursing and ambulance brigades were greatly
depleted. The initial slump was arrested by 1923, and by 1939 the number of first aid certificates awarded increased tenfold from 3,643 in 1921 to 36,354 by the end of 1939. From a
financial standpoint the organization was solvent and possessed considerable resources.

There was progress in other areas, most notably in the relationship forged with every
Workers' Compensation Board across the country, which began in Ontario in 1916. The
value of St. John Ambulance first aid training was quickly trumpeted by both the board
and labour groups. The various railroad special centres continued to train thousands of
workers every year, similar centres were established for the Department of National
Defence, Royal Canadian Mounted Police (RCMP), and the Bell Telephone Company. One
of the key areas of outreach in the post-war era was schools and school-aged children, an
initiative that yielded the first junior brigades and cadet Divisions. While cooperation was
established with the Victorian Order of Nurses, relations with the Red Cross became
strained, a problem that was not rectified until the beginning of the Second World War. In
terms of the structure of the Order of St. John in Canada, the most important development
was the creation of the Commandery in Canada. This replaced the Canadian branch of the
association, and with it a new more intimate relationship was forged between the association and brigade. The successes of this period do not fit into the traditional Great
Depression narrative. Some provincial councils such as Saskatchewan and Quebec suffered
greatly in the face of the economic crisis and there was a decline in the number of first aid

courses taken between 1931 and 1933, but on a national scale the reduction only amounted to 17 percent. Councils such as Ontario, British Columbia, New Brunswick, Manitoba, and Alberta all remained strong.

The continuing relationship with the railways helped to maintain a base of firm institutional participation throughout this period, as it had in the period leading up to the First World War. The interest of Prime Minister Richard Bedford Bennett, a subsequent crusade to Canada by Sir John Prescott Hewett from St. John's Gate, and a dynamic executive leadership at the national level brought about the establishment of the Commandery in Canada. In the lead up to the Second World War, as Canada began to emerge from the depression, growth within St. John Ambulance was robust, which helped prepare the Order for the work it would undertake during the Second World War. The establishment of the commandery afforded St. John Ambulance in Canada a new and more coordinated structure, and this was a factor in the growth of the association and the brigade between 1933 and 1939. An underlying tension between members of the association and brigade would persist throughout this period and this had a negative overall effect on the potential of St. John Ambulance in Canada. The establishment of the commandery went some ways to overcoming this tension, but it would take decades to build a truly unified St. John Ambulance.

Fostering a Peacetime Purpose

Immediately following the end of the First World War there was a precipitous decline in the number of first aid certificates being awarded. This is one of the best indicators of the level of interest in St. John Ambulance at any given time, as it is representative of the level of outreach undertaken by the organization and the overall fortunes of the association in particular. The reduction in first aid certificates awarded and courses being taken is understandable in the aftermath of the war and the influenza epidemic. Canadians had been subjected to an unprecedented series of crises, both at home and abroad and with the armistice and declining incidence of influenza by 1920, the sense of urgency that had driven everyone during the period from 1914 to 1920 lifted. The war highlighted the importance of first aid training and the usefulness of the brigade, but the return to peace, coupled with a brief economic downturn would have a negative effect. At the end of the war the brigade consisted of 89 ambulance and nursing divisions. By 1925 this had declined to 37.[1] This decline would continue into the 1930s and be a cause of concern for St. John Ambulance in Canada and at St. John's Gate.

The economic slump of 1920–1921 reduced the number of first aid classes offered, but as in the pre-war period the participation of Canada's major railways, the Canadian Pacific, Grand Trunk, and Canadian National, helped to maintain a solid core of annual institutional involvement, while individual non-centre related first aid courses being taken declined. This decline was only temporary and by 1924, as the economic situation improved and new company centres were opened the teaching of first aid increased.

Table 1

First Aid Certificates Issued, 1920–1925

Year	First Aid Certificates Awarded
1920	4,161
1921	3,643
1922	4,932
1923	5,180
1924	6,974
1925	6,933

One area that experienced no growth at all was fundraising and donations. The association relied primarily on interest earned from its foundation funds, totalling more than $200,000 plus an annual $5,000 grant from the Dominion government. During the war fundraising was channelled directly through the Red Cross, so as to avoid competition between it and St. John Ambulance, which had been united as by a joint committee for the duration of the war. Cooperation was cordial and effective throughout the conflict. In 1922 there was only $146.25 in donations for an organization that was expending $18,250.81 per annum. Most of the funds came from interest accrued on the foundation funds. Throughout the 1920s there were periods when no donations at all were recorded, and the association relied entirely on interest from its investments, the bulk of which were acquired at the end of the First World War through a transfer from the Joint Committee of the Red Cross. The brigade was in a similar position, drawing interest from its $100,000 foundation investments. The degree of solvency experienced by the various provincial councils was largely contingent on the number of first aid classes they offered. While the unification of fundraising with the Red Cross for the duration had served the broader cause well, it had a detrimental effect on the fundraising capabilities of the association and brigade for years to come.

As stated previously, the relationship between St. John Ambulance and the Red Cross had been effective during the period 1914–1919, but this would quickly deteriorate in the post-war era. Immediately following the Armistice, negotiations between the association, brigade, Red Cross, and Victorian Order of Nurses were opened in an effort to define roles and avoid duplication. The experience of wartime cooperation lead many to believe that coming to a peacetime agreement would be advantageous for all concerned parties and help them to better serve Canadians.

Early in 1919 an agreement was arrived at between St. John Ambulance and the VON, but no such agreement was reached with the Red Cross. The VON stressed that "coordination was the best policy,"[2] and one gets the impression that they were attempting to act as the mediator between St. John Ambulance and the Red Cross. There was discussion that the Red Cross should continue to be the collecting body, while the association would continue first aid training and the VON and brigade would undertake nursing duties. St. John Ambulance had gone into the meetings with a mandate to cooperate, following agreement in 1918 between the association and brigade that they "heartily approve of the proposed coordination of the work of the Canadian Red Cross Society, St. John Ambulance Association, St. John Ambulance Brigade, and the VON, under the direction of a National Committee."[3] By the end of 1919 no agreement had yet been reached between St. John Ambulance and the Red Cross, "matters have not yet reached such a point that anything definite has resulted."[4] This in part explains why the association was so slow at fundraising in the immediate post-war period, because they did not want to infringe on an area of responsibility that had been, in wartime, left in the hands of the Red Cross and it was assumed would continue to rest with them. Realizing that an agreement might be sometime in the making, the association decided to continue their work "without overlapping and duplication in the best interest of the people of this country."[5]

Assigning blame for the deterioration in the hitherto successful relationship is difficult. Part of it is related to the Red Cross commencing home nursing courses, and a more extensive program of first aid training to the general public. This began in 1923. There was also some disappointment on the part of St. John Ambulance officials that the wartime division of responsibilities was not maintained: St. John viewed this as "disinclination to cooperation,"[6] on the part of the Red Cross. It is uncertain how they came to the conclusion that the agreement would remain intact after the war. There was also a fear that the Red Cross would increasingly provide services that overlapped with St. John Ambulance.[7] The Red Cross was following the lead of the American Red Cross by entering the field. Of course in the United States, St. John Ambulance was not active and thus there was a role for the society to play in first aid training. To the Red Cross in Canada they were merely expanding to fill a need, although it was in an area already well served by St. John Ambulance, and in violation of a wartime agreement between the two organizations. The Red Cross was being opportunistic, but it was undertaking a step that it felt necessary to survive in the post-war era, and in theory at least, the wartime agreement had expired with the end of the war. It did not help that a mutually combative tone was taken by both organizations. Dr. Charles Copp, a future commissioner of the brigade, reflected the feeling of betrayal and anger "Are we not part of the Red Cross Organization of the Empire? If the Red Cross comes into the field [of first aid training] we will welcome them, but will beat them if we are true to ourselves."[8] One can only look at the deterioration in the relationship between the two organizations and regret that a more amicable agreement or parting could not have been achieved.

While at the national level the relationship became very bad, at the provincial and local levels there was still some cooperation. In Ontario, the Red Cross and St. John Ambulance would cooperate with the Ontario Motor League, forerunner of the Canadian Automobile Association, to set up a series of first aid stations along the No. 2 King's Highway, which connected Montreal and Toronto.

The growth of key special centres during the post-war period was an important development. The railways remained the strongest constant component of first aid subscribers and were recognized for having "done wonderful work in forming classes,"[9] throughout the interwar period. Such Canadian business icons as Bell Telephone (1922), Northern Electric (1928), Canadian Industries Limited (1929), Steel Company of Canada (1930), and even the Sunlight Soap Company of Toronto, although not a special centre, initiated widespread first aid training for employees. The federal government also continued to recognize the importance of first aid training through the establishment of special centres for the Department of National Defence and the Royal Canadian Mounted Police in 1922.[10] Colonel D.T. Irwin was the leading proponent of the DND Special Centre. A long serving artillery officer, Irwin had served in the Fenian Raids and although not a medical man was firmly devoted to the work of the Order. Commissioner Aylesworth Bowen Perry insisted that the newly formed Royal Canadian Mounted Police, which was established in 1920 through the amalgamation of the Royal North West Mounted Police and Dominion Police, be an active participant in first aid training. The Dominion Police was unique in that all members were required to hold a St. John first aid certificate. Certainly among many members of the new force there was a culture of first aid training:

> the Council desires to express its thanks to Commissioner Perry of the RCMP, for placing before the members of the force the importance of knowledge of first aid and the maintenance of high standard of efficiency.[11]

It was still in the non-governmental special centres that there was the greatest potential for growth. The railways continued to be a hub of St. John first aid activity, with ever increasing numbers earning first aid certificates. Employers and employees both supported first aid training; employers through covering the expense of courses and supplies, and employees through their earning of certificates and active participation.

First Aid Training, therefore may be said to result in the following advantages:
- The employee is trained to administer aid to himself and to others at work, at home, on the highway or elsewhere.
- He is taught that even the most trivial injuries are potential sources of danger, and therefore he takes fewer chances in allowing wounds to become infected.
- Due regard for fellow-employees, both as to their safety and the proper care of injuries they may receive, is stimulated.
- The first aid trained employee is less likely to become injured than the employee who has not been trained.
- First aid training promotes improved industrial relations, and stronger feeling of cooperation between the employer and employee generally results.[12]

The Bell Telephone Company of Canada was established as a special centre in 1922, at the request of its employees, "so that they might be able to render assistance to their fellow workers in an emergency."[13] Though not considered a heavy industry, Bell is an excellent example of the positive role first aid played in the daily lives of workers. Bell was different from other large Canadian companies in that it employed both men and women, who worked both inside and outside. The hazards Bell employees were exposed to ranged from electrocution, falling from telephone polls, being exposed to the elements, and all the seemingly innocuous yet potentially deadly dangers of the office.

In 1925 Bell had 4,080 employees and recorded 302 accidents, thus 7.4 percent of Bell's workers had an accident. For the next five years there was a gradual decrease to 6.3 percent in 1930, and by 1936 there was only a 2.1 percent accident rate among outdoor employees. In the period between 1922 and 1938 there was a 70 percent reduction in the number of accidents requiring hospitalization.[14] By 1932 all of Bell's outside workers held first aid certificates. An article about Bell's success noted:

> A man with First Aid training becomes accident-conscious, is therefore a more careful worker, and is one who understands the necessity of reporting even minor injuries, thus preventing infection or other complications, which would delay recovery and prolong the period of off work.[15]

Bell quickly became the proverbial poster child for St. John Ambulance first aid training. Hollinger Mining subsequently made it mandatory for all of its underground workers to hold a first aid certificate, this resulted in 2,277 men being trained over a three year period.[16] Other mining concerns such as the Consolidated Smelting Company of British Columbia also began to cover the cost of St. John Ambulance first aid training. Consolidated recorded that 91.93 percent of its employees held certificates at its Sullivan Mine in Kimberly, and that over a three year period it experienced an 80 percent reduction in shift loss because of accident or injury. What the railroads had discovered in the early part of the twentieth century was quickly being realized by other Canadian industries through the 1920s and into the period preceding the Second World War.

To bring first aiders together from all across the Dominion the Canadian branch held the first ever "Conference of First Aiders," on 17 October 1924 in Montreal and from 11 to 12 February 1925 in Toronto. These conferences brought together instructors, examiners, certificate holders, and the broader membership of St. John Ambulance in Canada to discuss and learn about first aid training techniques.

•   •   •

The association continued to log significant advances in first aid training for the public and special centres. The brigade sustained a decline in membership, and the chief commissioner for the Brigade Overseas at St. Johns Gate attempted to sound positive in his annual report for 1924:

> progress is slow compared with previous years of the war, but although a number of moribund Divisions have had to be removed from the strength during the year, the registration of four new divisions is a very hopeful sign.[17]

The registration of new divisions was a turning point for the brigade, and the post-war decline was arrested. In 1926 the lady superintendent of the Brigade Overseas, Ms. Lanctot Dent, visited Canada to help promote the work of the brigade and assess the situation.

The association and brigade had reached a highpoint by 1926,[18] having emerged from the post-war slump with increasing membership, a solid financial base, and increased interest in first aid courses. From 1926 until the end of the Second World War, every year but one was marked by a significant increase in the number of first aid courses taken and certificates awarded.

Table 2

First Aid Certificates Issued, 1926–1930

Year	First Aid Certificates Awarded
1926	7,373
1927	8,321
1928	7,937
1929	9,048
1930	12,855

In 1926 the Order undertook a crusade to the Holy Land, which saw members travel to Jerusalem to visit the St. John's Ophtalmic Hospital. Although no Canadians participated in the pilgrimage it had a buoying effect on the organization throughout the Empire.[19]

In the same year the Order was granted a new Royal Charter by King George V. This included altering the name of the Order from "The Order of St. John of the Hospital of St. John of Jerusalem in England" to "The Grand Priory in the British Realm of the Venerable Order of the Hospital of St. John of Jerusalem." This change acknowledged the fact that the Order was operating well beyond the shores of England, and that it was multifaceted in its membership, involving people from throughout the British Empire. The new charter also allowed for the expansion of the Order through the establishment of commanderies and priories in places outside the British Isles.

Sir Henry Pellat retired as deputy commissioner of the brigade in Canada, being replaced by Dr. Charles Copp in 1927. Pellatt would remain involved in the brigade, although, following the Depression, his failing financial fortunes forced him to focus on his personal affairs. With this the brigade lost one of its most stalwart and generous supporters.

The Quebec Provincial Council remained beset with problems. The Montreal centre of the association had to act as the provincial council beginning in 1927. Although Lady Drummond had been influential in bringing first aid to the women of the Canadian National Railway Company,[20] within Quebec there was little positive movement. There was concern that the association's involvement in the province was too focused on anglophones, "it was very difficult to say why the work had not taken root amongst our French Canadian citizens,"[21] although all materials and even the instructional film had been translated into French. Offerings of first aid courses in French were much more successful in New Brunswick. Throughout the early 1920s there was continuing friction between the association and the Quebec Safety Council, which was only overcome through the diligent work of Herbert Molson, whose generosity towards the Order was much more than just financial. By 1929 the situation had greatly improved under Molson's leadership.

Several provinces introduced first aid as part of their public (normal) school curriculum. The first to offer such courses province-wide was New Brunswick. This was followed by similar, but more limited programs in Ontario and Saskatchewan. The federal minister of Health, Dr. J.H. King had implored the association to "invade the schools of the country."[22] Interest among Workers' Compensation Boards remained significant. This was an impressive achievement given the ubiquity of such boards:

> every workman's compensation board in Canada but one has now adopted first aid regulations in connection with the administration of the new act. These regulations call for medical or nursing assistance under certain conditions, or qualified first aiders under others. This has been due entirely to the efforts of the St. John Ambulance Association, and it is gratifying to know that industrial employees generally will be benefited by the new conditions.[23]

Another Canadian first was the establishment of St. John Ambulance Ski Patrols. These were inaugurated in 1928 through the generosity of Herbert Molson. During the ski season members of the brigade would travel to the main ski areas in the Laurentians and set up first aid tents, which later became semi permanent first aid huts. These provided skiers with not only medical aid in the event of an emergency, but also shelter in a period before the construction of ski resorts in the area. St. John Ambulance was again proven to be an innovator and responded to fill a need as the country grew and changed.

The Canadian organization was not involved in the St. John's Ophthalmic Hospital in Jerusalem during the interwar period aside from periodic donations. Following an appeal from the grand prior in 1927, 20 guineas were donated to the hospital by the foundation.[24] During the 1931 centennial celebrations marking the establishment of the Order in England, Canada sent the second largest contingent of brigade members. It was also in the centennial year that the moratorium on members of the association being appointed to the Order of St. John was lifted.

Organizational Structure as a Platform for Growth

Since 1914 the Canadian branch of the St. John Ambulance Association was recognized as a Foundation of the Grand Prior in the British Realm. The administrative structure of the association included the General Council acting as the governing body, with subordinate provincial councils, special company councils and special centres under it. The General Council included one member from each of the provincial councils, a representative from each railway council, the director of ambulance, the president, vice-president, honorary treasurer, honorary solicitor, and three other members selected yearly. Provision was also made for representatives from various company centres and special centres to sit on the General Council when appropriate.

The Ambulance Committee, in essence the governing body for the ambulance brigade, was heavily dominated by members of the General Council, with all the senior officers serving as *ex-officio* members. There was clearly a desire that the Order in Canada would be a Dominion-wide organization that carried out the work of the association and the brigade under a single command structure. Nevertheless at the local level, ambulance brigade divisions and nursing divisions reported to London, and the feeling was that their relationship was most directly with the chief commissioner of the Brigade Overseas at St. John's Gate, and not with the headquarters of the Canadian branch.

Aside from the affairs of the brigade, the Ambulance Committee was responsible for approving provincial councils, company councils, special company centres, and local centres. The Ambulance Committee also had responsibility for issuing first aid certificates and ensuring that the standards of training and examination were maintained. The idea of devolving these responsibilities to the still young provincial councils was not considered.

Separate bylaws for the ambulance brigade were also appended, although it was intended to be subordinate to the association, this was clearly set out in section 2(d) of the act, and supported by the fact that the director of ambulance of the Canadian branch was head of the St. John Ambulance Brigade Overseas within the Dominion and that the affairs of the brigade were to be administered by the Ambulance Committee of the Canadian branch.[25] While this was a legal reality, it was not one recognized by members of the brigade at the local level. They felt equal to the association, and did not view themselves as a junior partner in any way.

The association throughout the British Empire was made up of priories, commanderies, and branches. The Grand Priory was the parent body. The first priory outside of England was the Priory of Wales, which was established in 1918. Becoming a priory or commandery required not only a significant membership, relative to population, but also that the national organization in a particular jurisdiction was responsible, mature, and on a firm financial footing. South Africa was the most independent of the St. John organizations in the Empire. It had become a commandery in 1927, followed by New Zealand in 1931, Canada in 1933, and Australia in 1946. Indeed South Africa would also be the first off the mark in becoming a priory, a status granted in 1943.[26]

The elevation of the St. John Ambulance Association in Canada from a mere branch, a status originally gained in 1910, to a commandery was directly tied to the visit of Sir John Hewett, Bailiff of Egle, and the improving fortunes of the Canadian association. In part this was precipitated by an increase in the number of first aid courses being taken across the country, the financial stability of the association, and the personal interest taken in the Order by the prime minister of the day, R.B. Bennett. Officials at St. John's Gate realized the golden opportunity that had been handed to them and were keen to capitalize upon it. The less public reason for the drive to establish a commandery was connected to the deterioration in cooperation between St. John Ambulance's two entities in Canada, the association and the brigade. Simply put:

> the relations between the Association and the Brigade have been lamentable as you know.[27]

Membership in the brigade had been on the decline since the end of the war, while the association had experienced growth. The view taken by successive presidents of the Canadian branch and officials at St. John's Gate was that if the Order in Canada was to be successful in the long term, both elements had to be active and growing.

Hewett was an Indian civil servant who held a variety of senior administrative posts which he discharged with distinction, being remembered as one of the fathers of India's industrial development.[28] Another significant project he is remembered for is his organizing of the 1911 Delhi Durbar for King George V and Queen Mary, the largest such spectacle ever to be orchestrated. Appointed Bailiff of Egle after many years of service to the Order, Hewett's 1933–1934 visit to Canada marked the third "Canadian Crusade," and would be the last of its type.

The slightly paternalistic attitude of St. John's Gate was not negative; it was seen as a natural way to promote the work of St. John Ambulance in Canada. London was the centre of activity of the Order and all major regulatory and structural decisions were made there. This was not the case of mother Britain sending out senior officials to direct affairs in the dominions and colonies, it was at the request of Canada that Hewett and his daughter came to promote the work of the Order. Canadian officials such as Cowan and Pellatt valued highly the advice they could receive from personages such as Hewett. St. John Ambulance in Britain was highly successful, financially stable, and much more established than in Canada. London also wanted to patch over the difficulties that had been experienced between the association and the brigade in Canada. The overall attitude conveyed by officials at St. John's Gate and Hewett himself was that while rules had to be followed they did not have to necessarily be uniform throughout the Empire. There was a sensitivity to local concerns and conditions that was always taken into consideration. In a confidential letter to the Earl of Scarborough, sub-prior of the Order, Hewett pled "there are certain changes which must, I think, be allowed, to bring the Regulations into accord with the feeling in Canada."[29] This was not the voice of a heavy-handed colonial bureaucrat enforcing sterile and distant regulations; it was an understanding voice laced with a desire for success in an unfamiliar environment.

Following the 1933 annual meeting of the Canadian branch of the association it was requested that a delegation be sent "by Chapter General to discuss the formation of a Commandery in the Dominion."[30] The branch felt somewhat ignored by London, there having been crusades to both Australia and New Zealand by Hewett in 1928. This feeling of isolation was compounded by the embargo that had been placed on the association nominating Canadians to be appointed to the Order. By December 1932 it was agreed between the Canadian branch and St. John's Gate that a delegation should be sent to Canada, the president of the Canadian association, C.G. Cowan viewed this as a turning point, the General Executive Committee of the association "desires me to express their deep appreciation for the Order's generous offer."[31] The generosity of London was more than figurative, as St. John's Gate agreed to cover all the expenses incurred by Hewett and his daughter during their cross-Canada tour. Although the association had a large foundation, totalling more than $225,000, following the war, there would be no large individual donations until the opening of the Second World War. From the standpoint of donations, the association's financial fortunes had suffered during the Depression, profits from fees and supplies in 1932 were down by 25 percent over the previous year, the total being $4097.29.[32] In laconic fashion the annual report simply noted "the need of careful husbanding of resources is evident."[33] The Canadian branch was in no position to cover the total cost for travel to and across Canada without having to eat into their nest egg, and this was not an option. Other Canadians helped to defray the costs, most specifically the various lieutenant-governors who placed their homes, offices, and cars at the disposal of Hewett. R.B. Bennett was equally generous allowing Hewett to use his personal railway car.[34]

Cowan in particular was aware of how effective a crusade from someone like Hewett could serve as a catalyst for building both the association and the brigade in Canada.[35] Hewett's visit to Australia and New Zealand had helped "to rally the interest and enthusiasm of the local toilers for the Order."[36] Cowan had been involved in the work of St. John Ambulance since the early days of the First World War, so he was well aware of what the organization was capable of, if only placed under strong leadership and motivated in a positive manner.

Hewett and his daughter Ms. St. John Atkinson sailed to Canada in grand style aboard the RMS *Empress of Britain*, Canadian Pacific's newest liner, arriving at Wolfe's Cove, Quebec City, on 26 October. Their two-and-a-half month itinerary was hectic and included visits to Quebec, Ottawa, Toronto, Vancouver, Winnipeg, Edmonton, Victoria, Vancouver, Calgary, and Montreal. Hewett would deliver twenty-four speeches, and even preside over an investiture in Vancouver. In Ottawa Hewett was hosted by the governor general and while in the provinces he was the guest of the various lieutenant-governors.[37] Within days of arriving Hewett remarked "our visit has created quite a little element of excitement,"[38] it was a trip that would almost wear out an energetic man who was renowned for rising at 4 a.m. daily to ensure he could maximize his output.

The original purpose of Hewett's visit was to meet with senior members of the Canadian branch at the federal and provincial levels to discuss the possibility of establishing a Commandery in Canada. Canadian officials of the Order had a different view of the visit, in that they believed that Hewett was coming to Canada to help found the commandery, not survey the state of affairs. The Canadians also desired to use Hewett to promote the Order and work of St. John Ambulance to the general public, not something that Hewett expected. While in Toronto he attended one reception where he shook hands with 1,600 people, the size of the crowds astonished him, and although unprepared for such duties he gladly obliged his Canadian hosts. Overwhelmed with the positive response, he commented: "the present state of my right hand is thus that it will be a physical impossibility [for Hewett to shake hands] and I shall have to put my hand in a sling."[39] Hewett was an enthusiastic promoter of the Order throughout the Empire, already replete with honours and recognition, his passion for St. John Ambulance was in seeing the good work of the organization spread farther and farther afield. Writing to Pellatt, former chief commissioner of the brigade in Canada, he expressed his excitement over his upcoming visit to the country "we are both looking forward most enthusiastically to our visit."[40]

Talk about creating a commandery was carried out with the aim of improving the place of St. John Ambulance in Canada and expanding the organization throughout the country. In his keynote address in Montreal, Hewett opened by saying "I have come as a delegation from the Grand Prior at St. John's Gate to discuss with the authorities of the Association and Brigade in Canada the improvement of arrangements so as to give the local authorities a position with respect to the Grand Priory more in accordance with the increased work than is the case at present."[41] Expanding and improving the association and brigade in Canada was the focus, not simply elevating the Canadian branch to a commandery; such a change would serve little purpose without a base of support and possibility for expansion.

The objectives of establishing a commandery in Canada were to better coordinate the work of the association and brigade, reignite interest in the work of the Order, and become a more active participant in the Order's work on an empire-wide basis. The draft regulations for the Commandery in Canada were based directly on those written for the commandery of South Africa in 1927. The word Canada was simply replaced wherever Union of South Africa appeared:

Objects of the Commandery
- to extend the influence of the Order
- to assist the maintenance of St. John Ophthalmic hospital at Jerusalem
- to assist in the maintenance, organization and administration of the St. John Ambulance Association, and of its ancillary, the St. John Ambulance Brigade Overseas,
- to cooperate in all other objects and purpose of the Order laid down in Statute 2

One regulation that was stressed was that "The Commandery shall in no circumstances whatever allow the work of the Order in its various aspects to be influenced by political considerations."[42] The work of the Order in Canada had always been non-partisan, with involvement from members of all major political parties. A close relationship had always existed with the Minister of Militia and Defence, regardless of political stripe, and many senators and MPs were similarly involved. There was perhaps a fear that because of the high profile support from Prime Minister Bennett, there might be the potential for politicization of the Order. Given that the leader of the opposition, and sometime prime minister, William Lyon

Mackenzie King was also a nominal participant in the work of St. John Ambulance it seems unlikely that there was any political innuendo in the background.

Although Hewett had been in Canada for little more than two weeks there were already open discussions about what was required to establish a commandery. "I was a little surprised to find that the Executives of the Association and Brigade brought forward so early in the tour a definite resolution in favour of the formation of a Commandery as one rather looked to this being a final act if all went well"[43] Hewett's correspondence leading up to his Canadian crusade leave the reader with the impression that he felt the Canadian branch held great potential but would require a significant amount of work to build. Throughout his tour of the country he would remark on the enthusiasm of those associated with St. John Ambulance.

At the meeting held at the Chateau Laurier in Ottawa on 15 November there was great momentum and an air of excitement. The governor general spoke at length expressing his belief that "the foundation of the new Commandery has been well laid,"[44] and that he would be honoured to accept the position of Knight Commander of the Commandery in Canada. R.B. Bennett was also present and spoke about his belief that the work of the Order was of increasing benefit to the Canadian people, and therefore he welcomed "the action taken to establish a Canadian Commandery."[45]

The question of honours emerged as one that had the potential to arrest the prompt elevation of the branch to a commandery, because of the overall membership of the Order. In the United Kingdom and other parts of the Commonwealth, the number of members the Order in a particular jurisdiction was viewed as representative of the devotion and interest in St. John Ambulance. Between 1919 and 1931 no Canadian appointments were made to the Order by the association due to Parliament's decision to prohibit the bestowal of honours on Canadian residents. This was lifted in 1931 through the efforts of the Earl of Scarborough and Duke of Connaught who implored Prime Minister Bennett to remove the ban. A full discussion of the history of the honour side of the Order is covered in Chapter Eleven.

There was a lingering fear on the part of Hewett that the resumption of appointments to the Order in 1931, with the approval of the Canadian government, was only temporary.[46] The association had ceased nominating its members for appointment to the Order following adoption of the Nickle Resolution in 1919, although members of the brigade continued to be awarded the St. John Service Medal and appointed to the Order. The brigade was able to do this because it reported directly to St. John's Gate and was essentially a division of a British organization. On the other hand, the association was incorporated by an act of the Canada's parliament, making it "Canadian," and thus subject to the Nickle Resolution. Understandably, the honours disparity between the brigade and the association was the cause of some friction. The association had been deprived of its key mechanism for rewarding exemplary acts and meritorious service over many years. Hewett emphasized that if St. John Ambulance in Canada was going to grow, appointments to the Order would have to be continued. The absence of association appointments to the Order for more than a decade meant that "in proportion to our population as compared with South Africa, New Zealand and Australia, Canada was far short of the requisite number to inaugurate a Commandery with a fairly full membership."[47] Buoyed by the enthusiastic response he received throughout his crusade, Hewett felt that although the number of members of the Order was small in Canada, that there was nevertheless a solid base for growth. With regularized annual appointments the problem of membership in the Order could be overcome in a matter of years. There was after all a backlog of worthy candidates dating back to 1920.

Throughout his tour Hewett used the media to promote the work of St. John Ambulance. His 6 November speech to the Canadian Club was broadcast on CBC Radio. With the help of M.A. Jamieson, the European manager of the *Montreal Daily Star*, Hewett was able to appear in that paper as well as others throughout Canada. Notices of Hewett's arrival were carried in most newspapers, which in part accounts for the large attendance at many of the events he was involved with. Such highly influential business leaders as Lieutenant-Colonel Herbert Molson, who held a special luncheon for Hewett and his daughter in Montreal that included the city's social elite, were anxious to help Hewett. The lieutenant-governors were similarly adept at arranging receptions and dinners to promote St. John Ambulance, and more promotion was obtained through official channels.

The Canadian crusade of 1933–1934 was a resounding success, having greatly stoked interest in the work of St. John Ambulance throughout Canada. Hewett was able to undertake a survey of the Dominion's major centres and highlight the potential of the organization at a time when such promotion was badly needed. On 8 December 1933, Cowan wrote to Sir Percival Wilkinson requesting that a petition be put forward to chapter general, "praying that a Commandery of the Order be established in Canada under the usual regulations."[48] A number of changes were made to the standard commandery regulations; taking into account local differences. These included using the calendar year as the fiscal year, only requiring the commandery general to meet once a year in view of the size of the country, and requiring the Knight Commander (governor general) to act on the advice of council and not on his own accord. Upon his return to England, Hewett reported to Chapter General on the success of his crusade.[49] One concern was that not enough women were involved in the work of the association.

Aside from the improving fortunes of the association, one of principal factors leading to the establishment of the Commandery in Canada was the long standing tension between the association and the brigade. The roots of the Canadian branch of the association can be most directly traced to the Dominion Council of the association, which was founded in 1897 and succeeded by the Canadian branch, founded in 1910 and incorporated by act of Parliament in 1914. The founding of the brigade came in 1909, although it continued to report directly to St. John's Gate in London. While the deputy commissioner of the Brigade Overseas in Canada — the nominal head of the brigade — was an active member of the association and sat on the executive, at the individual ambulance division and nursing division level, the relationship was far more directed towards affairs with the headquarters of the Brigade Overseas in London.

Both the association and brigade were integral parts of the Order, and thus it might seem counterintuitive that there was anything but a friendly rivalry between the two elements of the Order in Canada, however the divisions went much deeper, more because of social factors than an inability of the association and brigade to cooperate. During the First World War cooperation between the two elements had been highly successful and played a significant role in Canada's war effort. However through the 1920s and into the 1930s old fissures in the relationship began to appear.

The association was primarily composed of middle and upper-middle class citizens, and the executive level of the organization it was populated by members of the social, economic and political elite of the country. Lady Perly, Lady Drummond, Herbert Molson, Lord Shaughnessy, lieutenant-governors, senators, and senior military officers were all active in the affairs of the association. The brigade however was made up mainly by the labouring classes including factory workers, railwaymen, and clerical workers. Although it included a cadre of senior military officers, along with Sir Henry Pellat, one of Canada's wealthiest men, these people were only a small part of the brigade, holding senior positions, and were not your average first aider. One group that held membership in both the association and the brigade were medical doctors. Within both the association and the brigade they held such posts as senior instructors and examiners.

Regional factors also played a role in the relationship between the association and brigade. Although the brigade had been headquartered in Toronto since the First World War the association's headquarters had been moved to Ottawa in 1910 following the establishment of the Canadian branch. This had never sat well with members of the brigade in Toronto who felt that they were being abandoned by the association. The brigade in Toronto also tended to be highly critical of decisions taken in Ottawa. This was occasionally warranted, but was more often frivolous. The physical separation of the association and brigade also meant that the two were competing against each other for funds, a practice that would be firmly condemned by St. John's Gate as counterproductive and destructive.[50] There were few occasions when the brigade's annual report was included with that of the association but such reports were usually sent directly to London by the brigade without reference to Ottawa or the association.

Unfortunately for the historian, gauging the difficulties and level of tension is difficult. We are left with only anecdotal evidence and have to glean from certain comments — often what is not said — the state of affairs. In one letter Cowan, president of the Canadian association expressed his view of the situation and its cause:

> Frankly in my opinion membership in the Brigade has been made up too exclusively of English people of a certain class and that this has had the effect of keeping native born Canadians out of us. Under new organization I believe that we can attract more of our Canadian certificate holders into its ranks and I agree with you that the nursing divisions can be enlarged and strengthened.[51]

Cowan's circumspect use of the term "people of a certain class" reveals that he felt the problem was rooted in the brigade and not in the association. He was correct in his assertion that the brigade was heavily populated by British immigrants. One must be convinced that much of the difficulty was rooted in the class structure of the Order in Canada. It would be misleading to impose this dichotomy across the entire St. John Ambulance organization throughout Canada, and there were people such as medical doctors who were active in both, but this analysis held true in more locations than not.

Unlike Canada, Newfoundland did not experience any such tension between their branch of the association and ambulance brigade divisions. The comparison is not entirely equitable in that Newfoundland was a much smaller place than Canada, and its association and brigade were largely held together for many years by one man, Dr. Macpherson. Newfoundland also had the advantage of being a much smaller organization coupled with a relatively integrated membership.

The together but separate status of the association and brigade in Canada was often cited by officials in London as a reason St. John Ambulance as a whole in Canada was not more robust. There was also the structural problem in that the brigade in Canada had no national sub-divisions at the provincial level. Brigade divisions often made inquiries directly to St. John's Gate without reference to the Ambulance Committee in Ottawa. This was not an efficient or nationally focused governance structure. Sir James Hewett observed that "the Brigade will never really be successful in Canada until there is a separate Commissioner for each province, except the Maritime Provinces, where one would probably suffice"[52] During his visit to Canada, Hewett continuously attempted to promote better relations between the association and brigade:

> I have in every address that I have made in Canada expressed the opinion that the Brigade has a great part to play in Canada. But if it is to play it properly the senior officers of the Brigade must abandon, and make other members of the Brigade abandon, the sort of criticism of the Association, which we have ourselves heard them make and had to correct.... We think that our tour, which resulted in members of the Association and Brigade being brought together a public functions, may not only have resulted in their becoming more friendly towards one another, but also in the view of the public coming to regard them as integral parts of one organization working with a common aim.[53]

The creation of the commandery brought the association and brigade together on a governance level in a more intimate and well-defined manner than under the Canadian branch. All publications and correspondence were titled with "The Commandery in Canada" and included the name of both the association and the brigade. The headquarters of the brigade were moved to Ottawa to better facilitate coordination of work within the new commandery. Colonel Arthur E. Snell was appointed director of ambulance and made commandery commissioner (in charge of the brigade), while provincial commissioners were appointed in each province — though this would not occur in Nova Scotia and New Brunswick until 1940.[54] In 1941 Quebec would be given two commissioners, one for the English speaking divisions and one for the French-speaking divisions. This was a solid start to a new relationship, one that would take time to fully develop. Tension between the association and brigade continued into the 1960s, but with time it has been overcome.[55]

With the expected establishment of the commandery the Toronto *Mail and Empire* reported "Canadian First Aid to be Centralized,"[56] noting that the commandery was to be activated in the near future, and that the governor general had "graciously consented to become Knight Commander."[57] A brief history of St. John first aid training was included, the article also postulated that "In 1933 it seemed vital to have all St. John work concentrated in one organization and feeling this, officials from both association and brigade have been seeking for many months to bring their interests together and to establish some central control."[58] Throughout late 1934 in the approach to the first annual general meeting of the Commandery in Canada, headquarters prepared a "suitable article" on the establishment of the commandery to the Canadian Press.[59]

The creation of the Commandery in Canada also resulted in the creation of new positions within the organization. Governor General, Lord Bessborough, patron of the Canadian branch, was made Knight Commander of the Commandery in Canada; the president of the branch, Cowan, became lieutenant; R.E. Wodehouse was appointed to the new positions of hospitaller and almoner; Charles Gray became treasurer, and Alan T. Lewis was given the position of honorary solicitor. At this point no chaplain was appointed, as there appears to have been some difficulty in choosing a candidate. With the organization's elevated status an annual allotment of twenty-five appointments to the Order was set aside for Canada.[60] The formation of the commandery also resulted in much greater autonomy over nominations, which were now prepared in Canada for both the association and brigade and sent to London, where the only difficulty to arise was over the number of annual appointments, not the quality of candidates.[61]

The first meeting of the commandery chapter occurred on 1 November 1934 at Rideau Hall following an investiture of Order of St. John appointees in the ball room. The meeting was chaired by the Knight Commander, Lord Bessborough, One observer noted that "It is very clear too that the proceedings were very carefully thought out, and that everything went off without a hitch and with dignity."[62] Early in his term as Knight Commander, Bessborough took a very hands on approach, offering to help various lieutenant-governors with their work as it related to St. John Ambulance. Like others, he was optimistic that the new organization be successful. His enthusiasm went so far as to encourage the reorganization of Ontario's provincial council. Writing to Lieutenant-Governor Herbert Alexander Bruce, a long standing member of the Order, Bessborough suggested "It has occurred to me that perhaps you, as a Knight of Grace of the Order, might be willing to summon a meeting of the members at Government House, Toronto, at some time convenient to yourself, when the steps necessary to attain this end could be initiated."[63]

Following the establishment of the Commandery in Canada the number of citizens taking St. John first aid courses continued to increase, reaching a near threefold level of growth by the end of 1939. This was in part because of increased interest from special centres and better publicizing of the value and importance of first aid training. The increasing vibrancy of the Ottawa centre resulted in its establishment as an entity separate from the Ontario provincial council in 1929. Originally called the Federal District Centre, it was separated from the provincial council to allow the national capital to take full advantage of the presence of so many governmental agencies and to ease the bureaucratic imposition of the high degree of activity in Ottawa placed on the Ontario council based in Toronto. Federal District Centre was given the same status as the provincial councils in 1943.

Table 3

First Aid Certificates Issued, 1931-1939

Year	First Aid Certificates Awarded
1931	12,037
1932	10,581
1933	10,628
1934	12,733
1934	15,367
1936	17,866
1937	17,127
1938	27,902
1939	36,354

An increased public presence had been achieved through the use of radio and newspapers. Vancouver's CNRV ran a thirty-six-part series of St. John first aid lectures given by Dr. Lavell Leeson. These included instruction on home nursing, junior first aid, and senior first aid.[64]

In May 1933, the first cadet divisions were created. There had long been calls for "more active work amongst juniors"[65] to be undertaken. Juniors were defined as boys and girls under the age of 16. The inaugural division was founded in Manitoba: The 7 Oaks Cadet Ambulance Division. This was followed by divisions in Timmins, Vancouver, and Montreal. Cadets were instructed by members of the brigade in topics ranging from cleaning, cooking, and hygiene to fire fighting and swimming.

The forward looking nature of St. John Ambulance during this period was best demonstrated in the organization's response to increased automobile travel. In 1923 the association noted that "with the general adoption of the motor vehicle for purpose of transportation a danger has been introduced into the street traffic which is more serious and of greater menace than the railroad train."[66] The slogan quickly promoted was:

Every Motorist A First Aider[67]

In 1928, the Ontario Provincial Council proposed that first aid kits be placed in "motor camps" throughout that province. The provincial government covered the cost of the kits and they were placed in these early rest stops.[68] At the initiation of the Ontario Motor League, the forerunner of the Canadian/Dominion Automobile Association, St. John Ambulance in cooperation with the Red Cross set up first aid posts along the King's Highway No. 2, which linked Toronto and Montreal. Initially, twenty-two posts were set up, eventually expanding into the Niagara peninsula. In the first month of operation 106 cases were treated.[69] The British Columbia Council would follow the lead of Ontario and enlist the support of the provincial government to have first aid kits placed at stations along its principal highways. In 1937 a Ford delivery van was converted into an ambulance, which would be put into service in Ontario. Travelling more than 19,000 kilometres and treating more than 300 individuals. A second ambulance was added in 1939.

Nova Scotia experienced an increase in activity during the late 1930s. The provincial government made it mandatory for trainees in the Minors Apprentice Project to have a first aid certificate. The brigade also became much more active, becoming a fixture at the Nova Scotia Provincial Exhibition beginning in 1931. During the 1939 Royal Visit, the brigade in Nova Scotia rendered particular conspicuous service.[70]

In the lead up to the Second World War the brigade once again became a strong organization. During the golden jubilee celebrations marking the establishment of the brigade in England, sixty Canadian members travelled to London to participate. By 1939 the brigade in Canada had 2,773 members distributed across fifty-seven ambulance divisions and thirty-seven nursing Divisions. For the first time since 1919, the number of members and divisions exceeded the brigade's establishment at the end of the First World War. This was in part because of increased cooperation between the association and brigade in the lead up to the next world war. In 1939 alone seven new divisions, five ambulance and two nursing, were organized.

The five years following the creation of the Commandery in Canada were highly successful for St. John Ambulance. Both the association and brigade had weathered the preceding post-war slump and participation in first aid training was at an all time high. The worrying decline in the number of women taking home nursing courses[71] would be reversed early in the Second World War, when the VADs would also return. The pressures of war would also help to mend the relationship between the Red Cross and St. John Ambulance, as they once again joined together to serve King and Country. The commandery of Canada was in a strong position to make a significant contribution to Canada's overall war effort, as the Canadian branch of the association and brigade had during the last war. In terms of finances, structure, membership, and preparedness, St. John Ambulance had made significant advances in the interwar period, laying the foundation for the modern Priory of Canada.

Newfoundland

The association and brigade in Newfoundland did little work during the interwar period. Following the end of the First World War, Newfoundland's government faced a series of economic crises — it went broke — and the effects of significant manpower losses in the war had a profound effect on the development of the island right into the Second World War. There are many years where neither the association nor the brigade submitted annual reports to St. John's Gate in London. By 1924 the brigade in Newfoundland had been reduced to the Church Lad's Brigade, which had been one of the first groups to answer the call of King and Empire in 1914, and one nursing division operated in St. John's.[72] Dr. Macpherson continued to serve as deputy commissioner for the Brigade Overseas, he also directed first aid training classes for the association.

In 1926 Macpherson reported that "interest in first aid work is being revived and the prospects of an increased number of new classes are good."[73] That year saw twenty-six first aid certificates awarded. By 1930 this number had jumped to thirty-seven and the following year, forty-seven certificates were awarded. Throughout the 1930s periodic reports were sent to St. John's Gate related to the number of first aid certificates issued, but there was never any reference to the overall activity or financial status of the association and brigade. Sadly extant records and annual reports from this period fail to paint a full picture. At best it was a period of stagnation and decline for both the association and the brigade, although these outcomes were more tied to the hardships being experienced by Newfoundlanders as a whole, than on mismanagement or tension between the two groups.

SEVEN

RETURN TO SERVICE

The Second World War

Many Brigade people have given valuable service as instructors.
The Association has been recognized as the authority in
Canada on First Aid Training.
Air Raid Precautions Summary
Commandery Annual Report, 1942

By the end of the Second World War Canada had once again proven itself to be an effective military power, emerging as a mature industrial nation capable of participating on the world stage. The Royal Canadian Navy had grown to become the third largest in the world, the Royal Canadian Air Force was the fourth largest allied air force, and the Canadian Army had expanded significantly, playing an important role in theatres around the globe. Over the course of the war St. John Ambulance issued more than 450,000 first aid certificates and related awards, which in a country of only 12 million people meant that more that 5 percent of the adult population were qualified first aiders. The entire establishment of the RCMP and almost every combat soldier in the Canadian Army had also received St. John Ambulance first aid training by wars end.

We often forget the dark days of 1939, when the country was thrust into war once again, and the outcome was far from certain. In 1939 Canada was ill-prepared to enter an armed conflict — "the Armed Forces scarcely existed at the beginning of the war."[1] St. John Ambulance, however, was in fighting form and the growth of the organization throughout the 1930s, placed it in a strong position when war erupted that September. Both the growth of the brigade during the five years leading up to the war, and the establishment of the Commandery in Canada played a part in the contribution that St. John Ambulance would make to the overall war effort. The 1939 Royal Visit had provided the brigade with a much needed test of its abilities, with members of the brigade playing an active part in the celebrations surrounding the visit of King George VI and Queen Elizabeth. Members of the brigade saw service clear across the Dominion along the rail routes followed by Their Majesties. The brigade clearly demonstrated its usefulness on a nationwide scale, this was recognized not only by government officials but also by the King who approved a much increased honours list of 100 appointments and elevations in 1939. It would be the last festive national event the country would have until VE and VJ Days, which would follow six horrific years of war.

St. John Ambulance has thrived in times of external crisis. Whether it be armed conflict, natural disaster, or medical emergencies, the work of St. John has a pattern of expansion during tumultuous periods. Ever increasing numbers of Canadians were trained in first aid. Both civilians and those in uniform flocked to receive instruction in ever increasing numbers. It would be naïve to suggest that the work of St. John Ambulance in the lead up to the war was all in "preparation" for the conflict that broke out in September 1939 when Hitler invaded Poland. The growth was a confluence of factors including increased interest from industry, schools, and long-established partners such as the railways, Department of National Defence, and RCMP.

The Order entered the war with strength, in part because of the improving fortunes of St. John Ambulance in Canada and its increasing membership and involvement throughout the country. Dr. R.E. Wodehouse, lieutenant of the commandery provided strong leadership in the early part of the war. As deputy minister of the Department of Pensions and National Health, Wodehouse would ensure that St. John Ambulance was in a strong position to contribute to Canada's war effort The war would see St. John Ambulance lead by a series of strong forward thinking leaders who helped to maximize the reach of St. John Ambulance in Canada and overseas.

In retrospect, the immediate response of St. John Ambulance following the outbreak of war seems natural, but it was novel given how quickly volunteers were put to work. For its part, the federal government was slow to place the country on a war footing. Until early 1940, "no one anticipated a huge war effort."[2] In part the experiences of the First World War influenced the organization's response. At the national and provincial level, the leadership of both the association and brigade saw the war as an renewed opportunity to serve King and country and help to maintain the rapid growth that St. John Ambulance had enjoyed in the period immediately preceding the war.

As in the First World War, it was on the home front that St. John Ambulance would make the most significant contribution. Overseas 221 VADs would serve in Britain, France, Germany, Guernsey, India, Malaysia, and the Netherlands, working as nurse's assistants, ambulance drivers, and clerical staff. The organization was also maturing, relations between the association and brigade had become much more cordial and cooperative, and this was greatly enhanced by the war. Within the context of the broader Order, the Commandery in Canada was given much more autonomy from London. They were still required to report to St. John's Gate and follow the guidelines set out by London, but the Canadian war effort of St. John Ambulance at home and overseas was largely directed by officials in Ottawa and coordinated with St. John's Gate. This was in marked contrast to the work of St. John Ambulance overseas during the First World War, which was almost entirely directed by British officials of the St. John Ambulance Brigade. Leaders such as Margaret MacLaren, Kathleen (Kay) Gilmour, Wodehouse, and Alan Lewis were instrumental in carving out a Canadian contribution. Their leadership and the contribution of the whole St. John Ambulance organization in Canada were key to the establishment of the Priory of Canada in 1946 following the end of the war.

Before the outbreak of war, the brigade in particular began making preparations. As the situation in Europe escalated the brigade commenced a series of courses on air raid precautions, with twenty instructors being trained in Winnipeg and another thirty-six in Ottawa in 1938.[3] Throughout the war St. John Ambulance would cooperate closely with Air Raid Protection (ARP) committees at the provincial and municipal levels, with members of the brigade and association deeply involved in the first aid training offered to ARP volunteers. On the eve of war the brigade had strength of 2,773 members active in every province except Nova Scotia and Prince Edward Island. As an administrative preparation Allan T. Lewis was appointed sub-lieutenant of the commandery, making him second in-command of St. John Ambulance in Canada. Lewis would become involved in every facet of St. John Ambulance's war work, eventually taking charge as the lieutenant.

In light of the high degree of cooperation achieved between St. John Ambulance and the Canadian Red Cross Society during the First World War, it was natural that the two organizations would come together during the Second World War. The relationship between the Red Cross and St. John Ambulance at the national level had begun to deteriorate in 1923 when the Red Cross entered the field of home nursing first aid training, even though it had agreed that it would not enter the field of first aid training. The story at the provincial level was quite different. At that level, the two organizations cooperated effectively on projects such as Highway First Aid Posts in Ontario and British Columbia. It is certain that the difficulty at the national level was as much the result of personality conflict as competition between the groups in the first aid training field. At the national level animosity between the groups had begun to dissipate during the late 1930s when there was a substantial increase in the size of the brigade and in the number of St. John Ambulance first aid certificates issued annually. The success of both the Red Cross and St. John Ambulance in the five years preceding the war helped to alleviate some of the strain on the relationship.

Deputy Minister of Pensions and National Health Wodehouse who was then the lieutenant of the Commandery in Canada was anxious to see an agreement hammered out between the Red Cross and St. John Ambulance. As a senior bureaucrat, he had an intimate knowledge of how ill-prepared the country was for the challenges of war. Wodehouse was well aware of how much more effective the two organizations could be working together than independently, he also knew just how badly the services offered by St. John Ambulance and the Red Cross were going to be needed during the ensuing conflict.

On 20 October 1939 representatives of St. John Ambulance and the Canadian Red Cross Society met in a room at the Chateau Laurier in Ottawa. After a day of meetings, it was agreed that during the war the Order of St. John and Canadian Red Cross would cooperate in a number of fields:

- That the Red Cross Society will be responsible for the collection of funds and material together with the distribution of the same;

- That the Order of St. John will be responsible for the training of all male personnel in first aid as may be required for war service;
- That the Order of St. John and the Canadian Red Cross agree to set up a committee in the training of female personnel for volunteer aid detachments for war service, but that all qualified certificates in home nursing and first aid required by the Department of National Defence for war work be issued by the Order of St. John;
- That in the event of the Canadian Red Cross Society supplying ambulances and drives for Overseas, the Order of St. John will train the personnel of the same in first aid;
- That the Canadian Red Cross Society will pay the net cost of all aforesaid training by the Order of St. John, a budget for which will be resubmitted from time to time.
- That the Order of St. John and the Canadian Red Cross Society will set up a joint committee to explore the whole question of cooperation and the establishment and operation of first aid posts on the highways
- That a standing committee composed of members of both the Order of St. John and the Canadian Red Cross Society be set up to consider all matters arising from the fore-going plan of cooperation with the view to bring the efforts of both the Order and the Society into harmony for the duration of the war.[4]

The agreement was similar to the one arrived at in 1914, under the direction of Governor General the Duke of Connaught. Both groups were keen to repeat the successful work under-taken by the VADs during the First World War. St. John Ambulance was anxious to focus on first aid training in as many fields as possible, its area of proven expertise. The Red Cross looked to act as an umbrella organization that would not only raise money but coordinate war relief efforts including the provision of ambulances. Outpaced only by the Canadian govern-ment, the Canadian Red Cross Society was the most successful wartime fundraiser in Canadian history. Throughout the war the Red Cross made special war grants to St. John Ambulance, "which so materially helped in our increased work due to the war."[5] These funds helped cover the cost of training and other first aid related work, without which St. John Ambulance would have been forced to focus scarce resources on fundraising. The relationship between the two groups improved throughout the war. St. John Ambulance even arranged for additional lessons to be given to recipients of the Red Cross home nursing course so that they could obtain a St. John Home Nursing Certificate.[6] This was significant step forward given the rivalry between both organizations in the field of home nursing.

• • •

In every province ARPs were established along with comprehensive civil defence plans. ARP volunteers were responsible for assisting in the event of an emergency, instructing civilians on the use of gas masks, ensuring blackout restrictions were observed, and advising members of the public in making emergency preparations.

All the resources of St. John Ambulance were employed to assist with civil defence prepa-rations. "Many Brigade people have given valuable service as instructors. The Association has been recognized as the authority in Canada on First Aid Training."[7] On the west coast there was fear of attack from the Japanese Navy and Air Force, while on the east coast there was a constant fear of U-boat assault from the Kreigsmarine. Unlike the First World War, there was a constant fear of attack at home. Following the Japanese assault on Pearl Harbor every member of the brigade in Vancouver mustered to their various stations. Along with first aid training, members of the brigade and association were also enlisted to play a leading role in what was euphemistically called "casualty services."[8] In the event of a major catastrophe St. John Ambulance, along with police and fire authorities were to be the first responders. Thus, it was to the fields of first aid training and civil defence preparations that St. John Ambulance would direct much of its efforts during the Second World War.

In Ontario the brigade was made responsible for all ARP first aid training, while in Vancouver all 2,200 ARP wardens earned their St. John Ambulance First Aid Certificates.[9] In Vancouver the nursing divisions established a medical comfort depot, which looked after disadvantaged families that needed medical supplies. The depot was open day and night and was another St. John first. In the prairies, although there was a reduced risk of air attack, St. John Ambulance first aid remained popular. The brigade in Manitoba worked closely with the Manitoba Volunteer Reserve, the province's civil defence authority, and other provincial councils entered into agreements with their local ARP authorities to train wardens and volunteers. Early in the war a friendly rivalry developed between Winnipeg and other provincial capitals, it being noted in the 1940 annual report that Winnipeg "has the best record of any in war work [up to that point].[10] There ensued a unofficial contest to see which province could train the largest number of ARP personnel.

Training programs for the ARP volunteers were financed through funds raised primarily at the provincial level and through periodic grants from the Canadian Red Cross, which was the umbrella fundraiser for St. John Ambulance throughout the war. Unlike the First World War, the work being undertaken at the provincial level was being directed largely by provincial councils in concert with civil and military authorities. The federal cooperative structure of St. John was coming into being in a much more meaningful way than it had in the pre-war period. In May 1942 a two day conference was held in Ottawa for members of the brigade and association.[11] Hosted by Governor General the Earl of Athlone, a list of twenty-eight suggestions were developed to help enhance the war work of St. John Ambulance.

Blood grouping, sometimes know as blood typing would become one of the main focuses of the brigade in the later part of the war. The brigade continued to undertake training activities, especially in relation to the work of ARP committees, but the training of civilians in general remained the principal responsibility of the association. The contribution to the war effort through blood grouping will be examined further in this chapter.

Throughout the war Ontario's highway first aid program continued to operate successfully. As the program grew, Ontario was divided into eight districts, which treated an average twenty major accidents and 200 minor accidents per year. In 1938 the program that had been successfully pioneered by the Ontario Motor League, St. John Ambulance and Red Cross in Ontario was transplanted to British Columbia. In that province St. John Ambulance and the Red Cross worked with the British Columbia Provincial Police (BCPP) to maintain the first aid stations. An unexpected by-product of this new relationship was the training of all members of the BCPP by St. John Ambulance. The first aid posts were invaluable as indicated by the *Boston Bar Post*:

> An auto traveling along the Fraser Canyon Highway crashed over a steep bank injuring the four occupants. One man received back injuries; another head wound and fractured collar bone; one woman received a fractured ankle and wounds about the head and neck; while other injuries included a fractured skull and back abrasions. All four suffered greatly from shock, and after receiving First Aid treatment, were transported a distance of twenty-two miles to the hospital at Lytton.[12]

The lives of the occupants of the car were saved in large part through the presence of a St. John Ambulance-Red Cross first aid post and St. John-trained first aiders.

British Columbia also maintained an active St. John Ambulance Brigade Ski Patrol in the North Shore Mountains, following the example set by the brigade in Quebec, which had established the ski patrols in the Laurentian Mountains that were so popular with tourists.

All of St. John Ambulance's special centres remained active, although the pressures of war work had a particularly negative effect on the number of first aid courses taken by employees of Canadian Industries Limited:

> Increased activity in the manufacture of munitions and other essential supplies has resulted in longer and irregular working hours which interfered with our usual procedure of holding First Aid classes immediately after work.[13]

In spite of the pressures of war work, loss of volunteers through enlistment in the armed forces and the general stress of the war, St. John Ambulance would grow, offering first aid training to an ever-increasing number of citizens, both civilian and military.

In 1939 Canadian National Railways introduced a new type of folding stretcher specifically designed to remove passengers from sleeping cars, this was subsequently adopted by the CPR. At Northern Electric there continued to be a great zeal for first aid training with 1,300 employees holding valid certificates.[14] At the beginning of the war the RCMP implemented a new policy that all new recruits be instructed in St. John Ambulance first aid. To accommodate the increased number of classes being taken, several RCMP constables were trained as St. John Ambulance instructors. "All uniformed personnel of the RCMP are issued with a first aid manual and are expected to keep in touch with the subject."[15]

A number of new relationships were established during the war, including bonds with the Registered Nurses Association of Canada and the Canadian Nurses Association. In 1940 fifty nurses took exams and qualified as St. John Ambulance first aid instructors. "It is the intention of the nursing bodies that all graduate and undergraduate nurses should obtain the First Aid Certificate."[16] These same instructors were authorized to teach home nursing on behalf of

St. John Ambulance as the popularity of the program grew throughout the war.

In rural areas especially even the junior home nursing training course, "which has never been popular,"[17] gained a strong following. The war resulted in an ever increasing level of cooperation between members of the medical profession and St. John Ambulance.[18] Members of the Victorian Order of Nurses and the association rekindled an old relationship that had been forged in during the Influenza Epidemic, with VON nurses helping to train some St. John Ambulance instructors: "[T]hanks and paid tribute to the VON … found time to give SJAA much assistance."[19]

The number of first aid certificates and courses being given by St. John Ambulance exceeded all previous records in Canada in 1939, with 36,354 certificates being issued. By 1942 this number had jumped to 97,547, thus more certificates were issued in one year than during the entire First World War. First aid training on this scale was an immense undertaking, one that strained the resources of both the association and brigade, which despite losing many members, who enlisted or were commissioned in the armed forces, managed to increase overall membership throughout the conflict.

The brigade entered into a six-month membership drive in 1940, setting a goal of 3,000 members. Having seen over 400 members leave to enlist, its size had dropped to 2,300. By the end of 1940 the membership had almost doubled, with 4,000 members, 1,000 more than projected in the initial membership drive.

Despite war work, the brigade remained active at major public events such as the Calgary Stampede, various provincial exhibitions, and sporting events. New divisions were formed in every province except Prince Edward Island. St. John Ambulance was making a different sort of contribution in PEI where, beginning in 1944, public school teachers began to take first aid courses offered by the association. Being classified as a "vulnerable province" because of the threat of U-boat attack,[20] beginning in 1940 the number of first aid courses taken by islanders doubled.

A number of large-scale civilian medical emergencies were experienced during the war. In 1942 British Columbia encountered a health care crisis because of a lack of nurses and nurses' aids. The crisis eased when brigade nurses' aids took up temporary duties in a number of the province's hospitals, even undertaking some training activities with great success.[21] Ontario was hit by a similarly serious nursing shortage, and the provincial government authorized trained members of nursing divisions to serve in civilian hospitals as "semi-trained nurses,"[22] under the direction of a registered nurse.

In the summer of 1945 Manitoba experienced a medical crisis when an epidemic of dysentery broke out in the provincial School for Mental Defectives at Portage la Prairie. Eight nursing aids were sent to help minister to the needs of patients following an "emergency call"[23] from the premier for assistance. During the infamous VE (Victory in Europe) day riots in Halifax, St. John Ambulance was there to render assistance and first aid to the injured. The entire downtown core had disrupted, many of the injured were treated by members of the brigade, or whisked away to hospital in a St. John Ambulance.[24]

With the cooperation of the Canadian Press and other media outlets, the national headquarters attempted to heighten citizen's knowledge of first aid through newspapers and radio.[25] Federal District began advertising on the radio through CKCO, and the first printed advertisements for St. John Ambulance first aid training were posted in the cars of the Ottawa Electric Railway Company in 1942.

The work undertaken in the Maritimes was particularly successful in Nova Scotia, where there had been no brigade division since the end of the First World War. By the end of the Second World War, the province was home to thirteen nursing divisions. New Brunswick had a similarly successful record throughout the war, mustering three ambulance divisions and eight nursing divisions by war's end. It is curious that while Nova Scotia established many nursing divisions, it was unable to found even one ambulance division. One reason for this was the high proportion of the male population that enlisted in the Royal Canadian Navy, Merchant Navy, and Canadian Army.

Cooperation with the Navy League of Canada began in the early stages of the Battle of the Atlantic. The various Nova Scotia nursing divisions looked after survivors who arrived in Halifax. To assist in their work the Navy League requisitioned a large dormitory for the use of St. John Ambulance as a hospital ward. Many Halifax medical doctors and registered nurses freely volunteered their time and efforts to St. John Ambulance throughout the war.

Saskatchewan quickly became a leader in offering first aid courses. These were given to public school students and the province also became the first to see St. John Ambulance first aid become part of the hygiene curriculum in high schools, and all Grade 8 students earned their Junior First Aid Course certificates beginning in 1942. The province also ran a program of free classes for senior first aid, but this "did not prove entirely successful."[26] In Vancouver and Victoria similar schooling programs involving first aid training offered by St. John Ambulance were initiated in the early stages of the war. The other area that was particularly successful in British Columbia was in the field of industrial first aid training. In cooperation with the B.C. Workers' Compensation Board a new industrial first aid course was developed and approved.

Alberta experienced a steady rise in first aid course offerings, and was home to six ambulance and six nursing divisions by the end of 1945. The province would have one of the most active blood grouping programs in the country. Although there was great enthusiasm for establishing more divisions in rural areas, fulfilling these plans meant first overcoming the lack of first aid certificate holders. To that end, the association attempted to make inroads into areas outside Calgary, Edmonton, and Red Deer. Like British Columbia, Alberta soon became a leader in organizing industrial first aid "in isolated industries,"[27] such as mining.

The war resulted in the stabilization of the weak provincial council in Quebec, "never in the history of this Province has the Order of St. John become so integral a part of every day life."[28] This was a great development given the potential for growth in Canada's second most populous province. By the end of 1942 the brigade in Quebec was restructured by Lieutenant-Colonel Gaboury. The brigade structure was divided along linguistic lines to provide for more efficient training and to more fully involve French Canadians, who, while interested in the work of the brigade, naturally wanted to work in their own language. "The new Brigade units are now prepared to render very excellent assistance in case of any emergency in the Province."[29] By the end of the war Gaboury had helped established twenty ambulance and twenty nursing divisions made up of francophones, an unprecedented achievement that helped to fully involve French Canadians in the work of St. John Ambulance.

• • •

In 1942 Wodehouse resigned as lieutenant of the Commandery in Canada in response to the pressures of his work as deputy minister of pensions and national health. He was succeeded by Dr. Herbert Bruce, another highly distinguished man of public life, having served as inspector general of the medical services overseas during the First World War, as lieutenant-governor of Ontario from 1932 to 1937, and from 1940 to 1945 as a member of the dominion Parliament. Bruce served as the lieutenant of the commandery from 1942 to 1943 and resigned from the post when his duties as a member of Parliament began to interfere with his duties as lieutenant of the commandery. There was also some unease at having an active politician at the head of the organization. As the war dragged on Bruce became an outspoken supporter of conscription and critic of Prime Minister William Lyon Mackenzie King.[30] The press in French Canada attacked Bruce's views on the war and his desire to avoid any friction between anglo-phone and francophone members of St. John Ambulance played a role in his decision to step down. Bruce also felt that his talents were more useful as a parliamentarian and conscriptionist than as head of a charitable organization. Throughout his time as lieutenant, Bruce championed the importance of the nursing divisions and insisted that each province appoint provincial superintendents of nursing. He was also instrumental in the appointment of the first superintendent-in-chief of the nursing divisions in Canada, the principal nursing officer in Canada. Bruce was also a leading proponent of Gaboury's plan to establish francophone units of the brigade in Quebec.

Bruce was succeeded by Lewis, who had been the commandery's sub-lieutenant. A lawyer and adept organizer, Lewis would remain lieutenant of the commandery until 1946 when the Priory of Canada was established. Lewis helped to guide St. John Ambulance through its negotiations with the Red Cross and federal government on the blood grouping agreement, and it was in large part through his work that Canada was raised to a priory in 1946.

During the First World War, St. John Ambulance trained more than 200,000 members of the Canadian Expeditionary Force in basic first aid. This level of training was duplicated during the Second World War, during which St. John Ambulance trained members of the Royal Canadian Navy, Canadian Army, and Royal Canadian Air Force.

The work of Brigadier General R.M. Gorssiline, director general of medical services for the Canadian Army helped place St. John Ambulance at the forefront of first aid training throughout the conflict. Gorssiline had served as the first provincial commissioner for the brigade in Quebec from 1936 to 1942 and later served as hospitaller and almoner for the commandery. Having first been introduced to St. John Ambulance first aid training during the First World War, Gorssiline would be a staunch promoter of first aid training and the work of St. John Ambulance throughout his life.

By the end of 1939, St. John headquarters in Ottawa prepared a plan to offer voluntary first aid training to all combat members of the Canadian Active Service Force (army), which would be offered jointly by the association and brigade. By 1940, 100 percent of all stretcher bearers had taken the St. John Ambulance First Aid course, and the close relationship with the Royal Canadian Army Medical Corps was continued. By the end of the same year a new syllabus was developed for members of the Canadian military. As the war escalated the National Resources Mobilization Act was passed by Parliament. This act required all men over the age of sixteen to report for thirty days of military training. By 1942 the training period was extended to four months of military training. The training included twenty hours of compulsory first aid instruction provided by St. John Ambulance instructors. This did not qualify students for a first aid certificate, but it was sufficient time to teach the basics of battlefield first aid. Each person was also issued with an abbreviated first aid manual, which was given to all members of the military.

The RCAF made a special effort to train all its ground and air crew, "all RCAF personnel, officers and airmen, both ground and aircrew, are to be qualified to administer First Aid to the injured. This is also to include Officers and Airmen of the RCAF (WD)."[31] Of the three services, by the end of the war the RCAF had the highest number of first aiders amongst its members. Even the newly founded RCAF Cadet Corps (Air Cadets) were trained in St. John Ambulance first aid. [32] By 1943 all people entering the RCAF were trained in St. John Ambulance first aid. On a voluntary basis, this came to include persons trained under the extensive British Commonwealth Air Training Plan. There was such a demand for instructors that Bell Telephone lent its instructors to both the RCAF and RCMP.[33] Most members of the RCN were trained in first aid by the St. John Ambulance Association, the majority of classes taking place on Canada's East and West coasts, and even aboard ship. Halifax, Esquimalt, and St. John's Newfoundland were the principal RCN first aid training centres. Aboard ship sick berth attendants and medical officers gave instruction in St. John Ambulance first aid from St. John teaching materials. On Canada's East Coast the association took the lead in training because there were no brigade instructors in Nova Scotia, there being no ambulance divisions, only nursing divisions.

In the early stages of the war it was left up to the individual commanding officer to request first aid training from St. John Ambulance, and although somewhat haphazard, this system was effective, undergoing refinement as the war dragged on, with increasing involvement from officials of the Department of National Defence. By wars end a more coordinated national and provincial system was developed based on Canada's various military districts, with a focus placed on the main training centres.

To further facilitate the cooperation of the Red Cross and St. John Ambulance a joint board was established on 29 April 1943 under Order-in-Council 3439. Minister of National War Services Léo Laflèche was pivotal in facilitating the agreement. The St. John-Red Cross

Joint Board consisted of nine members, four each from the Red Cross and St. John Ambulance and a chair who was appointed by the minister. The chair was Morris Wilson the highly respected vice-president of the Royal Bank of Canada. The members from St. John Ambulance were Lewis, Senator Norman Paterson, R.V. LeSueur, and Lieutenant-Colonel Thomas Guerin. The Red Cross was represented by Jackson Dodds, Willis MacLachlin, Justice P.H. Gordon, and Leon Gerin-Lajoie.

The board met throughout the war coming to agreement on issues related to home nursing and first aid training. By 1944 it was agreed that all first aid certificates issued by St. John Ambulance and the Red Cross would be issued in the name of the joint board for the duration of the war to further emphasize the level of cooperation and to eliminate bureaucratic difficulties. In the provinces similar joint committees were formed between the Red Cross and St. John Ambulance to better facilitate war work at that level. Throughout the war the two organizations maintained an uneasy relationship, although Wilson's strong leadership helped overcome most difficulties.[34] Many held a concern that once the war concluded that the Red Cross would once again enter into open competition in the first aid training field.[35] A fear that was not totally unfounded.

There was perhaps no better example of the level of cooperation achieved between the Red Cross and St. John Ambulance than in the field of blood grouping and collection. While the Red Cross would become the national collector of blood products following the Second World War, St. John Ambulance played an important role in the wartime blood collection system.

One of the main activities undertaken by the brigade throughout the war was blood grouping, also known as blood typing. Following the First World War, techniques for transfusing, preserving, and storing blood became much more sophisticated and safe. With the development of a process for the drying blood — which could be reconstituted with distilled water — the ability to conduct transfusions near the battlefield became feasible, and thus there was a demand for blood donations. Part of the blood collection process is to determine the type of blood, there being four groups of blood, A, B, AB, and O, distinguished by the presence of different antigens and antibodies. When giving transfusions only certain types of blood can be given. Transfusing the wrong type of blood into a patient can result in an immunological reaction causing death, which makes the accurate grouping of blood a task of great importance. People with blood type O are "universal donors," because their blood can be given to anybody. Those with type AB are "universal receivers."

The purpose behind blood grouping was to provide the potential donor, civil defence authorities, and employers with a record of everyone's blood type. Persons being typed were pricked on the finger with a needle, the blood was then "typed," and the potential donor was issued with a wallet-sized card showing their blood type. In many cases employers also kept a register of their employees' blood types. If a typed individual was injured it allowed doctors to quickly ascertain what type of blood was needed, saving valuable time. In the event of a shortage of a particular type of blood, it allowed civil defence authorities to put out a call for a specific type of blood and receive donations quickly. This work was carried out by members of the various nursing divisions which coordinated blood grouping with the Canadian Red Cross Society.

Officials of both St. John Ambulance and the Canadian Red Cross realized that the "value of blood grouping on a large scale has been shown on many occasions,"[36] most specifically during blood drives and following large industrial accidents. An indication of just how revolutionary blood transfusions were in improving the morality of injured soldiers can be found by comparing treatment statistics of the two world wars. During the First World War, 75 percent of those who suffered from a compound fracture of the femur died, while in the Second World War 90 percent of the soldiers with the same injury recovered. Of those who received abdominal injuries during the First World War, 80 percent died as a result of their wounds, while during the Second World War 73 percent recovered. The increase in rates of recovery has been attributed to the use of blood transfusions.[37]

Early in 1942 the first blood grouping clinic was opened in Ottawa, being organized and financed by Dr. Kemp Edwards, district superintendent of federal district. Members of the Ottawa Central Nursing Division were trained in blood grouping and began by typing city police, firefighters, Air Raid Protection officers, and senior government officials. A special Red Cross blood donor clinic, staffed jointly by members of the brigade and Red Cross, was opened on Metcalfe Street in Ottawa. Members of the brigade were principally responsible for the typing of blood, and the Red Cross was responsible for taking blood donations. Given the close proximity of the clinic to Parliament all manner of senior officials and ministers of the Crown did their civic duty and had their blood typed. On one occasion Minister of Finance James Ilsley wandered into the clinic to be typed and make a donation. Ilsley had just delivered the 1944 budget, which increased income taxes, so he was not the most popular man in the country. The entire clinic was abuzz, as they had been warned by the chair of the clinic, Senator Norman Paterson, a close friend of Ilsley, that the minister was liable to show up to give a donation. A modest man, Ilsey never made a fuss about being a minister, and when asked what is occupation was he simply replied to the brigade member that he was "in the government."[38] Holding the syringe in her hand and attempting to be cheery the member replied "That's interesting. I wonder if you know Mr. Ilsley … we are expecting him this morning, and after what he did in raising our taxes we can hardly wait to give him the works!"[39] Anecdotal evidence suggests that the minister did not make his presence known until after he had finished giving blood, and only then when Senator Paterson greeted him as "Minister" in front of the unsuspecting brigade member. Throughout the war members of the brigade would type on average 30,000 people per year and cooperation with the Red Cross in this area would continue until 1951, when St. John voluntarily pulled out of blood grouping field, having typed more than 200,000 Canadians. The Red Cross would take over all blood related collection duties until 1998.

Volunteer Aid Detachments: The VADs

The enlistment of VAD volunteers and constitution of VAD units across the country did not begin until two years into the war.[40] Although preparations at the national level were begun in 1941, in the early years of the conflict the overwhelming focus was on ensuring first aid training was offered to as many Canadians as possible. As in the First World War, VADs were single women who held a St. John Ambulance first aid certificate, and in many cases these volunteers were also members of a nursing division of the brigade.

VADs were volunteers in the truest sense. Those who saw service overseas were unpaid, provided only with a uniform and small allowance for incidental expenses. While their travel and lodgings were paid for by St. John Ambulance it is incredible to think that these ladies spent two or three years as unpaid volunteers, many of whom stayed overseas for more than a year after the war ended.

St. John Ambulance worked closely with the Canadian Nurses Association, Canadian Hospital Council, Red Cross, and Royal Canadian Army Medical Corps (RCAMC) to develop the curriculum and criteria for VADs. The matron-in-chief of the RCAMC, Elizabeth Smellie was of particular assistance, working closely with Winnifred Kydd, the brigade's lady superintendent-in-chief. Smellie had previously served as chief superintendent of the Victorian Order of Nurses and had a strong respect for the work of St. John Ambulance. She and Senator Paterson worked to develop the VAD scheme for Canada, and it was largely through her efforts that St. John VADs were sent overseas.

VAD volunteers served as nurse's assistants, ambulance drivers, and clerical staff. They would see service in civilian and military hospitals in Canada, and some were even employed in liberated prisoner of war camps and concentration camps in Europe where they ministered to the sick. Along with the traditional duties of a nursing assistant and ambulance driver, some VADs served as physiotherapists, assisting those who had lost limbs or suffered serious injuries to their extremities. VADs took one of two training courses after being accepted into the program. "Course A" required 240 or more hours of work in a hospital setting while "Course B" required eighty or more hours of training in a hospital setting.

Ottawa and Federal District were the first to establish a VAD training centre. A teaching ward was set up, stocked with supplies, and made in every way identical to a regular hospital ward. There VAD volunteers were taught the basiscs of being a nurse's assistant. From the teaching ward VADs were dispatched to civil and military hospitals for hands on experience under the direction of registered nurses or members of the RCAMC.

In March 1942 Ian Mackenzie, minister of pensions and national health requested that St. John Ambulance send a delegate to England to study the civil defence preparations that had been put in place by the British government. Ms. Kathleen (Kay) Gilmour, lady district superintendent of the brigade in Ontario was sent. In 1943 Gilmour would succeed Kydd as lady superintendent-in-chief of the brigade. The 1942 visit to the United Kingdom gave Gilmour an opportunity to survey the success being achieved by British VADs. By 1943 more than 120,000 British VADs were serving throughout that country in civilian hospitals, first aid posts, and in air raid shelters.

Throughout 1942, Gilmour had observed a "steady increasing interest in a VAD programme."[41] As the shortage of nurses became more acute in Canada, the federal government pushed St. John Ambulance and the Red Cross commence a VAD program similar to that which existed during the First World War. One of the immediate results was the development of a

Canadian home nursing manual, with the assistance of the Canadian Nurses Association. The manual was written by Rae Chittick and J.M. Connal, acting for the Committee on Nursing Education of the Canadian Nurses Association. The new manual addressed specific Canadian situations and took into account Canadian public health policies. This was the first home nursing manual tailored for Canadian needs. By the end of 1943, in "preparation to meet requests for assistance, the Lady Superintendent-in-Chief [Gilmour] proceeded to England in December 1943 to complete plans for the sending overseas of members of the Nursing Divisions."[42]

Although Gilmour was the principal VAD officer overseas, the operations at home in Canada were directed by Lady Redfern the Dominion VAD Officer. She held this post until March 1945 when Hyacynth Willis O'Conner succeeded her. Their duties included vetting VAD applications forwarded from the provinces and perpetuating the VAD program in Canada.

The first major VAD recruitment campaign was inaugurated in 1943, with notices published announcing that VAD volunteers could serve in Canada or overseas. Gilmour travelled to almost every province and spoke to members of the brigade,[43] association, and general public on the importance of VAD work and the opportunities that awaited young women who wished to serve. One problem that initially arose in British Columbia, which would be encountered in every other province, was that large numbers of women volunteered for "service anywhere,"[44] not just in Canada. Under this recruitment plan, VADs were "trained for services in the RCAMC hospitals in Canada, as well as for civilian hospitals."

In February 1944, Gilmour and nine senior Nursing Division officers travelled to Britain to meet with the Joint War Organization of St. John Ambulance and the Red Cross.[45] The purpose of the trip was to determine what services they could best provide to the United Kingdom, and to gain ideas about how to expand the work and recruitment of VADs in Canada. So devoted were they to making use of their first aid skills, only three would return to Canada after the fact finding mission, the balance staying to serve in civilian hospitals, first aid posts, and air raid shelters until war's end. Even during the fact-finding stages of the visit members of the delegation became actively engaged in VAD work. By war's end 221 VADs would see service overseas.

In April 1944 the first request for Canadian VADs came in from the Joint War Organization. The notice requested "50 women motor drivers and one driver of a light mobile surgical unit."[46] The first contingent left Halifax for England on 5 July 1944.

Initially a temporary Canadian VAD St. John Ambulance Brigade headquarters was set up at No. 2 Cockspur Street in London, right next to the Canadian military headquarters. In late September 1944 more spacious accommodations were acquired through the help of the Canadian high commissioner. The new offices were located at 42 South Audley Street, near Grosvenor Square — not far from the high commissioner's home — provided a Canadian VAD headquarters until October 1946 when operations were concluded. Not surprisingly two regular visitors to VAD headquarters in London were Vincent and Alice Massey. Massey was serving as Canadian high commissioner to the United Kingdom and had always taken an active interest in the work of the Order of St. John. Another less distinguished but equally loved visitor was the VAD mascot "John." By wars end John had been given to an American soldier and was replaced by a lively Scottish terrier named "Jock" who would become one of the most photographed dogs in the history of St. John Ambulance, appearing in countless photos of VADs.

VADs were constantly on duty, whether it be in the air raid shelters of London, the civil hospitals surrounding the capital or in more exotic locations such as Gibraltar or Lisbon Portugal. One well known VAD was Constance (Conn) Hutcheon, who served as a VAD nurse and VAD quartermaster during the war. Renowned for being able to procure almost any item, Hutcheon embodied the ingenuity and resourcefulness of Canada's VADs.

VADs served not only in Britain and Canada, but also in Burma, Hong Kong, Gibraltar, France, Germany, India, Malaysia, and the Netherlands. One VAD spent three months offering relief to the sick at Bergen-Belsen concentration camp, which had been liberated by the British Army in April 1945. Another found herself on the island of Guernsey, which had been occupied by the Nazis from 1940–45. Others served in India and Malaysia treating released Commonwealth prisoners of war and interned civilians who had suffered so greatly at the hands of their Japanese captors.

Of the first VADs in Canada seventy-three were allotted to RCAMC hospitals in 1944, twenty-four of whom were withdrawn in late 1944 for service overseas. Their high level of training and professional demeanour was widely recognized, and the recipient hospitals "were pleased with the representatives."[47] VADs were recruited from every province that possessed a nursing division, and while the VADs tended to come from the provinces that had the largest nursing divisions there was still a good cross-country representation.

Table 1

VADs by Province from which they were Recruited

Provincial Council	Number of VADs Overseas
Alberta	6
British Columbia	56
Manitoba	35
New Brunswick	16
Nova Scotia	15
Ontario	49
Prince Edward Island	0
Quebec	16
Saskatchewan	4
Federal District	23

By the autumn of 1946 most VADs had returned to Canada, having spent more than a year after the cessation of hostilities away from home. Following victory in Europe many VAD drivers became welfare officers, charged with a variety of activities including assistance to returned soldiers, wounded servicemen, and civilians released from internment camps. In recognition of her outstanding services during the war in leading the VADs, Gilmour was awarded a rare honour, the Service Medal of the Order of St. John with Palms. The medal was presented by Governor General, Field Marshal Viscount Alexander of Tunis on 25 November 1946. It was not only recognition for Gilmour, but acknowledgement of the extraordinary services rendered by the VADs during the last part of the war.

Linen Guild

One endeavour that was a great success during the war that has today been largely forgotten was the Linen Guild. The guild was established in 1927 under the patronage of the Duchess of York, the future Queen Elizabeth, mother of Queen Elizabeth II. Initially it consisted of ten ladies, the president, and a chair.[48] The purpose of the guild was to raise money to purchase linens and bed clothes for the St. John Ophthalmic Hospital of Jerusalem. Funds were collected at St. John's Gate in London and various hospital supplies were purchased centrally and sent to Jerusalem.

The Canadian branch of the association had a history of sending annual donations to St. John's Gate to contribute towards the operation of the Ophthalmic Hospital, through the hospitaller, but it was not until 1937 that a branch of the Linen Guild was established in Canada. Other commanderies had established branches of the guild in Australia, New Zealand, and South Africa. By 1937 Queen Mary was the president of the Linen Guild, the Canadian branch of which was established under the direction of Lady Perley, wife of Sir George Perley. Lady Tweedsmuir, wife of the governor general was made president of the guild in Canada and Lady Perley was elected the first chair. The membership was limited to women and the first committee included seven members, including Senator Carine Wilson, Canada's first female senator, Thérèse Casgrain, and Willis O'Connor. Wilson and Casgrain were both prominent female rights activists. Willis O'Connor was the eminently well connected wife of senior aide-de–camp, Colonel Henry Willis O'Connor who served as the organizational mastermind behind the work of the guild. The other members of the inaugural committee were all the wives of prominent politicians, but the committee was far more than a social club, as they were effective fundraisers. In their first year they raised $250.98,[49] and throughout the war they would raise thousands of dollars for the ophthalmic hospital. In 1942 they donated more money to the hospital than the Commandery in Canada.[50] The presidency of the guild was taken over by HRH the Princess Alice following the departure of Lady Tweedsmuir in 1940. Throughout the war, Princess Alice proved a strong advocate for the work of the committee — not to mention a draw at fundraising events. While most of the events were afternoon teas, a skate-a-thon was also organized for the skating rink at Rideau Hall. Lady Perley resigned in 1944 and was replaced by Ms. Willis O'Connor who would continue in the post until 1967. In 1945, $909 was raised towards the purchase of items for the hospital. As we will see in subsequent chapters, the guild would eventually be renamed the Ophthalmic Hospital Guild, and the funds raised would be put towards covering the cost of sending a nurse to the ophthalmic hospital for a year.

• • •

With the victory over Germany and Japan, the war was over and Canada prepared to enter a new period of growth and prosperity. More than a million Canadians had entered the military over the period 1939 to 1945, 45,000 made the supreme sacrifice. St. John Ambulance had grown greatly over the duration, boasting more than 328 divisions and 8,410 brigade members by the end of 1945, a three–fold expansion. Women played an increasingly central role in the brigade's work, making up half of the total membership, and more than half of the divisions.[51] Brigade units had been set up in every province — save Prince Edward Island — in Nova Scotia were there had been only sporadic interest in the work of the brigade in the interwar period, thirteen nursing divisions were active. The association rendered equally important services throughout the war, most notably through the continued provision of first aid instruction, training nearly half-a-million Canadians in first aid through the war.

Table 2

Total First Aid Certificates Issued, 1938–1945

Year	Total Certificates Issued
1938	27,902
1939	36,354
1940	58,220
1941	66,843
1942	97,547
1943	88,752
1944	65,429
1945	42,571

The continued interest of industry and importance placed on first aid training by air raid protection officials throughout the war helped place St. John Ambulance on a solid footing in the post-war period. With the advent of the Cold War a new emphasis was placed on civil defence and again the value of the organization's first aid training was imparted to thousands of Canadians. The most conspicuous service was rendered by the 221 Canadian VADs who served overseas. Without financial remuneration these women served selflessly, tending to repatriated prisoners of war in Europe and the Pacific, alleviating suffering in a liberated Nazi concentration camp, driving ambulances, and providing comfort to the wounded in British hospitals. We can never quantify the contribution these ladies made in treating so many wounded. Aside from their skills as nursing aids, their smiling faces and cheery demeanour served as the medicine that nursed so many broken souls and bodies back to health.

Working with the Canadian Red Cross Society, St. John Ambulance recorded the blood types of hundreds of thousands of Canadians, once again demonstrating that the two benevolent organizations were capable of cooperating productively. The well-established relationship with the Department of National Defence and RCMP had expanded to include the federal and many provincial governments as well. The crisis of war had exposed an ever increasing number of citizens to first aid training giving them skills that were useful in any emergency, be it battlefield injury or car accident.

The efforts expended during the Second World War at the national and provincial level demonstrated to many St. John Ambulance volunteers that there continued to be a great deal of overlap between the work of the association and the brigade. Although a significant degree of integration had been achieved with the establishment of the commandery in 1934, at the provincial level there was still room for increased cooperation, and resistance to greater integration was still a factor in the dynamic between the two organizations. The elevation of the Commandery in Canada to the Priory of Canada aided in building of greater cooperation between them. Throughout the war the provinces had demonstrated themselves to be highly effective sub-divisions of St. John Ambulance and with this came a drive to give provincial councils greater autonomy within the broader St. John Ambulance organization in Canada.

EIGHT

GROWTH AND EXPANSION
The Establishment of a Modern Organization

If you never need what you learn in Civil Defence you lose nothing,
but if you never learn what you need, you may lose everything.
Defence Training Motto, 1954

The immediate post-war period was marked most notably by the establishment of the Priory of Canada. Along with other commanderies in Australia and New Zealand, Canada was raised to a priory in 1946. St. John Ambulance's relationship with the special centres remained strong. Although there was an initial post-war slump, it was short lived.[1] The country's population grew by 65 percent between 1946 and 1967, and St. John Ambulance first aid training outstripped this growing from 44,929 to 132,475 over the same period. The organization would mourn the passing of King George VI and celebrate the accession of a new sovereign head, Queen Elizabeth II. As Canada's industrial capacity continued to grow, so did the need for first aid training. Growth was significant at national and provincial levels. Indeed, the provincial councils became increasingly influential, building new headquarters and transforming into the backbone of St. John Ambulance as a national organization. One of the most important changes in first aid training implemented in this period was the gender neutralization of courses in 1951; men and women were no longer trained separately and coeducational classes were inaugurated.[2] In an era when many public schools throughout the country still had boys and girls enter through separate doors, this was an important step forward.

Post-war optimism was short lived and a new insidious menace emerged from behind what would become known as the "Iron Curtain." Just five years after the conclusion of the Second World War, Canada was again at war, this time in Korea alongside the United Nations. This conflict "weighed down by the more oppressive burden of the Cold War, made a profound impression on Canada."[3] A nationwide zeal for civil defence preparations and fear of atomic attack became focuses of governments and the Canadian public. Just as the two world wars brought St. John Ambulance and the Canadian Red Cross Society together, this new type of war saw the two organizations arrived at an agreement on first aid training and blood grouping.

In an effort to promote the growth of St. John Ambulance in Canada and to gain greater autonomy from St. John's Gate in London, negotiations were opened in early 1946 to effect the elevation of the commandery to a full priory. Lieutenant of the Commandery Lewis resigned from his post in July 1946 after the preliminary agreement was completed with officials in London. Lewis's resignation came about because of increasing business pressures brought on by the post-war boom. His leadership of St. John Ambulance in the last half of the war helped put it on a solid footing for the demands of peacetime life. He would be succeeded by Charles Gray who would remain at the head of St. John Ambulance in Canada from 1946 to 1960, overseeing the post-war growth and transformation of the organization.[4] The priory was formally established on 16 September 1946. Governor General Lord Alexander, up 'til then Knight Commander of the Commandery in Canada, graciously consented to become the first prior of the Priory of Canada, further cementing the relationship that existed between the Order and the office of governor general. Gray, lieutenant of the commandery, was given the new designation sub-prior, a term that would be changed to chancellor of the Priory of Canada in 1951. Priory Chapter, the governing body of St. John Ambulance, came into being, while other positions such as the hospitaller and almoner remained unchanged.

The first meeting of Priory Chapter was held on 25 November 1946 at Rideau Hall with the prior, Lord Alexander, presiding. Such meetings were usually preceded by an investiture ceremony,[5] but owing to continuing war restrictions on manufacturing on non-essential goods there remained a shortage of insignia. None of this dampened the atmosphere of confidence and anticipation as the priory was inaugurated.

One major change in policy that came about as the result of the establishment of the priory was that Canadians gained complete control over the appointment of officials to the association and the brigade. Previously appointments were vetted by officials at St. John's Gate. This was especially true of brigade appointments, which were closely scrutinized. With the establishment of the priory all senior appointments were now sent directly to the grand prior.[6] "On receipt of HRH's approval they will be immediately notified and such appointees will thereafter be reported to Council and Chapter General."[7] This change afforded Canada a much greater degree of independence, one that better reflected the maturity and abilities of St. John Ambulance in the Dominion.

Other changes were made to the structure of St. John Ambulance in Canada, most notably the previously separate elements of the association and the brigade. These came to be united under each provincial council beginning in 1946. At the provincial level the brigade had functioned separately from the association's provincial councils, although the councils had always included members of the brigade. The new provincial councils would have members from both organizations, however, the process was not simply one of adding a few brigade members to the existing membership of the association's councils.

The reorganization did much to place the brigade on an equal footing with the association, and streamlined the provincial operations of the two foundations. Nevertheless some in the brigade viewed them as an impingement upon their independence, and not all provinces implemented the change immediately. In 1946, Manitoba, Alberta, New Brunswick, and Nova Scotia were the first to experience amalgamation. Saskatchewan, British Columbia, Ontario, and Federal District would follow in 1947. Quebec was the last to amalgamate, holding off until 1949. Prince Edward Island, possessing no brigade at this time, was not faced with any change, and Newfoundland was constituted as an amalgamated provincial council upon its entry into Confederation and the Priory of Canada in 1949.

In the years leading up to the Korean War, the newfound zeal for civil defence was marked by typical St. John Ambulance innovations. A new first aid instructional film was prepared and released by the end of 1948. Canadian hospitals continued to experience a shortage of nurses, so members of the brigade coordinated with municipal hospital boards to provide badly needed volunteers. This effort would continue well into the 1950s, especially during the polio outbreaks, which were to grip much of the nation through the early part of that decade.

The Canadian West, always a hotbed of innovation, would experience a great expansion of first aid training. The president of Alberta's Council noted that St. John Ambulance, through its first aid training had grown "from a small unknown organization to an organization that is to become a necessity in the lives of every citizen."[8] With the development of the oil industry, the demand for first aid classes "increased almost beyond our ability to provide instructors."[9] Industrial first aid remained popular in British Columbia where St. John Ambulance worked closely with the province's Workers' Compensation Board, the Canadian Manufacturers' Association, and the Northern Interior Lumbermen's Association to ensure that there was a near total rate of first aid training among remote workers.[10] In Nova Scotia members of the brigade expended great energy blood grouping every member of the RCMP and armed forces. This was a springboard to the creation of first aid training programs at HMC's Dockyards in Halifax, HMC's Naval Magazine at Bedford, and HMC's Naval Armament Depot in Dartmouth. The 1947 Marian Congress (a conference of Roman Catholics) in Ottawa brought together brigade members from across Ontario and Quebec to treat more than 3,000 cases over the course of the week long event.

During the 1949 world Scout Jamboree, held in Ottawa, St. John Ambulance set up a thirty-bed field hospital, which treated 600 cases during the event. One of the most notable post-war service rendered by the brigade came during the S.S. *Noronic* disaster. On the morning of 14 September the S.S. *Noronic*, a Great Lakes cruise ship docked at Toronto, caught fire. The blaze spread throughout the old ship quickly trapping many passengers. Fire escapes were not properly marked and many of the crew failed to wake sleeping passengers. Of the 675 onboard, 139 did not survive. Members of the brigade were present at Pier 9 to help with the rescue effort; monitoring escape ladders, helping victims to safety, administering first aid, and offering blankets and warm drinks to the survivors.

Immediately following the end of the war the federal and provincial governments dissolved the Air Raid Protection committees that had been set up in every community across the country. With peace achieved there was no reason to believe that the skills of ARP volunteers would ever be needed again. Sadly, by 1947 the Cold War between the Soviet Union and Western democracies was underway. With this came the establishment of a nationwide civil defence program.

St. John Ambulance would play a prominent role in the implementation of civil defence plans and preparations, which were to be initiated in the event of atomic war. It was this threat of attack that once again brought the Red Cross and St. John Ambulance together.

The end of the war also brought a discontinuation of the St. John–Red Cross Joint Board, which was created in 1943. While the agreement had stipulated that it was to be in force for the duration of the war, relations had been cordial between the two organizations and there was an expectation, on the part of St. John Ambulance, that the agreement would be revised and renewed in the post-war period. The Red Cross had never been enthralled with the brigade's work in the blood grouping field and this was likely a factor, coupled with the Red Cross's desire to re-enter, more aggressively, the field of first aid training.

At the direction of Deputy Minister of National Health and Welfare G.D.W. Cameron, discussions between the Red Cross and St. John Ambulance began in early 1949.[11] By March of that year they had agreed in principal to meet and consider the establishment of a new agreement. Cameron was anxious to see the two organizations cooperate as the federal government planned to initiate a new civil defence in wake of the deteriorating international situation. So anxious were St. John Ambulance officials to enter into a new agreement that even before the meeting they offered to "speed up our retirement from the field of Blood Grouping."[12] Certainly on the part of St. John Ambulance there was a desire to cease competing the with Red Cross in the field of first aid training. The Red Cross was still in the process of establishing the National Blood Transfusion Service, and there was concern on its part that St. John Ambulance would want to continue blood typing. Understandably the Red Cross wanted to take over all blood donation responsibilities to eliminate any confusion in the public's mind about the new program and who was conducting it.

A new agreement signed on 25 January 1951, would become known as the St. John Ambulance–Canadian Red Cross Joint Operation Committee.[13] The mandate of the committee began:

> desirous of attaining the fullest possible cooperation one with the other in their similar fields of activity, in order to avoid duplication of effort and to supply services rendered by the parties in a manner most convenient and most suitable to individual needs and with the utmost economy and efficiency.[14]

In the agreement, St. John Ambulance conceded to "recede from the blood grouping and Rh typing fields," and thereby completely pull out of the blood field. The Red Cross would continue to offer first aid training to its own Corps, and continue its swimming and water safety programs. St. John Ambulance was made responsible for teaching first aid to industry and uniformed municipal employees, training of juniors, operation of patrols at public gatherings and in ski areas, and continued joint administration of the highway first aid posts. In essence the Red Cross agreed to leave the field of industrial/government first aid training while St. John Ambulance agreed to cease blood grouping, which by 1949 had developed into one of the brigade's major activities.[15] It was also agreed that joint advertising would be undertaken by the two groups and that there was great scope for cooperation in the field of nursing. These last two issues were left to be discussed in greater detail at a later date.[16]

Despite some initial difficulties the agreement ran smoothly. One early problem was the brigade in Saskatchewan's reluctantance to cease blood grouping, and despite the efforts of the national headquarters it would not be brought to an end until late 1952.[17] In this period the Red Cross withdrew from the Ontario Highway First Aid Post program that had been in place since 1928 in cooperation with the Ontario Motor League.[18] The agreement helped facilitate an amicable relationship until it was discontinued in 1978.[19]

On 6 February 1952 Sovereign Head of the Order King George VI died, largely on account of the toll the Second World War had taken on his health. Although he had spent less than two decades as head of the Order his service was conspicuous, especially during the war years when he and his consort Queen Elizabeth took an active role in the work of both the association and brigade. With the accession of Queen Elizabeth II to the throne the Order welcomed a new sovereign head. Chancellor Charles Gray represented the Priory of Canada at the Queen's Coronation. Almost simultaneous with the accession of a new sovereign came the appointment of a new prior and governor general. Lord Alexander, the first prior of the Priory of Canada, departed for Britain in 1952, being replaced by the first Canadian to be appointed to the post, Vincent Massey. A strong supporter of the work of St. John Ambulance, Massey had been appointed a Commander of the Order in 1934. Throughout his time as Canadian high commissioner to the United Kingdom, Massey and his wife Alice had been regular visitors to the VAD headquarters, which by war's end were not far from Massey's own home. One of St. John's own volunteers was taking up the priorship of Canada.

As the Cold War escalated the federal government placed an increasing emphasis on civil defence. Tens of thousands of Canadians had been trained by the Air Raid Protection committees that had been set up in every province early in the Second World War. Although these had been disbanded after the war, the government looked to reinvent them in the form of a civil defence program. In October 1949 the federal government appointed the first civil defence coordinator. The agreement between the Red Cross and St. John Ambulance was a by-product of the federal government's civil defence plans.

In 1951 the government enlisted the help of St. John Ambulance to train all civil defence officials and volunteers across the country. The organization became directly involved with the Civil Defence Health Planning Group at the Department of National Health and Welfare, and as the focus on blood grouping ceased it was quickly replaced by civil defence training. Realizing the potential participation in civil defence, Chancellor Gray commented "training for Civil Defence and the growing interest in such matters, had the effect of stimulating interest in first aid."[20] At the 1952 St. John National Conference, the main topic of discussion was civil defence and how to cope with the aftermath of an atomic attack. Much of this occurred in the period before the effects of fallout were fully understood, thus some of the training was overly optimistic in just what atomic injuries could be treated. A 45-minute skit on civil defence was created by members of the association and brigade. The skit "illustrates how varied and terrible would be the effects of a modern attack and the fact that proper organization can cope with almost any situation or number of casualties"[21] It would go on to be performed in every province as a method to encourage greater involvement in civil defence activities, bolster membership of the brigade, and introduce St. John Ambulance first aid training.

The mantra of civil defence quickly became "if you never need what you learn in civil defence you lose nothing, but if you never learn what you need, you may lose everything." St. John Ambulance worked with the federal government to create a civil defence first aid emergency pamphlet that was sent to all Canadian households in 1953.[22] A new booklet, *Fundamentals of First Aid*, was released in 1955 specifically to address the civil defence first aid needs of Canadians.

Federal authorities quickly realized that one of the most efficient lines of defence was women, and St. John Ambulance began cooperating in the provision of home nursing courses. In New Brunswick the provincial civil defence committee began coordinating plans with St. John Ambulance, the Red Cross, Salvation Army, RCMP, and Department of National Defence.[23] This multi-faceted approach would spread to most provinces by the time Civil Defence was renamed the Emergency Measures Organization in 1959. Preparation for the worst disaster imaginable became the focus of many civic organizations and it was quickly realized that a cornerstone to survival was having knowledge of first aid.

A year before the Cuban Missile Crisis, which took the world near to nuclear annihilation, Chancellor John Molson reflected on "survival planning,"[24] and what role St. John Ambulance would play following a national emergency. The aftermath of the Cuban Missile Crisis was a relaxation of the focus on civil defence by federal and provincial authorities. Nevertheless, St. John Ambulance remained active in the field. In Quebec the brigade was divided into seven areas to coincide with the province's Civil Protection Authority's emergency contingency plans.[25] The contribution to civil defence made by St. John Ambulance has rarely been acknowledged, yet it was a significant public service that again demonstrated the value of first aid training and the ability of the organization to work with a variety of partners.

Three Canadian disasters would ingrain St. John Ambulance in the minds of many Canadians; the Red River Floods of 1950, Hurricane Hazel, and the two Springhill Mining Disasters. Although Canadians are accustomed to severe weather, usually in the form of winter snow storms, the country has rarely been hit by massive flooding or hurricanes, least of all in central Canada.

In early May 1950 heavy rains caused the Red River to rise to his highest level since 1861. St. John Ambulance went into action nearly a month before the situation reached a crisis level, working in the community of West Kildonan establishing first aid posts and giving first aid to workers and volunteers engaged in the shoring up of dykes. By the first week of May the situation had become critical, with the Red River overflowing its banks. More than 70,000 people were evacuated and 1,000 square kilometres around Winnipeg would be transformed into a giant lake.

Responsibility for the overall relief activities, named "Operation Red Ramp" was left to

Brigadier General R.E.A. Morton, general officer commanding the Canadian Army's Prairie Command. Morton coordinated the volunteer relief efforts of various organizations including the St. John Ambulance Brigade, Red Cross, and Salvation Army.

Upwards of 5,000 members of the Canadian Army were put to work, and more than 500 St. John Ambulance personnel, 300 brigade, and 200 association, were put to work. Their duties ranged from maintaining thirty-five first aid posts set up along the dyke system and assisting with the evacuation of patients and the elderly from vulnerable areas, to working on the dykes and operating an emergency hospital at St. John House in Winnipeg. Members of the brigade played an important role in evacuating people to hospitals in Saskatchewan, Manitoba, and northern Ontario, not to mention the efforts put into running the fifty-bed emergency hospital that they set up at St. John House. The emergency lasted three weeks and throughout that period St. John Ambulance volunteers were active in every aspect of the emergency operations. The entire ordeal is estimated to have cost more than $700 million in 1950 dollars. It would not be until the 1996 Saguenay Flooding that this figure was exceeded.[26]

The next great test for St. John Ambulance abilities came following Hurricane Hazel. On 15 October 1954 Toronto and many of the outlying areas were hit by winds of 240 kilometres per hour and 210 millimetres of rain. The hurricane washed out bridges, backed up sewers, and swelled the Don and Humber rivers causing widespread flooding. When it was over the damage totalled $100 million, 2,000 were left homeless, and eighty-one had perished in the disaster. Included among the dead was one St. John cadet, Janet Crymble, who drowned in the flood waters. Throughout the crisis members of the brigade worked providing food and shelter to the homeless and displaced, and distributing blankets and badly needed supplies. Members of the association watched over children who had lost their parents and carried out similar duties in coordination with the brigade. The white cross had come to the rescue, providing a wide variety of services in the most significant natural disaster ever to hit Canada's largest city.

Two years later members of the brigade and holders of St. John Ambulance first aid certificates participated in the relief effort surrounding the first Springhill mining disaster which took place on 1 November 1956. An explosion was set off by coal dust trapping 127 miners in No. 4 colliery. Special rescue miners know as "draegermen" descended 1,675 metres to begin the rescue effort. All of these draegermen had been trained in St. John Ambulance first aid as part of a program supported by the Nova Scotia provincial government. Eighty-eight miners were brought to the surface alive, while thirty-nine did not survive. Members of the brigade helped to not only provide first aid at the pithead and look after those suffering from shock before transfer to hospital, but they helped to control the crowd that formed at the mine following the disaster.

When the second and most famous Springhill mining disaster occurred on 23 October 1958 the brigade was again on the scene providing assistance. The "Bump" as it became known trapped 174 miners in No. 2 colliery. Again draegermen trained in first aid descended, this time 4,200 metres below the surface, to begin the rescue operation. The entire ordeal became the first such event to be televised around the world. On 24 October, eighty-one survivors were brought to the surface. After five days of digging, another twelve were rescued. The last group of survivors emerged on 1 November. Throughout the event members of the brigade delivered first aid and helped transport survivors to hospital. Seventy-four perished in the collapse of the mine. The brigade also assisted in the recovery of bodies, having been trained as part of the Civil Defence program in such operations.

New fully bilingual and modernized brigade regulations were released in September 1952, and by November the Holger-Nielsen method of artificial respiration was implemented by St. John Ambulance. This replaced the Schafer and Silberstern methods, which had been adopted in the previous decade.[27] The first aid film strips released by St. John Ambulance remained popular until they were revamped in 1959.

In 1954 St. John Ambulance inaugurated the Save-a-Life Week campaign. The event was held in the third week of May, with a focus on first aid training and artificial respiration. This would later be adopted in other parts of the Commonwealth as an effective outreach method to introduce the general public to first aid training and to encourage new membership in the association and brigade. Save-a-Life Week would later expand to include public demonstrations of first aid and be coordinated with civil defence promotion. The success of this program and the high rate of first aid training among industrial workers brought visitors from the Priory of New Zealand who wanted to gain ideas on first aid promotion.[28] Along these lines Manitoba's Provincial Council undertook an aggressive information campaign during the last two years of the 1950s.[29] Developing a multi-panelled information display suitable for public areas, the Manitoba initiative would be duplicated across the country by the mid 1960s.

As the post-war shortage of nurses persisted into the 1950s members of the brigade and association remained active. At hospitals in Ontario, Newfoundland, Manitoba, and British Columbia members of the nursing divisions became more involved in public hospitals than they had been during the Second World War.[30] Nowhere was this more evident than when they participated in the various activities surrounding the spread of polio throughout Canada. Poliomyelitis is a viral infection that can cause paralysis or death because of respiratory failure. During the late 1940s and into the 1950s polio struck an increasing number of Canadians, many of whom were children. In Winnipeg in 1953 there was a serious polio outbreak and members of the St. John Nursing Division went into action. Working at Winnipeg General Hospital they admitted between 20 and 40 patients per day "many of the patients suffered from paralysis of the throat muscles and required very special individual care."[31] In cooperation with the Canadian Foundation for Poliomyelitis and Rehabilitation, nursing division members cared for thousands of polio victims. When the Salk Vaccine was introduced in 1955 members of the brigade were active in the mass vaccination that took place. In Winnipeg alone, brigade members were active at twenty-one of the city's twenty-two vaccination stations. During the 1959 Polio outbreak in Montreal, members of the brigade helped to administer 20,000 Salk Vaccines. This was in addition to the many other hospital duties that had been taken up by St. John Ambulance, which included sterilization of equipment.

As the 1950s drew to a close, members of the association and brigade came together in London Ontario to celebrate an auspicious occasion, the golden anniversary of the brigade in Canada. Along with the usual dignitaries were three distinguished guests, W.H. Pinnock, William Loveday, and F.H. Morton, all charter members of the first brigade division. The brigade had been founded on 3 May 1909, and that division would serve as the seed from which the brigade would grow in Canada, to involve 8,955 members by 1959.

Celebrations were held from May 2 to 4, and included a National Brigade conference, "The Brigade looks Forward," which sought to revitalize and expand the work of the brigade as it entered its next fifty years. Included with the conference was a banquet given in honour of the three charter members of the brigade. With Lieutenant-Governor John MacKay presiding, a special service of thanksgiving was held at St. Paul's Cathedral. As the brigade entered the 1960s, its membership would grow to more than 11,600, while the association experienced a steady increase in first aid course attendance. The old friction between the association and the brigade had, after two world wars and many projects, finally become little more than a joke between members. The successive changes to the structure of St. John Ambulance in Canada from a commandery into a priory, and the integration of the association and brigade in the provincial councils played a role in this transformation, but the credit truly lies with the individual volunteers of both foundations who took forward the ethos of cooperation in the service of humanity.

Royal tours have often served as the source of work for St. John Ambulance and this was no different in 1959 when the Queen and Prince Philip came to Canada to open the St. Lawrence Seaway. Members of the brigade served along the royal tour route like never before, reminiscent of the 1939 visit of King George VI and Queen Elizabeth, the brigade helped with first aid, especially in dealing with over-excited onlookers. That same year Federal District, in cooperation with the Ontario and Quebec provincial councils, rendered a variety of services to the Conference of Ontario Handicapped Groups, which was held in May of that year. In an age long before wheelchair accessibility and motorized wheelchairs many of the conferences delegates required the assistance of St. John Ambulance to get around. For the first time St. John Ambulance began advertising the benefits of first aid on television. Beginning in December 1959 a one minute advertisement was run on the CBC's main network from coast to coast. The following year saw the number of first aid certificates and other awards jump by 23 percent and the campaign was judged to be a success.

After more than forty years of service to the Order, fourteen of which were as chancellor, Charles Gray stepped down from his post in June 1960 at 83 years of age. Gray had worked in many posts dating back to 1916.[32] In every sense, he was the builder of the Priory of Canada and this was recognized by people throughout the Order of St. John around the Commonwealth. Scarcely two months after his retirement Gray died following a short illness on 21 August 1960. It came as serious shock to all members of the organization. Highly respected and well known, "he would be the first to say that this development [of St. John Ambulance in Canada] was the outcome of the devoted service of St. John members, from coast to coast but they, in turn would affirm that his leadership played a vital role in making this fine record possible."[33] On 23 June 1961 a commemorative plaque was placed in the council chamber at St. John's Gate in London, honouring Gray's contributions to the Order in Canada and internationally. He was the first Canadian to be so honoured. We can only speculate that had he lived it seems likely that Gray would have been made a Bailiff Grand Cross, especially when one considers that he helped to create the largest priory of the Order outside England.

The 1960s saw a deepening of the relationship with the Department of National Defence, with 19,480 first aid certificates being issued to all three services in 1960 alone. The participation of the other special centres remained strong and in 1961 the Ottawa Civil Service Centre was inaugurated to help in the training of public servants. Under Molson's leadership St. John Ambulance made a presentation to the Royal Commission on Health Services "The Hall Commission" and outlined the role and contributions of St. John Ambulance. In May 1962 the first life-sized training doll arrived in at St. John headquarters. Named Resusci-Annie, the 15-kilogram doll was ideal for teaching mouth to mouth resuscitation. One doll was subsequently distributed to each provincial council, marking the beginning of a new type of first aid training in Canada.

Another prominent retirement occurred in 1963 when Superintendent-in-Chief Margaret MacLaren, who had served in the job for 18 years, stepped down. A veteran of the Second World War, it was largely MacLaren's organizational genius that facilitated the work of the VADs. She was the first Canadian woman to be made a Dame Grand Cross of the Order, being invested by Governor General Georges Vanier on 3 July 1963. After a five month illness the most familiar female face of St. John Ambulance died on 1 October. Within two months of her death the Margaret MacLaren Bursary Fund was established to provide student nurses with financial assistance. The Margaret MacLaren Memorial Library was also established in her honour. Opened by Mme. Vanier in October 1964 the library was relocated to St. John House when the headquarters moved in 1978.[34] MacLaren was immortalized in an oil painting depicting her in full uniform with decorations.

Although St. John Ambulance had grown from a branch to commandery, to priory, the act governing the organization dated from 1914 and had never been updated. This caused a number of inane legal difficulties that had the potential to become increasingly serious as the organization grew. In 1951 a proposal was made to St. John's Gate in London to alter the act, but this was found to be unacceptable in view of the proposed governance structure. By 1963 the matter had been left to the skilled legal mind of Brigadier General G.E. "Ted" Beament. A veteran of the Second World War, Beament was a highly respected lawyer who devoted much of his life to St. John Ambulance. It was his legal skills that helped create the new bill, *An Act Respecting the General Council of the Canadian Branch of the St. John Ambulance Association*, Bill S-5. Up to this point a number of legal anomalies caused the existence of both a General Council of the association and the Priory Council, even though the two bodies carried out similar duties and had shared senior memberships. The legislation sought to allow the corporation (St. John Ambulance) to act as a trustee for the priory. With this change the

General Council of the Canadian branch of the St. John Ambulance Association became St. John Priory of Canada Properties, which acts as a holding trust for the priory, under the direction of the priory.[35]

Senator John Kinley, a long-time member of the Order introduced the bill on 26 February, "This bill has great importance because of change and growth and because of the success and progress of the order of St. John."[36] The bill sailed through the usual readings, and after being scrutinized by the Standing Committee on Banking and Commerce was read for a third time on 12 March 1964, with Royal Assent being granted on 21 May.[37] Beament was subsequently appointed vice chancellor of the Order, the first to hold the post. He would go on to serve as chancellor from 1975 to 1978, and was appointed a Bailiff Grand Cross in 1995. He remains one of the few persons appointed to the Order of Canada in recognition of his service to St. John Ambulance.[38]

As the country approached the centennial of Confederation opportunities for St. John Ambulance to render training and volunteer services were boundless. During Save-a-Life week in 1966, the one millionth Canadian to participate in the save-a-life program was presented with his certificate. Prime Minister Lester B. Pearson presented John R. Matheson, who happened to be registrar of the Order, with his certificate at a special ceremony on 18 May.[39] It was also in May 1966 that "Heart-Lung Resuscitation" was approved by St. John Ambulance. With this training, materials and manuals were updated and new training courses were developed in the ever changing field of first aid training.

In January 1965, following three months of negotiations, an agreement was signed at Government House between the Boy Scouts Association, St. John Ambulance, the Red Cross, and the Royal Life Saving Society of Canada. St. John was given responsibility for training 300,000 boy scouts in first aid, while the Red Cross and Royal Life Saving Society were to teach swimming and water safety.[40] The following year a similar agreement was made with the Girl Guides and by 1967 the Navy League had entered into a first aid training agreement with St. John Ambulance. A significant amount of effort was put into revitalizing the declining home nursing program and in 1965 the first entirely Canadian home nursing manual was released. Officials at the federal and provincial levels hoped that *Patient Care in the Home; A Textbook of Home Nursing*,[41] would serve to increase the number of home nursing courses taken, history would prove this effort futile in the wake of sweeping social and health programs that were introduced to Canadians in the 1960s. One way of explaining the decline in this program was that citizens became lazy and less concerned with prevention of health problems because treatment was no longer a financial burden.

During the major centennial celebrations on Parliament Hill and at EXPO 67 in Montreal the brigade was active providing first aid services at every event. Over the six months in which EXPO was open the brigade treated 39,000 visitors, with over 40,000 volunteer hours given. St. John Ambulance was honoured on 1 September 1967 when Governor General Roland Michener proclaimed it St. John Ambulance Day at EXPO. Michener ably summarized the ethos of St. John Ambulance:

The name of St. John is synonymous with a high standard of First Aid and with the virtues of charity. It has transcended nationality, race colour and religion. It is our greatest wish that St. John Shall remain in all the countries of the Commonwealth as symbol of its motto — for the service of mankind — and as a practical example of doing things for other people and doing them for nothing.[42]

The preparations to involve the brigade in EXPO 67 dated back to 1965, and it remains the largest and longest public event that St. John Ambulance has ever participated in. The three millionth St. John Ambulance first aid certificate was awarded as part of the EXPO celebrations, being presented to St. John cadet Wayne Dorion of Lachine, Quebec.

It was not only EXPO 67 that consumed the energies of St. John Ambulance. The Royal Tour of 1967 involved volunteers from across the country, and at the Pan American Games in Winnipeg St. John Ambulance set up twenty-five first aid and two mobile first aid posts. This latter contribution was undertaken entirely by Manitoba's provincial council without external support. In Canada's centennial year Priory Historian G.W.L. Nicholson completed the first comprehensive history of St. John Ambulance in Canada. The first copies of *The White Cross in Canada* were presented to Governor General Michener.

The 1950s and 60s was a period of great expansion for St. John Ambulance in Canada. This growth was felt at both the national and individual provincial level. As the provincial councils became more established and successful many began the construction of new headquarters. The first to undertake such a project was Alberta, which opened its new provincial headquarters in 1955. This was the first time in the history of St. John Ambulance in Canada that a building was purpose-built for the needs of the organization. New buildings would subsequently be erected in Vancouver, Victoria, Winnipeg, Toronto, and Montreal. First aid training had also been brought to Canada's north, with more than 1,500 certificates issued in 1965. This was a significant achievement, one that would not have come about without cooperation from the RCMP.[43]

It is remarkable to consider that by 1967 St. John Ambulance in Canada was being funded primarily through public donations. Following the end of the war the organization would engage in a national annual fundraising campaign. The campaign in 1946 was not terribly successful, which was understandable given that throughout the war years the Red Cross had been the umbrella fundraiser for St. John Ambulance. In 1947 the national fundraising campaign grossed $645,415.04, which was an immense sum.[44] There was a high degree of cooperation between national headquarters and the provincial councils throughout these campaigns, with a significant portion of the funds going directly to the provinces. In 1954 St. John Ambulance began participating in the Community Chest fundraising campaign as well.[45] Every year the Community Chest would provide St. John Ambulance with a significant grant. By 1967, 45 percent of an annual budget of $1.27 million dollars, came from the Community Chest. This was the single largest source of revenue for St. John Ambulance followed distantly by first aid training fees at 20 percent and the annual grant from the federal government at 8 percent. This funding system allowed St. John Ambulance to focus on the provision of first aid training and brigade members for public events, rather than expending significant resources on fundraising activities. It also allowed for significant expansion of the work done by the organization throughout the post-war period leading up to Canada's Centennial. Sadly it was not an arrangement that would survive the 1970s.

Newfoundland

During the Second World War the association and brigade again became active in Newfoundland. Although there is scant record of how many first aid courses were taken over this period a single reference to Newfoundland in the 1946 annual report of the Brigade Overseas confirms that training did take place throughout the war. Members of the brigade and association who had served during the war were made eligible for the war services certificate that was issued by the Priory of Canada. The year preceding the Dominion's entry into Confederation saw seventy-two first aid certificates issued. The Newfoundland Provincial Council was created in April 1950,[46] thus transforming the branch that had been established in 1910 into an integral part of the Priory of Canada. By 1960 the size of the brigade in Newfoundland had increased from the two divisions that predated Confederation, to thirteen divisions. The number of islanders taking first aid training ballooned to 3,400 in 1967, surpassing the number trained over the course of the entire first three decades of the association's establishment in Newfoundland. In honour of his contribution to St. John Ambulance and Newfoundland, Dr. Macperson, who had founded the brigade in the province, was made a Knight of Justice. At a ceremony held at Government House in St. John's, Lieutenant-Governor Sir Leonard Outerbridge, himself a long-time supporter of St. John Ambulance, invested Macpherson as a Knight of Justice.

NINE

THE FIRST CENTURY COMPLETE

From National Centennial to the Order's Canadian Centennial

We must continually review our programmes to ensure
we are keeping up to date in meeting modern needs.
Chancellor Beament, 1976

The 1970s would see a transformation in the programs offered by both the association and the brigade. Indeed, 1974 brought about the amalgamation of the association and brigade into St. John Ambulance. The introduction of a wide variety of health and social services had a profound effect on the perceived need for programs such as home nursing. As Canadians became comforted by the presence of a comprehensive publicly funded health care system St. John Ambulance had to re-tailor its home nursing and non-first aid training programs to better meet the needs of the general public. The 1970s would also see the introduction of audio-visual materials to assist in teaching first aid. St. John embraced the new technology as it revamped its entire compliment of first aid training. Early in 1961 Chancellor Molson expressed great concern that "new blood was not being infused into the Ambulance and Nursing Divisions fast enough to replace older volunteers. Recruitment of younger men and women is desirable."[1] Future chancellors and senior officials took this matter seriously and through the late 1960s and 70s ensured that as older members retired from active participation in St. John Ambulance they were replaced by younger, more active volunteers. This transition sustained the progress made in the early post-war period and demonstrated that St. John Ambulance was able to adapt. It was, however, not seamless or without difficulties. There remained the solid support of the special centres and a great boom in first aid training was initiated as a result of federal workplace legislation. As the federal government increased its requirement for first aid training, it effectively ceased investing any energy in the Civil Defence/Emergency Measures Organization that had been so key to the growth of St. John Ambulance in the immediate post-war period. This period would see an end to the highly successful agreement between St. John Ambulance and the Canadian Red Cross, followed by the aggressive entry of the latter into the field of first aid training as the former approached its centennial year.

St. John Ambulance continued to grow and evolve in the euphoria of Centennial Year. All first aid courses and teaching materials were reviewed and updated in 1968. Throughout the late 1960s and into the 1970s there was a decline in the home nursing program. Initially the brigade was slow to react to changes related to gender roles and the massive transformation being experienced in the field of health care. In some areas such as Nova Scotia this had a particularly negative affect on the nursing divisions of the brigade and their membership.[2] Through the revitalization of all St. John first aid and home nursing courses[3] the decline in home nursing was reversed by 1978. In 1968, numbers for St. John Ambulance first aid training dipped only slightly from the high of 1967, and were about to skyrocket as the federal government imposed a variety of new safety regulations. St. John Ambulance and its instructors were very nearly overtaxed, but this did not elicit any complaints.

During one of the first OXFAM marches held in Canada, St. John Ambulance operated seventeen first aid posts and treated 5,000 marchers along their sixty kilometre route in Ontario. Shortly after Dominion Day 1968, the federal government released Treasury Board Circular 1968/48.[4] This outlined that all buildings used by the federal public service had to not only to possess first aid kits, but that during normal office hours there had to be present at least one trained first aid attendant.[5] This would be the first in a series of new regulations intended to make the workplace a safer environment. It had the effect of increasing the number of first aid certificates awarded to the point where records were broken annually from 1969 to 1983. With strong support from the federal government, the special centres, and St. John's other traditional supporters, the organization was in an ideal position to conquer the 1970s. Through the prudent leadership of Chancellor Nicholson and his successors in the position, Roch, Beament, Laurin, and Dubuc, St. John Ambulance excelled in providing first aid to an ever greater number of Canadians in all areas of the country. The grand designs of these leaders would have come to naught without the dedication and devotion of a growing pool of St. John Ambulance volunteers who involved themselves in the work.

Canada's Workers' Compensation Boards had historically been strong supporters of St. John Ambulance first aid training. Indeed, for some workers in British Columbia such training was made mandatory by the board. In 1969 the WCB endorsed St. John Ambulance as their single national first aid training agency, much as the Department of National Defence and RCMP had been doing since 1922. This year also saw the opening of a new St. John headquarters in Montreal. The prior of the Order, Roland Michener, presided over the ceremony unveiling the beautiful and modernist building, which had been funded through an anonymous donation of $600,000.

As snowmobiling became more popular throughout Canada in the early 1970s, St. John Ambulance began to work closely with the provincial government in Quebec and with the Ontario Federation of Snowmobile Clubs and the Ontario Motor League to develop a snowmobile first aid kit. Elements of the standard first aid courses were also slightly augmented to address the particular first aid needs of these early snowmobilers.

The first issue of *St. John Today* issued in 1970 boldly announced "ST. JOHN READY FOR THE SEVENTIES."[6] This spoke to the confidence felt by St. John Ambulance members. Their commitment to first aid would be proven in a rather curious way — through a study undertaken by Ontario's Workers' Compensation Board. The First Aid Community Training for Safety (FACTS) study was undertaken in Orillia, Ontario. The study was a "world first safety research project to measure the effect of extensive First Aid training on the accident rate."[7] Other organizations such as Bell Telephone had discovered in the 1930s that the higher the rate of first aid training among their workers the lower the incidence of minor and serious accidents. The WCB in cooperation with the association began a two-year blitz to saturate the community with first aid training. Throughout the study it was often joked that Orillia was going to become the safest place in the world to work and live. The claim was not far off the mark and when the study was released in 1972 it found that "First Aid trained employees experience significantly reduced accident rates, by as much as 30–40%."[8] The findings would even make its way to the United Nations.

The skills and fortitude of St. John Ambulance were put to the test on 5 July 1970 when Air Canada Flight 621 crashed at Toronto's International Airport. The DC-8 lost an engine and burst into flames on the runway killing all 109 passengers and crew. Within twenty minutes St. John Ambulance volunteers were on the scene to assist with the recovery effort. Over a twenty-two day period, ninety-two members performed 2,000 hours of work, assisting in classifying and transporting the remains of victims away from the crash scene.

Chancellor Nicholson pushed forward with a new national plan for St. John Ambulance and this would become the template for the great rate of growth that was experienced by the end of the decade. Following the centennial there had been a steady decline in brigade membership as an older generation of volunteers retired from service. Had a comprehensive plan to deal with attrition been in place this would not have been a serious problem, however no contingencies were made as the pace of membership had grown through the 1960s. In consultation with the provincial councils, and even through a youth essay writing contest, an action plan was put in place to reverse the declining numbers. In many ways the association had the opposite problem, a growing membership and number of instructors by a ballooning demand for first aid courses. Bell Telephone revamped its first aid training system along the lines of that used by its sister corporation, American Telephone and Telegraph. The innovation was to allow Bell employees to take first aid courses during company time.[9] There had long been a near 100 percent participation rate by Bell's outdoor employees, but this new "study at work" program brought St. John first aid training to a whole new segment of their workforce. In New Brunswick other fields were entered as well. Cadets were introduced to a new and specialized form of care, when they were trained and then placed in charge of babysitting children with cystic fibrosis. The relationship would continue for many years, the project having been successful.[10]

Training of Air Canada employees began as part of Canadian National's Special Centre, before the two transportation gains were partitioned. The forerunner of Air Canada, Trans-Canada Airlines, had long had a relationship with St. John Ambulance, but this was on a less formal basis. Flight and ground crew would all be trained by members of the association in a specially tailored standard first aid course. Another great advance was the introduction of a new Canadian Labour (Safety) Code in 1971. The new "Federal Regulations Respecting First Aid" required that wherever groups of up to five employees are working in an isolated area that at least one must have knowledge of life saving techniques, and in groups of fourteen or less at least one employee must have a valid emergency first aid certificate.[11] This had the effect of increasing the number of first aid certificates issued between 1971 and 1972 by more than 21,000 a 15 percent increase in first aid certificates. Such increases became the norm throughout the decade and into the 1980s; never had there been such a persistent demand for St. John Ambulance first aid training.

The Queen honoured the Order by appointing Chancellor Leonard Nicholson a Bailiff Grand Cross of the Order in 1971. He was subsequently invested by the sovereign head of the Order at Buckingham Palace. Like the two previously appointed Canadian Grand Crosses, Nicholson had devoted much of his adult life to the work of St. John Ambulance and participating in the organization at the senior most level with great passion and devotion. In response to his appointment Nicholson modestly replied, "I feel that my elevation to this highest grade in our Order was not a personal honour alone, but an honour earned for Canada and to be shared with all St. John People."[12] Nicholson remains one of the most highly decorated chancellors in Canadian history.

The 1970s saw an expansion of St. John Ambulance in Canada's north. In March 1972 a territorial council (equivalent to a provincial council) was created in the Northwest Territories. Even the St. John Standard First Aid Manual was translated into Inuktitut.[13] Dr. Ali Uygur, territorial surgeon, spent more than a year working on the project that would bring first aid training to a whole new group of Canadians. Training in this hitherto neglected area would grow significantly as a result of the efforts of the Territorial Council.

St. John Ambulance would receive a grant of $300,000 from the federal government in 1972 as part of the expanding field of first aid training for public servants. This was part of the association's "Federal Intensive Project," which sought to take advantage of the new federal requirements for first aid. There remained, however, difficulties in the attrition rate being experienced by the brigade, which had shrunk by 700 members or 6 percent. While this may not sound like a significant figure, senior brigade officials knew that demographics were not on their side, and without a concentrated effort to increase the brigade's membership it would be in serious trouble by the dawn of the 1980s. Chancellor Nicholson opened 1973 with his call for "good communication between all levels to lubricate our relationship and reduce causes of frictions."[14] This had a dual meaning. In part it was directed to members of the association and brigade, who he wanted to see working in harmony, despite the boom for the association and difficulties for the brigade. The message was also a call to take advantage of every opportunity given to St. John Ambulance in this period of great first aid training expansion. He was disappointed with the lack of brigade membership growth, which inspired a new strategy for building up the brigade. Plans were adopted to design new uniforms for female members of the brigade and to engage in more outreach activities to gain new membership. Small changes, like the more functional and modern uniforms that moved the organization out of the 1930s, had a significant effect in attracting more women to the brigade. In 1972 newly appointed Chancellor Redmond Roche, a former chief commissioner of the brigade would expend great efforts to reverse the decline in brigade membership. The home nursing program would also be completely revamped and a new combined first aid and home nursing training program was developed by Dr. L.J. Calvert.

Canada's smallest province celebrated the centennial of its entry into Confederation in 1973, and with this came the establishment of the Prince Edward Island Provincial Council. Although the association had been sporadically active on the island since the 1930s, a consistent organization failed to take root. In founding the council there was the additional problem of negotiating with the Red Cross, which had been the island's major supplier of first aid training since the end of the Second World War.

The first large-scale project undertaken with the Red Cross since the end of the Second World War was inaugurated in late 1973. With the growth of multimedia training techniques both the Red Cross and St. John Ambulance saw an opportunity to bring basic first aid skills to a broad audience.[15] Both organizations were being forward thinking in their desire to integrate these new learning techniques with traditional methods, "such an approach to training would be feasible and serve a most useful purpose."[16] Given the immense cost of writing, producing, editing, and distributing such programs in the era before video recording, an application was submitted to the federal Department of Health to underwrite some of the start-up costs. Once completed the program became know as the "There's No Place Like Home for Health Care." St. John Ambulance had also developed a smaller scale multimedia training course called SOFA, Safety Oriented First Aid. Both programs were milestones in the history of first aid training in Canada.[17]

In Quebec, the province's Civil Protection Authority encouraged the establishment of more brigade units, and gave them increasing responsibility over ambulatory services on the provinces highways.[18] This program had been initiated in 1966 with three ambulances and would grow to twelve by 1973. The ski patrol brigade units remained popular and widely supported throughout the province.[19] Although St. John Ambulance in Quebec had been successful in working with the provincial government on a number of projects it began to experience difficulty in 1973, partly as a result of a decision taken in 1970 that saw the association and brigade divided into separate administrative bodies. This was highly inefficient and caused friction between members of the organizations. "Quebec council has been challenged by unsatisfactory financial results on its current operations"[20] The approaching 1976 Olympics in Montreal would help to overcome many of these difficulties and see the council recover and expand in the province that had the largest brigade membership.

The appointment of a new grand prior came in 1974 following the death of Prince Henry Duke of Gloucester. He had served as grand prior of the Order since 1939, having succeeded Canada's former governor general, Prince Arthur Duke of Connaught. Prince Richard Duke of Gloucester was born in 1944 and would go on to study at Cambridge where he earned his degree in architecture in 1969. Following the death of his brother HRH Prince William in an air crash, Richard became commandant-in-chief of the Ambulance Corps of the brigade. He acceded to the dukedom in June of 1974 and was appointed grand prior shortly thereafter. It was also at this time that the association and brigade were united into one foundation called St. John Ambulance. This reflected the reality that both the organizations had been functioning in Canada as one since the creation of the Priory of Canada in 1946.

In an effort to improve the popularity of the home nursing program the curriculum underwent a major change, bringing it up to date with not only the practices of the 1970s but also current Canadian health policy. The program was renamed "Patient Care" and grew to include a more significant section on child care. The health care field beckoned as the publicly funded health care system began to experience growing pains. Chancellor Beament noted, "The restraints now arising in government spending on the delivery of health care make more than ever more evident, the need for a vastly increased amount of training in patient care in the home."[21] It was a field that St. John Ambulance knew well and was eager to capitalize upon the expected demand. Although it had the potential to become the single largest training program, it would never reach its full potential, despite an immense amount of effort, innovation, and expertise invested by St. John Ambulance. The introduction of publicly funded universal health care meant the younger generation of Canadians no longer felt it necessary to learn much more about health than they were taught in school. In case of illness the immediate reaction was increasingly to go to the doctor, the visit was after all "free." For the previous generation a visit to the doctor was an expense that was to be avoided, save the most serious situation. Of course without proper training a patient risked becoming gravely ill, but that is why the St. John Ambulance home nursing and later patient care courses were so valuable. It would be one of Beament's great disappointments that more could not be done to vastly increase the success of the program.

The Order saw the implementation of the new Royal Charter in 1975.[22] The Priory rules and regulations were greatly streamlined and updated. One setback that occurred in 1975 came when the provincial government in British Columbia authorized community colleges to begin teaching first aid. Initially this had a negative affect on the training activities of the association but it was short lived. A new publicity campaign was undertaken throughout 1975 with four thirty-second televisions ads being run on all the major Canadian networks in both official languages. They featured real life situations where St. John first aiders were able to save a life or assist the injured. This was part of the broader St. John National Awareness program that included not only television ads, but radio spots, articles and adverts in newspapers and magazines, the holding of a public relations conference for St. John volunteers, and the production of the first ever public relations manual. The program was a great success in getting St. John Ambulance into the public's mind. Midway through his term as chancellor, Beament offered some timeless direction "we must continually review our programmes to ensure we are keeping up to date in meeting modern needs."[23]

The twenty-first Olympics came to Canada in 1976 being held in Montreal, with some events taking place in Kingston. More than 350 brigade members from all across Quebec and seventy-five from Ontario participated in the two week event. Before the opening of the games St. John Ambulance first aid training was given to 6,000 members of the Olympic Organizing Committee or COJO. It was a banner year on another front as well. Funding for the joint St. John-Red Cross project that had been turned down in June of 1975, was granted following a subsequent submission in 1976. The federal government pledged $1 million towards the development of "There's No Place Like Home for Health Care" program. The grant called for the program to be released in 1979. St. John Ambulance had found a friend in federal Health Minister Marc Lalonde who was excited about the project. "As a private citizen I have had many opportunities to be in touch with the excellent work carried on by your Order especially as the father of four children and a wife who loves skiing."[24]

While the two organizations where in the middle of working on the program, senior officials at the Red Cross indicated that they were interested in getting into the field of first aid. This ambition had been regulated by the 1951 agreement creating the St. John Ambulance–Canadian Red Cross Joint Operation Committee, and the Red Cross wanted to amend the text. Throughout 1976 discussions were held between the two parties but no agreement was reached. As if predicting a negative outcome the 1976 annual report noted "it is to be hoped that 1977 will see the matter brought to a conclusion satisfactory to both organizations."[25] On two occasions previously the Red Cross had withdrawn from agreements with St. John Ambulance and it seemed likely that history would repeat itself.

Two special Canadian appointments were made in 1976. Kathleen Gilmour, the indefatigable veteran of the Second World War and former superintendent-in-chief was appointed Canada's second Dame Grand Cross of the Order, in recognition of her lifetime of service. It was a fitting mark of recognition, one that was celebrated by all members of the Priory of Canada. The other appointment saw Dr. (later Sir) Conrad Swan, a Canadian who was serving as a herald at the College of Heralds in London, was appointed genealogist of the Order at St. John's Gate.

Over the course of 1977 a series of five meetings were held between St. John Ambulance and the Red Cross. This was done under the neutral chairmanship of Rocke Robertson, a highly respected medical doctor and former chancellor of McGill University. The meetings were held in an effort to "renegotiate and amend as appropriate the 1951 Agreement to provide for the reasonable aspirations of each organizations in a manner consistent with the public interest."[26] On 2 August 1977, without warning, the Red Cross gave its necessary notice terminating the agreement six months hence, thereby dissolving the Joint Committee and accompanying agreement in February 1978. Despite the efforts of Robertson to get the Red Cross back to the table he was met with no success through 1978 and 1979. In a bizarre twist, St. John Ambulance and the Red Cross continued to cooperate on the "There's No Place Like Home for Health Care" program. For either party to have withdrawn from the partnership in this project would have resulted in an immediate cessation of funding from the federal government.

As part of the effort to keep St. John Ambulance in the public mind a new strategy for future growth was mapped out with four areas of focus: growth, quality, financial independence, and improved image. The earlier attempts to improve brigade membership had been successful and by the end of 1978 the membership was up to a new record of 12,261. Billboards emblazoned with the white cross and "ISN'T IT ABOUT TIME YOU TOOK A FIRST AID COURSE, St. John Ambulance," went up in 200 communities across the country. New partners were also being sought out. One was the University of Regina, which implemented a comprehensive first aid training program with St. John Ambulance. In Quebec the first ever braille standard first aid text book was published in French. This year would also witness the presentation of the five millionth first aid certificate, and with the number of certificates issued per year on the rise it would be only another three-and-a-half years until the six millionth first aid certificate would be presented.

During a royal visit in 1978, the Queen opened a new St. John Ambulance Building in Deer Lake Newfoundland. Her Majesty then proceeded to Edmonton where she opened the 11th Commonwealth Games. Not surprisingly upon arrival in Alberta, she was again greeted by members of the brigade, 250 of whom provided first aid services throughout the event. As St. John Ambulance grew into a larger organization, both at the national and provincial levels, there was an urgent need for a new national headquarters. Most provincial councils had either built or purchased new buildings by the mid 1970s, yet the national headquarters remained in its wartime home at 321 Chapel Street in Ottawa.[27] A new, significantly larger building was acquired at 311 Laurier Avenue. The structure had previously served as a barracks form the Canadian Women's Army Corps and Canadian Provost Corps. It also briefly served as the opulent Richelieu Club from 1922–1928 before being occupied by the Grey Sisters for 14 years. The original structure was built by George Goodwin and dated from 1884; understandably the noble old edifice required a significant amount of work before it was suitable to carry the designation St. John House. The newly appointed prior, Edward Schreyer, opened St. John House on 26 January 1978.

As the end of the decade approached the new chief commissioner of the brigade, Yvette Loiselle began planning for the future. The first woman chief commissioner of a brigade anywhere in the Commonwealth, Loiselle had been an active member since 1944. Her goal was to encourage the brigade to grow until there was one brigade member for every 1,250 citizens, a target of 19,200 at the time. This would mean increasing the size of the brigade by over 6,000 members. Although this goal would not be reached during her time as chief commissioner, the brigade continued to expand. The gender differentiation that had been part of the brigade since its founding would largely be discarded by 1979, and the gradual removal of gender specific tasks — which was well under way — would be greatly accelerated.

The most dramatic service rendered by St. John Ambulance in the 1970s came at midnight on 10 November 1978 when a Canadian Pacific freight train derailed in Mississauga, Ontario. The train was laden with explosives and poisonous chemicals, most notably toluene and chlorine gas. The derailment of the 106 car train resulted in the explosion that sent a fireball 1,500 metres into the air. Once the civil authorities learned of the train's cargo they decided to immediately evacuate the city. A total of 250,000 residents had to leave, making it the largest single evacuation in North American history[28] until 2005. St. John Ambulance volunteers were on the scene and assisted the police and fire officials with the evacuation, especially the work involved in moving people out of hospitals and nursing homes. A total of 470 St. John Ambulance volunteers participated in the evacuation. So successful was the operation that it would become the mass evacuation model studied by municipalities around the world. Scarcely three months later members of St. John Ambulance volunteers again found themselves assisting with disaster when a coal mine in Glace Bay, Nova Scotia collapsed. On 24 February 1979 No. 26 colliery suffered a cave-in that took the lives of twelve miners. St. John Ambulance volunteers were on the scene to assist with the recovery effort. It was a sad but fitting way to begin the year which marked the 70th anniversary of the brigade's founding in Canada. Celebrations were held in London, Ontario to mark the event, even William Loveday, then 89 years of age was present to participate.

Leading up to the centennial year preparations to implement the "There's No Place Like Home for Health Care" program escalated. The project consisted of thirteen films about first aid instruction and home health care. Produced in both English and French, the content was developed by St. John Ambulance's chief nurse consultant Margaret Hunter and Janet Chatterson of the Red Cross. The program would be tested in Ontario and Prince Edward Island before its formal release. It was "designed to teach home healthcare skills to the general public," and to teach them how to look after those who were sick or convalescing at home.[29] The government "hoped this can lead to a decrease in the use of acute care institutions, plus a reduction in total health care spending."[30]

By December 1979 the research stage had concluded after a period of trial testing and the program was released in mid 1980. Developed to be a modern equivalent to the home nursing program, "There's No Place Like Home for Health Care" was popular and successful. Once again St. John Ambulance and the Red Cross had demonstrated that they could cooperate on a major project that was national in scope. Despite the success, the Red Cross would withdraw from the program in 1983.

With the first native language first aid training manual having been developed and the growth of first aid in Canada's Arctic St. John Ambulance volunteers began taking a greater interest in the affairs of Canada's northernmost reaches. Special survival cairns, containing first aid supplies had been placed throughout Canada's north in the 1970s as a precautionary measure to aid those in distress. In 1980 the Yukon branch of the Alberta Council helped to provide 40 volunteers for the VI Arctic winter games.

Throughout the early 1980s the demand for first aid training remained unabated. Coupled with this, St. John Ambulance continued to stimulate the promotion of health care.[31] This was most specifically done through a joint health care program that was being developed with the Red Cross. It was also in this period that the marketing department of St. John Ambulance was created. Its goal was to publicize the work of St. John Ambulance and to better market first aid products and training. In a way it is amazing that the organization had functioned for so long, and so successfully, without a department dedicated solely to the promotion of the good works undertaken. In the area of promotion a thirty-second television ad was filmed featuring comedians Luba Goy and Dave Broadfoot, from the television show, *Royal Canadian Air Farce*. They extolled the virtues of first aid in a humorous manner. The advertisements were run on all the major Canadian networks. In January 1982 a new Standard First Aid Oriented text book was released to update the first aid training program.

In 1982, a year after her retirement as commissioner-in-chief of the brigade, Loiselle was made a Dame Grand Cross of the Order. That was also that the year the cadets celebrated their sixtieth anniversary in Canada. As well, new "Lifesaver" and "Home Health Care" brochures were released in the spring. These were distributed to pharmacies and other outlets related to health care. As part of the 12th Commonwealth Games in 1982, twenty members of the brigade from Alberta travelled to Brisbane to work with members of the Australian brigade during the event, proving the work of St. John Ambulance was not limited to Canada alone.

As part of the ongoing commitment to developing a new health care courses a generous grant of $1.5 million was given to St. John Ambulance by the J.W. McConnell foundation in 1982. The funding went towards the development of a healthcare for seniors program and "to provide Canadian seniors with the information and skills necessary to continue living health and productive lives."[32] It was under the direction of a future chancellor and lord prior of the Order, Eric Barry, that this unprecedented grant was obtained. A national project team as well as provincial coordinators from each council worked to put the program together.

Working alongside the Canadian Heart Foundation, St. John Ambulance also continued to perfect its CPR courses, which had been inaugurated in 1979. The First Aid Updates Video Cassette Program was completed in 1983 with the release of twelve training videos touching upon pertinent first aid situations.

Centennial

Although he desperately wanted to live to participate in the St. John Ambulance Centennial Celebrations, William Loveday, the last surviving charter member of the brigade died in January 1981 at ninety-three years of age. Having devoted seventy-four years of his life to the work of St. John Ambulance his dedication remains a potent reminder of the influence one volunteer can have on an organization like St. John Ambulance.

Many plans across the country were made for the centennial of St. John Ambulance in Canada. Tracing its founding to the inaugural first aid class held in Quebec City in 1883, the slogan "First With First Aid to Canadians for 100 Years," was adopted. Indeed it was true, for 100 years St. John Ambulance had been the main, and in many cases sole, provider of first aid training. The celebrations included many banquets and publicity events in every province right down to the unit level. In speaking about the success of the Centennial year, Chancellor Dubuc remarked:

Special it was indeed, for our Centennial Year marked a long period of progress and achievement for St. John in Canada, and provided us with the confidence that our second century will bring even greater opportunity for service to our fellow Canadians.[33]

One of the most popular elements of the celebrations was the presence of a knight on horseback — bearing the white eight-pointed cross on his chest.[34] It was not all parties and revelling, the association went national with the innovative program, "What Every Babysitter Should Know," which was pioneered by members of the association in Toronto. The most important centennial souvenir was of course, the new first aid manual titled *First Aid Safety Oriented*. The quality of St. John Ambulance's audio visual training tools had been recognized the world over, with the Priories of New Zealand and Australia making use of the Safety Oriented First Aid Course materials.

The fifth triennial conference of the Brigade Overseas was held in Toronto, with delegates focusing on the "relevance of the present work of St. John to the 1980s."[35] By the beginning of the centennial year, the brigade in Canada had grown to nearly 15,000 members with 608 divisions treating 200,000 cases annually. This included the crusader and cadet divisions, which helped to bring the value of first aid to the younger generation. One special visitor was the matron of the St. John Ophthalmic (Eye) Hospital, Ruth Parks, who also paid a visit to Toronto to help celebrate the Centennial.

Included in the events marking the Centennial was the release of a commemorative stamp in honour of St. John Ambulance by Canada Post and the striking of a Centennial medallion by the Royal Canadian Mint, for sale to the public. To mark the Centennial, Colonel Strome Galloway, a long time member of the association, updated G.W.L. Nichoson's *The White Cross in Canada*. The book was published in both official languages and was a great success.

One of the highlights of the year was the investiture held by the grand prior at St. Bartholomew's Church in Ottawa. There on 5 June, HRH Prince Richard Duke of Gloucester invested Loiselle as a Dame Grand Cross of the Order. It was the first time that such an investiture was held by a grand prior in Canada. It was well deserved recognition for a lady who had done so much to modernize the brigade in Canada and, perhaps more important, served as a role model for other women first aiders. Loiselle embodied many firsts for St. John Ambulance and her achievement was celebrated. Following the investiture a parade was held on the grounds of Rideau Hall where the prior, Edward Schreyer and the grand prior conferred.

Ophthalmic/Eye Hospital

Priory support for the St. John's Ophthalmic Hospital[36] in Jerusalem had been steady in the post-war period, with financial support emanating from national headquarters through the hospitaller, in addition to donations made by many provincial councils. In 1970 alone, as part of the Miles for Millions fundraising drive, a total of $34,360 was raised, exceeding the target of $30,000.[37] Interest in the work of the hospital was significant and only needed stimulation to yield results.

Support also came from the Linen Guild, which was established in Canada in 1937. A group of eminent women who were involved in the Order, the guild initially raised funds for linen and bedclothes, but would later go on to more involved projects as we will see in the following chapter. Hospitaller, Dr. Brian Liddy headed the project to send a Canadian ophthalmologist to work at the hospital for twelve month period. The Priory had never before sent a medical doctor to work at the hospital, although a Canadian had previously spent three years there. Dr. W.F. Thompson of Moncton New Brunswick served as registrar of the hospital from 1924 to 1927, and returned in 1945 while working for the Anglo-Persian Oil Company. After retiring home to Canada after a life abroad, Thompson reflected "There was no lack of material to occupy the staff all day and even in the evenings and the theatres were kept busy all the time during the "dry" season."[38]

After conducting a nationwide search in which applications and letters of reference flowed in from across the country Dr. Lawrence Brierley was selected to serve at the hospital. Brierley, who was accompanied by his wife and family, would serve a full year at the hospital before returning to practice in Canada. Seven other Canadian doctors would be dispatched to serve at the hospital for a year at the expense of St. John Ambulance Canada.[39] It was an important step in elevating the Canadian contribution to this foundation of the Order of St. John by physically having a representative participate in the hospitaller work that finds its roots in the eleventh century and the Blessed Gerard.

It is tempting to look upon the period between 1968 and 1983 as the golden era of St. John Ambulance in Canada. First aid training ballooned from 99,453 to 355,293, and brigade membership grew from 8,726 to 14,884. Grants from the federal government and private foundations for specific projects reached unprecedented levels and fostered unique developments in the field of first aid and health promotion. Unquestionably it was a period of great growth and many successes. There were setbacks, most specifically the withdrawal of the Red Cross from the Joint Operation Committee and the failure of the home nursing or patient care program to meet its potential. External factors had a great deal to do with the successes, notably the wiliness of federal and provincial governments to mandate first aid training and the availability of large amounts of grant money for pilot projects. It was a confluence of strong dynamic leadership in a time of great opportunity that produced success for St. John Ambulance in this period. The 1980s and 1990s would see the number of first aid certificates issued annually approach the 800,000 mark. The significant government support, from both federal and provincial agencies had the unintended effect of making St. John Ambulance more reliant on government support than it had ever been. This likely affected the amount of effort put into soliciting new non-governmental partners. In the following decades Canada would experience economic stagnation and deep government cuts, developments that would have a profound effect on the fortunes of the St. John Ambulance into the new millennia.

TEN

THE ORDER OF ST. JOHN IN CANADA TODAY
1984–2007

I want to thank the volunteers for their
incredible dedication to serving their communities.
E.H. Rector, New Brunswick Council
9 May 1996

The period between 1984 and the 125th anniversary of the inaugural first aid courses being held in Canada saw St. John Ambulance's ethos of innovation continue. Through the Therapy Dog Program and service rendered during the Westray Mining Disaster, Ontario–Quebec Ice Storm and World Youth Day 2002, the work of St. John Ambulance has continued to be prominent in the public eye. Nevertheless the recent history of St. John Ambulance in Canada has been one of extremes. Over the course of this period at the national level, and in some provinces, there were great financial difficulties and parts of the organization faced insolvency. Not since the establishment of the Canadian branch of the St. John Ambulance Association had the Order come so close to a calamity of such proportion.

The historian has not been afforded the invaluable asset of hindsight in writing this chapter. A judicious and tempered assessment requires a distance of three or four decades from the actual events of any period, thus the intent of this chapter is to outline the major events in the history of St. John Ambulance through this period, substantial historiographical analysis will be left to future work. The records from this period are substandard at best, there being entire years when annual reports were not published. Even the content of annual reports became more focused on photos and less concerned with actual content beginning in the late 1990s. Some of the reports issued between 1998 and 2003 were full of the usual optimism and euphemistic language, which taken at face value gave an unrealistically rosy view of the state of affairs at a time when at the national level there was a financial crisis. We are still emerging from the difficulties of the late 1990s and this has hampered the expansion of the Order in Canada over the past decade. St. John Ambulance has not been the only organization faced with such difficulties. Other traditional allies such as the Victorian Order of Nurses faced near extinction and the Canadian Red Cross was forced to enter into bankruptcy protection in the same period. This period saw the backbone of St. John Ambulance remained strong with a stable pool of volunteers and a high annual rate of first aid training.

The 1990s was a period of financial restraint throughout Canada, with significant cuts to all government and social services at the provincial and federal levels. As Chancellor Johnston noted in 1997, "health related and social service charities have been particularly squeezed, as funding cuts to health care and social supports have left their clients more needy and vulnerable than ever."[1] The 1970s and early 1980s had witnessed a boom in first aid training through a series of provincial and federal programs that sought to spread first aid to their respective employees. Significant grants were garnered from the federal government and a private foundation to aid in program development, yet this form of funding would largely disappear by the 1990s. In the federal government's zeal to restore the finances of the nation they cut the historic annual grant to St. John Ambulance that had been in place since the First World War, and the investments held by St. John Ambulance yielded smaller returns, further hampering the ability of the organization to get its message out to the general public and modernize. Nevertheless, the number of Canadians trained by St. John Ambulance actually grew over the period 1984 to 2006, from 353,493 in 1984 to more than 600,000 in 2006.

Throughout the 1980s and 1990s the number of annual appointments to the Order increased at a rate that outpaced its ratio to membership growth; it would not be until 2003 that this situation was rectified. A significant change came in 1990 when the Order was formally incorporated into the Canadian honours system as a Canadian order. These issues of honours policy are thoroughly examined in Chapter Eleven.

The year following the St. John Ambulance centennial celebrations brought the Queen to Fredericton, New Brunswick on 25 September 1984. There the sovereign head reviewed members from all twenty-four divisions of the brigade in the province. At the national level new plans were put in place to expand first aid training for both the brigade and association. The innovative Ski Patrols, which were established in Quebec in 1928 and formed into Ski Patrol divisions in 1969, would celebrate their silver anniversary and the brigade in Canada would celebrate its seventy-fifth anniversary, with more than 14,000 members. Although there had been a slight decline in brigade membership over the previous year the number of brigade divisions had increased, which was viewed as a positive sign for future growth. Cooperation with the special centres — the Department of National Defence, RCMP, Via Rail, Canadian National Rail, Canadian Pacific, the federal government, Northern Telecom, Canada Post, Bell Canada, and Eaton's department stores — remained strong, making up 56 percent of the first aid courses taken by Canadians. New partnerships were built with such organizations as the Independent Druggist Association (IDA), which distributed 100,000 copies of St. John Ambulance's *Healthy Aging Handbooks* in 1985 alone. The following year a new audio video series was developed under the title *St. John Ambulance Presents*. Dating back to the earliest first aid silent film, St. John Ambulance has embraced the latest technology in an effort to bring first aid knowledge to the widest possible audience. Indeed, the St. John video on CPR would go on to win the "Apple Award" at the National Educational Film and Video Festival in Oakland, California.

In Western Canada, St. John Ambulance was particularly busy throughout 1987. The year opened with the fifteenth Winter Olympics in Calgary, and St. John Ambulance was present with eighty-two brigade volunteers who would treat more than 2,500 patients over the event's two week run. As the brigade celebrated the anniversary of its founding in 1887, 42 Canadians travelled to the United Kingdom to participate in the centennial celebrations. On 20 June 1987 40,000 brigade members from all over the world and 120,000 other St. John Ambulance supporters gathered in London to celebrate a century of service and achievement. The brigade's centennial year also included notable service rendered following the deadly Edmonton Tornado of 31 June 1987, which claimed the lives of twenty-seven people and injured more than 300. St. John Ambulance volunteers sprung into action with fifty members of the brigade, who worked alongside Edmonton's Emergency Medical Services, police and fire departments ministering to the injured and homeless.

Throughout the 1980s there was an increasing demand for cardiopulmonary resuscitation (CPR) training and St. John Ambulance was able to capitalize on this. A new CPR course was devised in 1987 "due to recent changes in the first aid protocols for rating choking victims and for performing artificial respiration and cardiopulmonary resuscitation."[2] These changes in training came at a significant cost, but they helped to keep St. John Ambulance first aid training the most up-to-date in Canada.

Although the brigade began to suffer a membership decline, dipping below 11,000 in 1989, the number of active hours grew by 17 percent.[3] New inroads were made when Queen's University inaugurated the first university campus brigade division in Canada. Chancellor McEachren noted "as we begin a new decade I am confident in our ability to meet the challenges presented by the changing demands of life in the 90s."[4] The 1980s were a period of the most significant changes in course development in the history of St. John Ambulance up to that point. The development of the highly popular CPR training booklet *Heart Start* brought first aid training to an increasing number of Canadians.

During the 1990s St. John Ambulance was further transformed. This was particularly evident with relation to the brigade, as part of a broader effort to stabilize and increase membership. A new brigade training system was implemented in 1993 to "ensure that the training received by each member is appropriate for the services provided."[5] One of the most controversial changes made was outlined in 1992, "as the Brigade moves ahead in the 90's, it will gradually shift in focus from its hierarchical structure to the function of the individual member as a community service volunteer."[6]

The brigade, which had been structured along the lines of a military organization since its inception, was being transformed. The focus was less on uniforms, ranks, and traditions and more on the potential it offered as a pool of able volunteers backed by the association. Membership in the brigade rose from 11,000 in 1994 to 12,000 in 1995. National Commissioner Harold Richardson noted that it was experiencing "increased and improved communication in all areas of the brigade across the country."[7] By 1996 the brigade had been renamed "Community Service Units," a title which bore little connection to the historic service of the St. John Ambulance Brigade. The Community Service Units are covered under the broader designation, "Volunteer and Community Services."

Today all St. John Ambulance volunteers, whether they provide community services along the lines of the old brigade, or first aid training like the old association, are considered to be part of St. John Ambulance. Nevertheless the old designation "brigade" persists in relation to St. John Ambulance's provision of volunteers for public events.

In response to shrinking health spending and reduction in health services St. John Ambulance launched a "Training For Life" program, which was a comprehensive health program for all ages. With the assistance of the prior of Canada Ramon Hnatyshyn, the successful program was launched in March 1993. Chancellor Eric Barry would set a goal of training one million Canadians in CPR by the end of 1995. Although this target would not be reached over the period 1990 to 1997 the number of Canadians taking St. John training had increased by more than 30 percent from 600,000 to 799,862.

St. John Ambulance was a pioneer in the creation of computer-based first aid instruction. Beginning in 1995 members of the RCMP and Ontario Provincial Police had the option of taking the Standard Level Computer-based Recertification program on a computer. This allowed officers to carry out the theory portion of their recertification on a computer at their detachment. A multimedia project was also started with the Canadian Coast Guard. Ten separate simulated emergency scenarios were developed. When completed the program was used by rescue specialists who determined the best course of treatment/action.

A period of self examination began in 1996 in an effort to identify gaps in health related services and seek out new partners. A plan to develop a standard first aid CD-ROM was created and partnerships were entered into with several manufacturers of inline skates. Well beyond Canadian shores and in one of the most volatile countries in the world, St. John Ambulance, working alongside the RCMP, helped to train Haitian police and firefighters in first aid. This project was undertaken with the support of the Canadian International Development Agency (CIDA). It is interesting to note that members of the Haitian Police continue to wear their St. John Ambulance first aid training qualification badges. An unintended by-product of this project was the training of a number of hospital nurses and medical staff.

In May 1996 the New Brunswick Provincial Council announced that it would close its ambulance service throughout the province in the coming September. As the longest running and most successful ambulatory care program in the history of St. John Ambulance in Canada this was a setback to the confidence of the organization. In all twenty-six emergency ambulance services and eight patient transfer services were discontinued. A drop in the number of volunteers and the introduction of new care standards by the provincial government made maintaining the service unfeasible. Under the new regulations the province required that two certified emergency medical technicians be present at each ambulance call, and the most that St. John Ambulance was able to guarantee was one. This was a trend that had ended St. John Ambulance ambulatory services in other provinces over the preceding decades.[8] With the end of this service the province redoubled its efforts in the field of first aid training. The vice president of the volunteer board, E.H. Rector, graciously acknowledged the service of so many St. John Ambulance volunteers, "I want to thank the volunteers for their incredible dedication to serving their communities. For decades, these individuals have given their time and energy to ensure their neighbours have a free ambulance … their contribution has always exceeded the call of duty."[9]

One of the great innovations pioneered by St. John Ambulance in the 1990s, which continues to be a success, was the creation of the Therapy Dog Divisions. Begun in February 1992 by James and Doreen Newell, from Peterborough, Ontario, the program started with eight dogs. Initially there were some barriers related to hygiene, liability insurance, dog behaviour, and, most important, acceptance by patients. St. John Ambulance developed a St. John Therapy Dog test to determine if a dog is of sound temperament. The dogs provide affection and comfort for the sick, bedridden, elderly, and lonely.

In 1993, Gentle Jenny, a therapy dog, became the first non-human to receive a service award certificate from St. John Ambulance.[10] Gentle Jenny spent over 450 hours as a therapy dog working with patients in nursing homes and hospitals.[11] The first therapy dog division was formed on 1 June 1994 as the Trent Hills Therapy Dog Division.[12] The program has become so successful that special awards have been developed for the dogs. A red tag is awarded for 75 visits, silver tag for 150 visits, and a gold tag is awarded for 250 visits. In 1995 therapy dog volunteers were recognized as members of the brigade and have thus become an important part of the St. John family. As of 2007 there are 2,200 therapy dogs and handlers, there being a strong demand in many communities for this most unique service.

Not unrelated to the development of therapy dog divisions was the creation of a St. John Ambulance *Pet First Aid Manual* and pet-related first aid kits. Endorsed by the Canadian Veterinary Medical Association and the Canadian Federation of Humane Societies, the manual was released in 2003 and provides valuable information on treating an injured pet.

In an effort to revitalize St. John Ambulance in the face of steeply declining revenues, a new vision was adopted for the organization at the national level. Without a steady revenue stream — which was garnered from investments, sale of first aid products, first aid training services, and donations — St. John Ambulance would be unable to continue its valuable work. Throughout the 1990s various cost-cutting measures had been implemented at the national level, including the reduction of the staff at the national office from sixty-nine to twenty-six. Between 1995 and 1997 St. John Ambulance's national revenue declined by 25 percent. Beginning in 1996 an implementation task force considered the options and in September 1997 all councils were informed of the plan to create a new arm of the organization. St. John Ambulance was divided into two parts, a charitable part under the name St. John Ambulance, and a business trust, which was titled St. John Enterprises (SJE).

Table 1

Roles and Responsibilities

St. John Ambulance (Charity)	St. John Enterprises (Business Trust)
Community Services	Training
Fundraising	Sales of Products
Public Relations	Operations
Order Matters	Net Income to Charity

The program began in October 1997, "in the face of declining revenues due to aggressive competitive activity, increasing scrutiny of charitable originations by Revenue Canada, and spiraling operating costs, the reorganization was initiated to structure and manage St. John Ambulance in a way that maintains and improves the products/services while increasing cost effectiveness."[13] To help ease volunteers and staff into the changes "Focus on change," a special newsletter, was to be published every six weeks.

Historically there had been a great deal of duplication of services at the national and provincial levels and the development of a national marketing plan held great potential. Understandably some provincial councils refused to participate in the program, viewing it as a power grab by the struggling national headquarters. St. John Enterprises was intended to become "the premier provider of top quality safety and health products, service training that meets all customers' expectations."[14] When it began in January 1998 only six joined: Saskatchewan, Ontario, Federal District, Quebec, British Columbia, and the Greater Toronto Area. On the surface the plan sounded good, yet it would turn into an unmitigated failure that would take St. John Ambulance at the national level to near bankruptcy. One early indication of difficulty was the fact that the 1998 Treasurer's Report, which was issued as part of the 1998 annual report, contained no figures whatsoever. This would be the last annual report published until 2003.

Large amounts of money were put into developing CD-ROM multimedia publications focused on first aid and babysitting. The expenses of SJE outstripped revenue as the project got underway. This problem would persist until the organization essentially ceased to operate in 2002.

The number of Canadians given St. John Ambulance first aid training in 1997 reached a new high of 799,862 and membership in the brigade had been constant at 12,500. Amidst the financial problems St. John volunteers again went into action during the Ice Storm that gripped much of Quebec and Ontario. It was one of the largest undertakings of the brigade in recent history. Volunteers worked moving patients out of nursing homes and providing supplies and first aid treatment. "[E]mergency services coordinators quickly realized the value of trained volunteers, and assigned St. John volunteers crucial jobs."[15]

A New International Structure for the Order

It was not only St. John Ambulance in Canada that was being restructured, but the governance structure of the Order of St. John at the international level was significantly altered in 1999. Since the Royal Charter of 1888 the Grand Priory of the Order — which was not an organization of the Order, but was the Order itself — served as the parent body for all the priories around the world. Based at St. John's Gate in London, the Grand Priory also served as the priory for England, thus the Priory of England was the senior parent body, with subordinate priories in Australia, Canada, New Zealand, Scotland, South Africa, the United States, and Wales. The organization was structured along the lines of the old British Empire with England at the centre as the imperial power, and the outlying colonies and dominions as junior partners. While the overbearing attitude of the Grand Priory had long since disappeared, the structure of the organization was still hierarchical and did not reflect its international and equal composition. Major decisions were made by the grand prior on the advice of the Chapter General, which was made up largely of British officials of the Order.

The significant changes to the Order in 1999 resulted in the creation of a separate priory for England and the Islands — to operate on an equal basis with other priories — the establishment of the Grand Council of the Most Venerable Order of the Hospital of St. John of Jerusalem, which is served by the small secretariat of the Order. The old Chapter General was in essence replaced by the Grand Council, and the eight priories of the Order were placed on an equal footing.

The Grand Council is the governing and legislative body of the Order worldwide. The council makes recommendations that pertain to the affairs and work of the Order, ensures that priories and commanderies observe the statutes of the Order and assist with strategic planning on a worldwide basis. The Grand Council is also responsible for establishing new commanderies and priories; suspending and dissolving existing ones; proposing changes to the statutes and regulations of the Order; and, through the Honours and Awards committee, developing policy related to appointments and promotions within the Order. The Order has thus developed a confederal structure, with the sovereign head and grand council uniting the various priories around the globe.

These changes to the governance structure of the Order fully reflect the equality of the eight priories while simultaneously maintaining the unity of the Order through the sovereign head. The idea for developing a confederation of priories was first developed following the Second World War in April 1947. Officials at St. John's Gate in London realized that as the dominions (Australia, Canada, New Zealand, and South Africa) became more independent and completely separate from the United Kingdom, they would need a mechanism to modernize the governing structures of the Order to better reflect their independent and equal status:

> It is self evident that these six priories [Grand Priory, Scotland, Wales, South Africa, New Zealand, Canada, and Australia], whilst in all respects absolutely loyal to the Sovereign head, and his representative the Grand Prior, will not remain satisfied indefinitely with a

subordinate position, and to have their purely internal affairs under the control of the Order in this country.[16]

In many ways the modernization of the Order's governance structure in 1999 was long overdue, especially when one considers that such plans were initially considered more than half-a-century earlier. The original 1947 proposal was only circulated to senior officials at St. John's Gate, with Secretary-General W.G.B. Barnes noting that the other priories would have to "be accepted not as Subordinate bodies, but as the equals in all respects of the Order in this country [England]. With the Sovereign Head and his representative the Grand Prior as the connecting links."[17] Since 1999 the new structure has proven to be successful. Indeed the second lord prior to hold office under the new structure, Eric Barry, is a Canadian and past chancellor of the Priory of Canada.

The St. John Eye Hospital

As one of the foundations of the Order, the St. John Eye Hospital, formerly known as the St. John Ophthalmic Hospital,[18] has been supported by St. John Ambulance in Canada since the establishment of the commandery in 1934. Located in East Jerusalem, the hospital sees more than 64,000 patients each year and performs more than 4,500 major eye operations.

At the end of the First World War members of the Newfoundland divisions of the brigade endowed a bed in perpetuity to serve as a lasting reminder of the service given by Newfoundlanders. Historically, Canadian support of the hospital had been in the form of donations made to St. John's Gate and transferred to the hospital through the purchase of supplies and equipment. Renewed Canadian interest in the hospital resulted in Canadian Ophthalmologist Dr. Lawrence Brierley going to the hospital in 1979 to practice for a full year. The program of selecting and sending a Canadian doctor, under the auspices of the priory hospitaller continued until 1993, when Dr. Mathias Fellenz served, though his term was cut short. His predecessor Dr. George Beiko, was the last Canadian to spend a full year at the hospital, having served there from 1992 to 1993. He has continued his service to St. John Ambulance over the years most recently as the priory hospitaller. In October 1991 the Priory of Canada presented Sir Stephen Miller, hospitaller at St. John's Gate, with a cheque for $119,000 to endow a bed in the hospital.[19]

Another contribution made by the Priory of Canada was the funding of a Canadian nurse to work at the hospital for a year. Although the project was triumphed as a 1983 centennial project, the idea was first promoted by the redoubtable Kay Gilmour in 1977. Following her death, plans for the project were continued by Dr. Helen Mussallem. The Kay Gilmour Memorial Project was founded and would play a role in revitalizing the Linen Guild. Since 1937 the guild had been sending funds annually to the hospital to cover the cost of various hospital supplies. One way which members of the Linen Guild — renamed the Ophthalmic Hospital Guild in 1984 — felt that they could increase interest in their activities was to move from simply making a donation to sending a person, the embodiment of hospitaller work. Funds were raised through skate-a-thons, bake sales, special Christmas card sales, and the publication of recipe books. The guild was also responsible for holding a competition and selecting a suitable candidate.

Under the leadership of Mussallem the Kay Gilmour Memorial Project was a success, and responsibility for the sending of a Canadian nurse to the hospital would fall to the Linen Guild. Between 1984 and 1993 a total of six Canadian nurses were sent by the Ophthalmic Hospital Guild.[20]

The first Canadian nurse sent to work at the hospital for a year was Kendra Napp. A night nurse from Stanton Yellowknife Hospital in the Yukon, Napp served at the hospital from 1984 to 1985. It was a significant undertaking for both Napp and St. John Ambulance given that the guild was responsible for raising all the funds to cover the nurse's travel, salary, and incidental expenses. Myrna Hamson, who served as a Canadian nurse at the hospital from 1985 to 1986 noted that "The Hospital is very clean, well-managed and has a staff that truly cares about the health and well-being of the 50,000 people it helps each year. The St. John Eye Hosptial is truly an oasis in a desert of need."[21] The most recent Canadian nurse to serve for a year at the hospital under the patronage of the guild was Heidi Bartsch who worked there from 1992 to 1993. Because of a shortage of funds "recruitment of a Canadian nurse has not be encouraged."[22] Since 1994 the guild has awarded the Guild Bursary for Nursing annually, which is awarded to a student nurse at the hospital in Jerusalem. The bursary is colloquially known as the Canadian Shield.

A Canadian doctor has not been sent to the Hospital in recent years for a variety of reasons, most notably the fact that since the early 1990s there has been an acute shortage of ophthalmologists in Canada. It was also found to be administratively difficult and cost prohibitive to cover the salary of a doctor for a year, and thus it was decided to "focus our support towards a program of hospital medical staff development."[23] In 1997 Hospitaller Brian Leonard made arrangements with the University of Ottawa Eye Institute for a position to be set aside for two years to allow for comprehensive advanced ophthalmic training of a candidate from the St. John Hospital in Jerusalem, this was to include a stipend. Unfortunately this project was never implemented. As the financial status of St. John Ambulance in Canada improved there was a renewed focus on contributing to the hospital. Since 2001 the Priory of Canada has provided $120,000 in funding annually to support the work of Dr. Maram Isaac, a pediatric ophthalmologist who practices at the Hospital in Jerusalem.[24]

Maintaining the historic and highly symbolic connection to the St. John Eye Hospital in Jerusalem is an important part of the Order and it is hoped that in the years to come an even greater focus will be placed on enhancing the highly important contribution made by the Priory of Canada to this element of our hospitaller tradition.

• • •

The period between 1999 and 2001 was marked by declining revenues, although the number of St. John Ambulance first aid training courses taken by Canadians remained almost constant. The decline of the technology sector of the stock market hit St. John Ambulance's investments particularly hard. An extraordinary move was taken in 2001 when national headquarters took control of Quebec's council because of the impending insolvency of the organization in that province. In July 2002 the national headquarters of St. John Ambulance vacated St. John House at 312 Laurier St. in Ottawa. Home of the national headquarters since 1978, the operations were moved to an office tower outside downtown Ottawa.[25] The sale of the St. John House yielded some needed funds. It was nevertheless a blow to many volunteers and staff. Through the personnel cuts of the 1990s an increasing portion of the house went unused, and the capital cost of maintaining and upgrading the structure was cost prohibitive.

In 2003 under the chancellorship of Jeffrey Gilmour a significant investment was made in Project Unity, a system to coordinate and monitor volunteers and community services. This was an important step forward in modernizing the business operations of St. John Ambulance. The organization had been one of the first to embrace computerization in 1985. It was also at this time that a comprehensive review of St. John Ambulances governing structures and decision-making processes were reviewed and completely revised. Then Vice-Chancellor René Marin and an eight member restructuring task force[26] developed a new strong governance model "to ensure the stability of St. John Ambulance as a national organization."[27] The result of the task force's work was the adoption of an accountable, transparent governance structure. In the wake of the financial difficulties experienced this was a long overdue change. Marin, who had become known as a no-nonsense administrator during his time as chair of Canada Post in the 1980s was an ideal leader for the group.

During the July 2002 visit of Pope John Paul II to Canada for World Youth Day, 1,200 St. John Ambulance volunteers participated in activities across the country with 650 members providing patient care, while others served as drivers and supply organizers. With more than 900,000 worshipers attending the event there was no shortage of work. St. John Ambulance volunteers even assisted in the operation of four field hospitals that were set up, treating patients primarily for heat exposure-related ailments.

In 2003 the St. John Canada Foundation was established "to assist our organization financially, helping to ensure we will continue to meet our training and community service commitments throughout Canada."[28] More prudent stewardship of St. John Ambulance's national assets and investments was made a priority.

During the 2003 SARS outbreak, St. John Ambulance volunteers worked long hours to assist health authorities in Toronto. A series of severe wildfires in Alberta and British Columbia saw St. John volunteers working alongside emergency officials to assist firefighters and other volunteers. During the Ontario Blackout in which 10,000,000 Canadians were without power, St. John Ambulance volunteers delivered assistance to the elderly and vulnerable throughout the province. When Hurricane Katrina struck the United States in August 2005, St. John Ambulance Canada worked closely with the Priory of the United States and Canadian Red Cross Disaster Relief Fund to provide medical supplies.

In 2006 and 2007 more than a million-and-a-half Canadians received St. John Ambulance first aid training. With 25,000 volunteers and 552 community service units in every province and territory across the country, St. John Ambulance is a vibrant and growing organization. Today St. John Ambulance continues to provide panoply of training courses and first aid products. The number of courses has grown from the traditional Standard First Aid and Home Nursing First Aid to fifteen different courses, ranging in length and detail. These include, Emergency Level First Aid, Standard Level First Aid, Level A "Heart Start," Level B "Heart Saver Plus," Level C "Basic Rescuer," Level D "Child and Infant," Medical First Responder, Automated External Defibrillation, Workplace Hazardous Material Information Systems (WHIMIS), We Can Help, What Every Babysitter Should Know, The Lifesaver, First Aid on the Farm, Instructor Certification Program, and Instructor–Trainer Certification Program. In an effort to improve St. John training a new training methodology was introduced for the first time since the 1980s. With this and many other efforts the organization looked forward to its 125th anniversary and the mission to bring training to an ever increasing number of Canadians.

The historic relationship between St. John Ambulance and the Department of National Defence has provided countless tens of thousands of members of the Canadian Forces with high quality training and saved thousands of lives. As we have seen, this relationship was forged by Colonel Ryerson, founder of the St. John Ambulance Association in Canada, and Major-General Jones, surgeon-general of the Canadian Expeditionary Force during the First World War. Their desire to see all members of the military trained in first aid and receive high quality treatment in all settings lives on to this day. In 2006 more than 50,000 Department of National Defence personnel were trained by DND's St. John Ambulance instructors. In the words of Surgeon-General Hilary Jaeger, "the success of the military first aid program continues to be directly linked to the excellent working relationship that exists between my office and the St. John Ambulance National Headquarters staff, and the ongoing cooperation received from St. John Ambulance's provincial councils."[29]

In an innovative effort to expand the reach of St. John Ambulance first aid training and first aid products in 2006, St. John Ambulance entered a partnership with the American Health and Safety Institute in the United States. Profits realized from this endeavour are put towards funding the St. John Eye Hospital in Jerusalem, continuing a long tradition of hospitaller work in the Holy Land.

St. John volunteers remain active across Canada at local and national events. From the Formula 1 Grand Prix Auto Race in Montreal and Rolling Stones Concerts held in Halifax and Regina to the Canadian National Exhibition in Toronto and Calgary Stampede, a strong commitment to community service continues. St. John Ambulance has not limited itself to only assisting Canadians but has also looked beyond our shores to help those in need. In 2006, St. John Ambulance Canada in cooperation with the Canadian Emergency Preparedness College, helped to train six members of the brigade from Sri Lanka in emergency preparedness.

Working with the federal government, St. John Ambulance became a partner in Public Safety and Emergency Preparedness Canada's "72 Hours" program. In cooperation with the

Salvation Army, St. John Ambulance launched the "72 Hour Emergency Ready Kit," to encourage Canadians to become more self-sufficient immediately following an incident. More than 30,000 St. John Emergency Ready Kits were purchased in 2006 as part of this program. As citizens become more attuned to the need to prepare for an emergency it is certain that St. John Ambulance will be called upon to render important training services not unlike those rendered as part of Air Raid Protection committees and civil defence authorities during the Second World War. It is an area that contains much potential for introducing increasing numbers of citizens to the benefits of St. John Ambulance first aid training and related programs.

ELEVEN

THE ORDER OF ST. JOHN

An Order of Chivalry

After careful consideration our Government has concluded
that appointments in your ancient Order are not subject
to the restriction of the resolution.
R.B. Bennett to the Earl of Scarborough
21 June 1931

Beyond being a charitable organization — operating arms — in the form of the Order of St. John Foundations — St. John Ambulance and the St. John Eye Hospital — the Order of St. John is an order of chivalry that is part of Canada's national honours system. In countries where priories exist, such as the United Kingdom (England, Scotland, and Wales), New Zealand, and Australia, and in a number of other countries, the Order is integrated into respective national honours systems, the exception to this is the United States. The Queen is sovereign head of the Order in all these jurisdictions, much as The Queen is head of the Commonwealth, and the Order retains its international dimension. In Canada, the Order is formally known as the Most Venerable Order of the Hospital of St. John of Jerusalem, and consists of five grades: Bailiff/Dame Grand Cross; Knight/Dame of Justice or Grace; Commander; Officer; and Serving Brother/Serving Sister.[1] There is also the Service Medal of the Order of St. John, which is awarded for twelve years of service with St. John. These are the honours of the Order that comprise part of the Canadian honours system. Other awards such as the St. John Lifesaving Medals, Priory Vote of Thanks, the Chancellor's Commendation, Provincial Commendation, and Donats are institutional awards and have no official status within the national honours system. However, they are important tokens of recognition that cannot be overlooked.

This chapter examines the "honours system" side of the Order of St. John: The method of appointment, alterations made to the Order and other logistical details that make up national honours in Canada and throughout the Commonwealth. The insignia of the Order, certificates, robes, and heraldry are examined separately in Chapter Twelve.

No other charitable organization in Canada has its awards included in the national honours system in the manner of the Order of St. John. This distinction is in large part because of the special relationship that the Order has had with the Crown in the United Kingdom, and with Canada since 1883.[2]

There has often been some confusion between the "Order of St. John" as a charitable organization and the "Order of St. John" as a part of the honours system. In the broadest sense "orders" can be divided into four principal categories; religious, military, chivalric (honours), and fraternal. In the past century a fifth category, that of orders of merit has been developed. The Order of St. John began as an order devoted to nursing pilgrims in the Holy Land — hospitaller work — and defending the Holy Land from Muslims. The Order of St. John was thus both a religious and a military order, and has grown to become what can today be classified as a charitable order that also embodies the chivalric tradition, comprising part of the honours system. Orders as "honours" are societies of honour that are instituted or sanctioned by the state, usually to recognize exemplary service of the highest calibre over an extended period of time. Orders are usually divided into several different grades/levels to allow for recognition of those who have rendered service at different grades and with varying degrees of responsibilities. Today the Order of St. John is both a charitable organization and an order of chivalry.

• • •

A proper discussion of the Order of St. John as an honour bestowed upon Canadians cannot be undertaken without briefly examining a history of honours.[3] In Canada the fount of all honours is the Crown, and at various times in our history the flow of honours has been restricted or reduced to a trickle. This was the case from 1918 to 1931, 1935 to 1939, and 1945 to 1967. The Order of St. John, however, managed to circumvent parts of the government policy that prohibited the bestowal of honours. Through clever manoeuvering and bureaucratic disinterest, the Order managed to get around certain rules — thus Canadian appointments have been made to the Order without interruption since 1931.[4]

Canadian policy towards honours was closely related to the growth of national autonomy and the desire to establish a domestic identity for institutions such as the honours system. Before 1967, Canada, like most countries in the Commonwealth, utilized British honours to recognize both members of the military and civilians for valour, bravery, meritorious service, war service, and long service, and this array of honours also included the Order of St. John. Canadian military men received such honours as the Victoria Cross, Distinguished Service Order and Military Medal, while women serving as nurses were eligible for the Royal Red Cross, which, despite its name, was not associated with the Red Cross. Those who worked with the St. John Ambulance in Canada were eligible for the Order of St. John. It was not, however, the military honours that caused Canada to place strict restrictions on what honours could be bestowed upon Canadians. Civil honours, most specifically peerages and knighthoods, became highly controversial in the first decades of the twentieth century. Canadian men of public life had a long tradition of being knighted, often appointed to the Order of St. Michael and St. George or more regularly being made Knights Bachelor. Canadian difficulties with honours arose not so much because of the number of awards or structure of the honours system, but because of who was receiving civil honours and how they were recommended to receive those honours. It was the issue of who controlled the flow of honours: although emanating from the Crown these were awarded primarily on the advice of politicians such as the prime minister of the United Kingdom, the colonial secretary, and, to a lesser degree, the prime minister of Canada. It is instructive to examine how Canada came to gain control over the flow of honours to Canadians and to then place an almost total restriction on all official honours in Canada. Strangely, for much of the period that honours were restricted in Canada, the Order of St. John circumvented the rules and in some ways served as the *defacto* national order, for service not only to the Order, but to the country as a whole.

The history of honours in Canada takes us back to the period preceding Confederation. As Canada grew in size, influence and confidence, so grew the desire to become more autonomous in many spheres and this included honours. The Order of St. John played no appreciable role in the controversy surrounding honours; indeed, it was because of an approach made by the Order to R.B. Bennett that the federal government resumed allowing appointments to not only the Order of St. John, but to all British honours of the period. Bennett had been involved with the association towards the end of the First World War[5] and would retain a lifelong interest in the work of the Order.

Before Confederation, the British government did not feel obligated to consult the colonial governments of British North America before conferring an honour upon a resident of what would become the Dominion of Canada. The system was simple: The governor or governor general would suggest to the colonial secretary that a particular person be recognized; if the colonial secretary approved the nomination, it would be put forward for the approval of the British prime minister and ultimately the sovereign. Recommendations did not have to originate with the governor or governor general. In theory, they could have originated from any member of the general public, though in practice it was unlikely that the colonial secretary would have acted upon the recommendation of, say, a Mr. Morency of Bytown, Canada West. Similarly, the colonial secretary could suggest that a particular person in a colony be recognized, and of course the governor of the colony in question, as the local authority, would always be consulted.

Residents of Canada were eligible for most British honours — save those that did not apply to Canada.[6] In the pre-Confederation period, relatively few honours were bestowed upon Canadians. Those awarded were usually knighthoods bestowed on judges and senior colonial politicians. There were no junior civil awards or long service medals for the local constable. The Order of St. John was informally part of this system before the 1888 Royal Charter, but it was not an officially recognized honour, and the insignia of the Order were not supposed to be worn at public functions, being intended for use within the Order alone. This was similar to the insignia and aprons worn by members of the Masonic Order, Loyal Orange Lodge, and Knights of Columbus. Unlike these groups, the insignia of the Order of St. John was designed to be similar to that used by the British orders of chivalry; that is, it consisted of a neck or sash badge accompanied by a breast star. The first Canadian to be appointed to the Order was Sir Allan Napier MacNab, premier of the Province of Canada[7] from 1854 to 1856, aide-de-camp to Queen Victoria and long serving member of the Legislative Assembly of Canada. MacNab was made a Knight of Justice in 1842, and subsequently appointed as a Bailiff Grand Cross on 20 August 1855.[8] MacNab also served as the senior official of the Order in Canada, holding the title of "Preceptor." Although there is not a great deal of documentation about MacNab's role, he seems to have held this position from 1849 until his death in 1862. MacNab's appointment was followed by another premier of the Province of Canada, the Honourable Sir Étienne-Pascal Taché, who was made a Knight of Justice on 18 January 1858.[9] Two other Canadians, Warren Hastings Ryland and Alexander Bell were appointed Knights of Grace on 8 June 1859; however, there were few subsequent Canadian appointments until after 1888.[10]

Following Confederation, a general convention emerged whereby the prime minister of Canada submitted his honours lists to the governor general, who vetted them and submitted them to the sovereign. The governor general — who was then a British official — also nominated Canadians for honours, usually without the knowledge of the Canadian prime minister. Awards for members of the military were submitted by the general officer commanding the Canadian militia to the governor general for transmission to London, although there were some instances when the prime minister nominated senior Canadian officers for honours. The Order of St. John worked outside of this paradigm, with nominations emanating from Canadian officials of St. John Ambulance being transmitted to the Grand Priory in the British Realm at St. John's Gate, London.

Following the 1888 Royal Charter, the Order became a British order of chivalry recognized by the Crown. Appointments to the Order were sanctioned by and made in the name of the sovereign, with the grand prior acting as the conduit. Before the Royal Charter, appointments were simply made by the grand prior as titular head of the Order. This method of effecting appointments in the name of the sovereign head of the Order, who is the sovereign, continues to this day, although a number of significant administrative changes have occurred since 1888. Nominations have always emanated from officials and members of the Order of St. John (since 1935 at both the national and provincial level, being coordinated by St. John headquarters in Canada), and the Order has never been subject to the same political involvement that the various British orders of chivalry, such as the Order of the Bath, the Order of St. Michael and St. George, and the Order of the British Empire were. It was this direct relationship with the sovereign that allowed the Order to function in Canada during the various periods of honours prohibition. Beginning in 1896, appointments to the Order were published in the *London Gazette,* just as all other British honours. This administrative fact played a significant role in the Order's continuance in Canada after passage of the Nickle Resolution, which virtually discontinued the bestowal of honours in Canada.

From 1888 until the restructuring of the Order in 1926, Canadians were appointed as Knights/Ladies of Grace, Honorary Knights of Grace, Esquires, Honorary Serving Brothers, and Honorary Associates, most being appointed at the Knight/Lady of Grace grade and as Esquires: at this time Esquires were equivalent to Officers of the Order in the current grade structure. St. John was also the first order to be awarded to Canadians in which women were included.[11] The total membership of the Order was small, never exceeding ninety members: thirty-one Knights of Grace, sixteen Ladies of Grace, eighteen Esquires, two Honorary Serving Brothers and twenty-three Honorary Associates. Even during the heavy days of the First World War, when St. John's Ambulance work reached a feverish pace, there were fewer than ten appointments per year to the Order, primarily at the Knight and Lady of Grace grade, with a corresponding number of Esquires to attend to the newly appointed Knights of Grace.

•   •   •

For the broader British honours system in Canada, the process of informal consultation functioned fairly well until 1901, when controversy arose over the knighting of Thomas Shaughnessy, president of the Canadian Pacific Railway. The governor general, Lord Minto, suggested to the prime minister that Shaughnessy be knighted for his services during the 1901 Royal Visit of the Duke and Duchess of Cornwall and York (the future King George V and Queen Mary). Sir Wilfrid Laurier opposed the idea on the grounds that Shaughnessy was unpopular with Canadians and certainly no friend of the prime minister. Minto, however, disregarded Laurier's advice and sent the nomination forward.

Laurier was furious when Shaughnessy was knighted, and it did not help that he learned of the appointment from a newspaper and not the governor general. By 1902, Laurier had drafted an official policy on honours in Canada. It set out that all honours, save the Royal Victorian Order and Order of St. John, had to be approved by the prime minister before any list could be sent from the governor general to the King. The governor general and the British government took their time in replying to Laurier's policy, and while they agreed that the prime minister should be involved in reviewing the honours lists and submitting names, they maintained that the governor general would retain the right to nominate Canadians. This policy remained in place until the Nickle Resolution.

The First World War brought much social and constitutional change to Canada, and the nation's policy towards honours was affected. Before the war there had been some opposition to titular honours such as peerages and knighthoods, but aside from the Shaughnessy case, it had been fairly muted. Honours were viewed as necessary, even if they were used as tools of patronage from time to time. This prevailing attitude changed during the First World War following several high-profile controversies. In 1914, a private member's bill was introduced in the House of Commons, one which sought to abolish peerages and knighthoods in Canada, but not other honours. This proposal was poorly received and promptly defeated. By 1917, however, the mood had changed.

In particular, two very public scandals over honours induced Parliament to examine the issue. The first involved the 1915 appointment of the Canadian minister of militia and defence, Sir Sam Hughes, as a Knight Commander of the Order of the Bath. Hughes had been pilloried in the press over his mishandling of the Canadian Expeditionary Force, most specifically his involvement with the purchase of the Ross rifle. The more serious outrage occurred in 1917 when Sir Hugh Graham, owner of the *Montreal Star* and a staunch imperialist, was elevated to the peerage as Lord Atholstan — against the advice of the Canadian prime minister and governor general. Graham's peerage was so controversial in part because of his jingoist views and because of an increasing suspicion among Canadians of peerages and knighthoods. There was also the perception that Graham had done nothing — either in Canada or Britain — to warrant such an appointment. The reality of Graham's generous philanthropic services throughout the war was conveniently ignored by many.

This was the only time in Canadian history that the British government ignored advice from both a governor general and prime minister. Whitehall's disregard of Ottawa's wishes was related to the fact that the British prime minister, David Lloyd George, was selling peerages and knighthoods to raise funds for the Liberal Party.

Although the general public was unaware of this, all the evidence now points to Graham having bought his peerage. He was a close friend of Lord Northcliffe and Lord Beaverbrook, who had been involved in similar dealings.

Apart from these events, there was an underlying naïveté about honours in Canada. Peerages and knighthoods were thought to be the same thing — both hereditary — and there was similar confusion regarding the other British orders of chivalry. For instance, when the creation of the multi-level Order of the British Empire was announced in 1917, Canadian newspapers announced that 300 Canadians were going to be knighted with the new Order. This was obviously not the case.

In March 1917, following Graham's elevation to the peerage as Lord Atholstan, Sir Robert Borden drafted a new government policy stating that all honours must be approved by the Canadian prime minister, and that no further hereditary honours (peerages or baronetcies) were to be awarded to Canadians. Only a week after this policy was drafted, William Folger Nickle, the Conservative-Unionist MP for Kingston, introduced a resolution in the House of Commons requesting that the King cease conferring peerages to Canadians. Nickle had no trouble with knighthoods or other honours — only those that had a hereditary quality. Nickle's resolution was in fact very similar to Borden's new policy. After lengthy debate, the House of Commons adopted a resolution placing power over recommendation for all honours in the hands of the Canadian prime minister, while at the same time asking the King to cease awarding hereditary titles to Canadians. This is what came to be known as the Nickle Resolution, even though Nickle himself voted against the version eventually adopted.

Although the Nickle Resolution was adopted, the debate was far from over. Some military awards were conferred, but Borden did not send forward any further recommendations for honours, as he thought the issue was still too contentious to test the new protocol.

Throughout late 1918 and most of 1919, the British press was littered with reports about people purchasing honours. Although this was a problem confined to Britain, many people assumed that the practice was followed in Canada as well. Fearing that an avalanche of knighthoods was to accompany the newly created Order of the British Empire, Nickle introduced another motion in April 1919. This one called for the King to "Hereafter be graciously pleased to refrain from conferring any titles upon your subjects domiciled or living in Canada." Nickle was now going after both peerages and knighthoods, a departure from his original opposition to only hereditary honours. Following another lengthy debate that in many ways mirrored the one in 1918, the House of Commons voted to create the Special Committee on Honours and Titles, which held several meetings and eventually submitted a report to Parliament that called for the King to cease conferring all honours and titular distinctions, save for military ranks and vocational and professional titles, upon residents of Canada. It also recommended that action be taken to extinguish the heritable quality of peerages and baronetcies held by Canadians. The committee approved of the continuance of naval and military decorations such as the Victoria Cross, Military Cross, and other decorations for valour and devotion to duty: No reference was made to the Order of St. John, possibly because the number of annual appointments to the Order was comparatively small, plus the additional fact that appointments to the Order were never made on the advice of the Canadian government: The chain of command and responsibility being directly linked with London, rather than Ottawa. The final part of the report affirmed the committee's desire to see that no resident of Canada be permitted to accept a title of honour or titular distinction from a foreign (non-British) government. Parliament passed a motion of concurrence with the report and it was adopted.

There has, invariably, been some confusion about the Nickle Resolution and the report of the Special Committee on Honours and Titles. Neither was a statute, and neither had any standing as anything more than a recommendation — as Prime Minister Bennett would demonstrate, with respect to the special committee's report, in 1933. The Nickle Resolution served as a policy document on how a prime minister could submit honours lists, and while it requested that no further hereditary honours be bestowed, it did not prevent Canadians from accepting other honours, whether a knighthood or the Order of St. John.

The House of Commons adoption of the Nickle Resolution in 1918, and the report of the Special Committee on Honours and Titles in 1919, brought the award of honours in Canada to a near-complete end. This included the appointment of Canadians to the Order of St. John. The annual reports of 1918–1922 do not reveal that the new prohibition on honours had a significant impact on the work of St. John in Canada. It was a concern that one of the historic mechanisms used by St. John, dating back to the revival of the Order — the bestowal of honours — had been prohibited. As worthy cases for appointment to the Order arose St. John volunteers and even non-St. John personnel began to write to the prime minister to find if there was a way to circumvent the restrictions placed on honours. After all, the Order conferred no title, precedence, or privilege, yet it was an important tool for recognizing the good works of those who were contributing not only to St. John and their communities, but to the well-being of Canadians in all parts of the country.

Following the adoption of the special committee's report by the House of Commons in May 1919, officials of the Order of St. John contacted Prime Minister Borden to ask if the prohibition on honours would include them. "The question is submitted whether appointments to the Order of the Hospital of St. John of Jerusalem in England may now be made compatibly within the resolution of the House."[12] The deputy minister of justice reported, "I think it very doubtful that they can be regarded as within the strict letter of the resolution [Nickle Resolution]."[13] While officials discerned that the essence of the prohibition on honours should not extend to the Order of St. John, just as it did not extend to decorations such as the Victoria Cross and Military Cross, it was decided to be politically prudent to leave the honours issue in abeyance and not to allow the Order of St. John to resume appointing Canadians, lest it be perceived as a new government policy to reinstate honours: such a topic would be a Pandora's Box in any general election. After 1919, no further Canadian appointments were made to the Order of St. John. Indeed, so concerned about the situation were St. John officials that they ceased printing the list of members of the Order in the annual report from 1920 until 1931.[14]

Despite this attitude, some Canadians were not satisfied with the restrictions placed on the Order. Montreal lawyer Bernard Rose wrote to Prime Minister Arthur Meighen in September 1921 to nominate Madame Dumont Laviolette to be appointed to the Order in recognition of her "splendid patriotism," and her volunteer efforts during the First World War.[15] Meighen obviously weighed the question as he referred it for a detailed examination by the Department of External Affairs, which worked closely with the Department of the Secretary of State on issues related to honours. An October 1921 memorandum noted "the Canadian Government has adopted and acted on the view that it is no longer able to recommend the awards of Honours or decorations." The memorandum tacitly acknowledged that "Awards under this Order are not made in pursuance of official recommendations [i.e., not on behalf of the Dominion government.] It is understood that Officers of the Order themselves make the recommendations as the result of information which they secure."[16] The Department of External Affairs was more concerned that the prime minister was unable to make recommendations than the fact that honours in Canada were effectively banned. Meighen simply replied to inquiries related to the Order of St. John and future appointments that "I find on investigation in the Governor General's office that appointments to the Order of St. John of Jerusalem are included within the prohibition."[17] This advice was contrary to that given in 1919 by the deputy minister of justice. Meighen may not have known of the earlier memorandum, as it does not appear in his papers. No reason for the change in official advice can be found, although it was likely related to persistent misinterpretation of the Nickle Resolution and the related parliamentary report. In April 1924, a short note was placed on the 1919 memorandum from the deputy minister of justice, which simply states "these orders were against the intention of the resolution,"[18] on this; Canadian appointments to the Order continued to be prohibited.

Despite the opinion of the Dominion government, appointments to the Order of members of the St. John Ambulance Brigade continued sporadically. The 1927 annual report notes that seven Serving Sisters were appointed, along with the bestowal of nine Service Medals.[19] For the brigade, honours continued to flow, in large part because it was administered from Britain, while honours for the association had come to a complete halt in 1920 and would not resume until 1931. The disparity of honours between the brigade and association was the source of some friction, however, the association was careful not to voice its frustration too loudly for fear that the government would become involved in the affairs of the brigade.

Neither Prime Minister Meighen nor William Lyon Mackenzie King submitted honours lists for British honours, although it was well within their power to do so. Both leaders hesitated because the issue remained contentious, and Mackenzie King in particular had little interest in such devices. The prohibition was not complete however, as Canadians living in other parts of the British Empire were still eligible to be awarded honours. The best example was Dr. George Washington Badgerow, a world-renowned otolaryngologist (ear, nose, and throat doctor). Badgerow was born and trained in Canada, although he made his home in Britain. Throughout the First World War and until his death he was involved with the Order of St. John and was appointed an Officer of the Order in recognition of his service. In 1926 the British government requested permission from the Canadian government to allow Badgerow to be knighted. Two years later the Canadian government responded that the award could go forward because Badgerow, although born in Canada, was a resident of Britain and was being rewarded for services he performed in Britain. Thus the prohibition was incidental, and Bennett would prove that there was no legislative prohibition at all, but a series of prime ministers who had no interest in honours lists.

Prime Minister Bennett broke the moratorium on the bestowal of honours that had existed in Canada between 1919 and 1933. In fact, Bennett adhered perfectly to the Nickle Resolution and had eighteen Canadians awarded knighthoods and 261 appointments to the various non-titular grades of the British orders of chivalry, including appointments to the Order of St. John — other than for members of the brigade. This action played a leading role in the re-establishment of honours in Canada.

The subject of honours had long percolated in the back of Bennett's mind. He had always seen them as a useful tool in building greater sense of citizenship and for rewarding exemplary service. Some credit is owed to Donald James Cowan, member of Parliament for Port Arthur, Ontario, for it was he who began pushing for Canadian appointments to the Order to be resumed. In January 1930, Cowan wrote to Prime Minister Mackenzie King with a letter nominating Ms. T.N. Andrew to be made a Lady of Grace of the Order of St. John in recognition of the leading role she played in the "organization work for the new hospital"[20] in Port Arthur. Mackenzie King replied in due course that "I had occasion ... to secure an opinion from the Government authorities and was advised that this title fell within the scope of the Resolution of the Commons, and that it would therefore, not be possible to have it conferred."[21] In famous Mackenzie King fashion, he was confusing the issue of titular honours, such as peerages and knighthoods, with non-titular honours such as the Order of St. John. This was an excuse that Mackenzie King used regularly to deal with questions relating to honours, even though various government officials advised him that he had the power to end the prohibition on honours in Canada.[22] Cowan would bring this case to the attention of Bennett following the general election of August 1930 that saw Bennett's Conservatives defeat Mackenzie King's government.

Two months after being sworn in as prime minister, Bennett received a letter from the sub prior of the Order, the Earl of Scarborough. In the letter, Scarborough noted the "disabilities from which our members are suffering in the Dominion [of Canada] compared with those in other parts of the Empire."[23] Attached to the letter was a memorandum in which Scarborough ably provided a synopsis of the work of St. John, and why the Nickle Resolution should not apply to the Order in Canada. He requested:

> having regard to the foregoing it is submitted that the Prime Minister might be pleased to ask the legal advisors of the Canadian Government to reconsider their opinion on the point, or alternatively that he might favourably consider the introduction of a short measure freeing the Order of St. John from this restriction.[24]

Bennett responded "I agree with the reasoning of the memorandum. I shall be very glad to discuss the matter with H.R.H. the Duke of Connaught, Grand Prior of the Order, on Wednesday next."[25] Bennett was in London to be sworn into the Imperial Privy Council by King George V, and it is entirely possible that the King played some role in orchestrating Scarborough's letter. It will be remembered that the Duke of Connaught had served as governor general of Canada from 1911 to 1916 and was familiar with Canadian affairs. He had a keen interest in securing a more positive position for the Order of St. John in his old dominion. Bennett met with Connaught on 22 October and assured him that he intended to reintroduce Canadian appointments to all British honours over his term as prime minister, and that the Order of St. John would be included in this plan.[26] While still in London, Bennett made his decision and again wrote Scarborough:

> I saw the Duke of Connaught after I had received your last note, and I told him that after thinking the matter over, I had concluded that it was absurd that you have been treated as you have, and I will take an early opportunity to arrange matters to, I hope, your satisfaction.[27]

Upon his return to Canada, Bennett was consumed with other issues and the Great Depression was gripping Canada hard. As the centenary of the re-establishment of the English tongue of the Order of St. John was approaching, officials in London and Canada were anxious to see the honours side of the Order of St. John reinstated in Canada.[28] One St. John official confided "I have had no direct information regarding this and am somewhat perturbed, [with Bennett] as well we all hoped that the rule would be abolished, or at any rate relaxed."[29] Scarborough again put pen to paper and pressed the prime minister, "the Order is celebrating the centenary of its revival in England, the week of June 22–27 … how splendid it would be if an announcement could then be made that the embargo had been removed so far as concerned the Order of St. John."[30] Bennett came through on 21 June in a cablegram:

After careful consideration our Government has concluded that appointments in your ancient Order are not subject to the restriction of the resolution of the House of Commons, and we will accept responsibility for any Canadian appointment that may be made. I earnestly trust that your Centenary celebrations may be the most successful and worthy of the great traditions of the organization.[31]

The Duke of Connaught, Earl of Scarborough, and members of Chapter-General were elated, as were the sixteen Canadians who could now be appointed to the Order during the centenary celebrations.[32] Scarborough noted "It was a great joy to get your cablegram … your decision could not have reached us at a more opportune moment."[33] With this, the appointment of Canadians to the Order resumed after more than a decade.

To avoid any controversy or reopening of the debate on honours the Canadian branch noted that "appointments to the Venerable Order … were not subject to the resolution of Parliament [the Nickle Resolution] with regard to titles and honours in the Dominion, since they confer no rank, title, or precedence upon their recipients."[34]

In recognition of his pivotal role in allowing the resumption of Canadian appointments Bennett was appointed a Knight of Grace in 1932, receiving the notification of his impending appointment on 20 October. He was subsequently invested with the insignia of the Order by King George V at Buckingham Palace.[35] Bennett was nominated by Cowan, president of the Canadian branch, who had encouraged Scarborough to engage Bennett on the issue of resuming Canadian appointments to the Order.[36] The resumption of Canadian appointments to the Order and the newfound support played a part in the establishment of the Commandery in Canada in 1933.

During his crusade to Canada, Hewett felt that it was "essential to build up the Organization of St. John in the Dominion; that owing to the action of Parliament some years ago in proscribing the granting of honours to Canadians practically no one in Canada had received recognition … for several years."[37] Both Canadian members of the association and officials at St. John's Gate in London felt that if the Canadian branch was to successfully become a commandery and grow, that appointments to the Order would have resume. There was also a realization that a balance of honours would have to be achieved in terms of gender, linguistic group and region. [38]

Spurred on by the success of the Order of St. John, in November 1931 Bennett asked the governor general to make enquiries as to how the government could resume issuing biannual honours lists for other British orders of chivalry such as the Order of the Bath, the Order of St. Michael and St. George, and the Order of the British Empire, thus completely reviving the hitherto moribund honours system in Canada. The first to be recognized was Sir George Perley, who was elevated from a Knight Commander of the Order of St. Michael and St. George to a Knight Grand Cross of the same Order in the 1932 New Year's honours list.[39] Bennett would continue drawing up honours lists until he was defeated in the 1935 general election.

In 1933 for the first time ever, the King's birthday honours list published in the *Canada Gazette* included the heading:

THE KING has been graciously pleased to sanction the following promotions in and appointments to the Venerable Order of the Hospital of St. John of Jerusalem.[40]

The list included sixty-two appointments to the Order that had been made in 1931, 1932, and 1933. This would be the last time until 1991 that appointments to the Order would be published in the *Canada Gazette,* although the appointments of Canadians to the Order have continued uninterrupted since 1931. The following two years brought more appointments, seventy-six and thirty-six respectively, including to Vincent Massey, who was appointed a Commander in 1934. Massey would go on to become one of the greatest Canadian promoters of the Order and St. John Ambulance, not to mention Canada's first native born governor general and Bailiff Grand Cross of the Order.

In terms of the broader honours system in Canada, Bennett's policy was non-partisan and designed to avoid the political imbroglio that honours had traditionally precipitated in Canada. For the Order of St. Michael and St. George, and the Order of the British Empire, Bennett solicited nominations from the lieutenant-governors and other officials, and then personally selected each candidate. Unlike previous lists, Bennett's were largely non-partisan and well distributed among the provinces and between the sexes — a novelty for the period. Among others, Bennett's lists recognized Sir Frederick Banting, the co-discoverer of insulin; Sir Ernest MacMillan, the noted composer and conductor; Sir Thomas Chapais, the esteemed historian; and Sir Arthur Doughty, the dominion archivist. At the non-titular level, Lucy Maud Montgomery was made a Commander of the Order of the British Empire and Lester Pearson was made an Officer of the Order of the British Empire. Public reaction to these awards was muted.

The method by which Canadians resumed being appointed to the Order was not dissimilar to that used before 1919 by Canadian officials of St. John. A person could be appointed to the Order after twelve to fifteen years of voluntary service;[41] they were almost invariably admitted as Serving Brothers or Serving Sisters. Officials from St. John's headquarters in Ottawa would collect names from the provinces and vet them and forward them to secretary of the Order of St. John at St. John's Gate. The Canadian nominations were then reviewed by the Honours and Awards Committee and sent to Chapter General for approval. Nominations were then approved by the grand prior and sanctioned by the sovereign. Any person involved in St. John was capable of making a nomination; however, Canadian nominations seem to have largely emanated solely from senior officials of St. John at the federal and provincial levels.

When Mackenzie King was re-elected prime minister in 1935, the brief revival of British honours came to an end; this did not, however, include the Order of St. John in Canada.

Mackenzie King adhered to Bennett's interpretation of the Nickle Resolution and the report of the Special Committee on Honours and Titles. Although he had a strange phobia of honours — despite ending up the most honoured Canadian politician in our history — he could stomach the Order of St. John because he was not responsible for it, appointments were listed in the *London Gazette* and it was non-controversial. Although Bennett had approved the publishing of Canadian appointments to the Order of St. John in the *Canada Gazette,* Mackenzie King put a stop to this. With no government apparatus involved in the nomination process, it was not as though he had any real ability to prevent the appointment of Canadians to the Order.

Canada entered the Second World War with no government policy on honours, other than to allow for the bestowal of gallantry and valour awards. Canadian appointments to the Order of St. John continued, and no questions were raised by government officials.

In essence, they saw it as a British order to which Canadians were appointed. The appointments were sanctioned by the sovereign and published in the *London Gazette,* as all honours in Canada had been since before Confederation.[42] Given that the federal government was at no time involved in the appointments, they felt nothing could be done to prevent Canadian appointments. The reality was that the Order of St. John was awarded throughout the Commonwealth, the King was sovereign head of the Order, and Canadians were appointed by the King on the advice of Canadian officials of the Order, making them as "Canadian" as those appointments made on the advice of the federal government of Canadians to the Order of the British Empire throughout the Second World War. Nevertheless neither the secretary of state nor the prime minister had to take responsibility for the Order.

Following the establishment of the commandery, Canada was allotted an annual quota of twenty-five appointments to the Order.[43] As the commandery grew, this relatively small number — which for the years immediately following the resumption of Canadian appointments to the Order was full of retroactive awards — was no longer sufficient to recognize the quality and quantity of work being undertaken in Canada.

In 1946 the commandery of Canada was raised to a priory. With this came a number of changes important to the Order. The governor general was promoted from Knight Commander of the Commandery in Canada to being prior of the Priory of Canada, a much more elevated status. Indeed, one of Governor General Lord Alexander's first acts was to host an investiture in the Ball Room at Rideau Hall.

Administratively the Second World War brought about changes to Canada's annual allotment of appointments to the Order. The overall number of annual appointments to and promotions within the Order was limited, there being a set number of living Bailiffs/Dames Grand Cross, Knights/Dames, and Commanders. Although there was no restriction on the total number of Officers and Serving Brothers/Serving Sisters, there was an overall limit on the total membership of the Order. Before the war, the number of Canadian appointments had been small, numbering thirty-five promotions and admissions per year.[44] This was the number agreed upon in 1931 when Canadian appointments resumed,[45] and while special allowances for an increased number of annual appointments were made during the War — in light of the increased activity and work of St. John — following the end of hostilities, it was expected that the old quota of thirty-five would be resumed. The sub prior of the Order in Canada, writing to the secretary-general noted "we must have an increase in the number we are recommending ... that this be raised to at least one hundred immediately."[46] The allotment structure for the other dominions had been set in 1943, while Canada's allotment had not changed since 1931.

Table 1

Worldwide Appointments to the Order, 1946

Realm	Number of Annual Appointments/Elevations (Brackets denote actual number of appointments/elevations made in 1946)
England (including Wales)	(494)
Australia	25 (57)
Canada	35 (34)
New Zealand	10 (41)
South Africa	30 (30)
Colonies	Counted in as part of the Grand Priory (numbering appointments 75 in 1946)

These numbers caused Canadian officials of the Order some concern. Australia and New Zealand had been permitted to greatly exceed their allotment/quota. To allay Canadian concerns, the offer was made to increase the number of Canadian appointments/elevations to fifty, half of the requested allotment.[47] Brigadier Barne, secretary-general of the Order attempted to explain that the quotas were going to be reviewed in January 1948, "You will I am sure realise that it is necessary for us to keep Subordinate Establishments on the same lines otherwise we run into all sorts of trouble."[48] Gray was not satisfied with this bureaucratic answer and took particular exception to the term "Subordinate Establishments." In his terse reply, Gray expressed his frustration, "In the year 1946 we actually instructed more people in the subjects taught by St. John than in England and yet the number of Honours normally available is considerably less than ten percent of the number granted in the British Isles ... We in Canada feel, perhaps mistakenly that we are not subordinate, but rather a partner in the organization."[49] Nearly two months later Gray had still not received a reply from St. John's Gate on the issue and decided to act unilaterally. "We will be submitting a list for approximately one hundred honours from the Dominion of Canada."[50] In fact only eighty-three appointments and elevations were proposed by Canada in 1948, so perhaps Gray feared he had been too vigorous. Barne replied that Canada would be permitted to submit Gray's list, but noted that as this exceeded Canada's allotment of fifty appointments/nominations by

thirty-three and that for 1947 Canada would only be able to submit twenty-seven names —
having deducted the unilateral increase from the annual allotment. This approach did not
impress Canadian officials of the Order, but they realized that despite having a strong case for
a significant increase in Canada's annual allotment, officials in London had ultimate control
over the numbers. In 1949 the Investigation Committee, which was charged with developing
allotments for the entire Order throughout the Commonwealth, arrived at a new and complex
system for calculating the number assigned to each priory and commandery.[51] The worldwide
membership was revised to 300 Knights, 100 Dames, 800 Commanders, and an unlimited
overall number of Officers and Serving Brothers/Serving Sisters. There were, however, restrictions placed on the number of Officers and Serving Brothers/Serving Sisters appointed
annually. As in the past the Knight/Dame and Commander grades could only be filled when
vacancies occurred. Canada was now limited to forty-eight Knights and Dames, and ninety-
six Commanders. It was allowed to appoint seventeen Officers and forty Serving
Brothers/Serving Sisters per annum.[52]

Gray was still not satisfied with this, given the great increase in St. John activities that
followed the end of the War there was a need for more honours. While attending the Coronation of Queen Elizabeth II in London, Gray had occasion to meet with his old friend, Lord
Bessborough, who as governor general had been instrumental in the establishment of the
Commandery in Canada. Bessborough agreed to bring up the issue of Canada's allotment with
Lord Wakehurst, lord prior of the Order.[53] Bessborough's intercession had some effect as in
1953, the Canadian establishment was increased to sixty Knights/Dames, 120 Commanders,
plus annual maximum appointments/elevations to thirty Officers and sixty Serving
Brothers/Serving Sisters.[54] From this point onwards, officials at St. John's Gate were more
receptive to Canadian concerns about the annual allotment.[55]

• • •

The broader issue of Canadian policy towards honours evolved lethargically. With the beginning of the Korean War, cabinet was once again faced with making decisions about honours
in Canada. It elected merely to institute a policy similar to that used during the Second World
War, which allowed for members of the Royal Canadian Navy, Canadian Army, and Royal
Canadian Air Force to accept British gallantry decorations and the non-titular levels of the
British orders of chivalry. However, in contrast to the Second World War, civilians who made
an important contribution to the Korean War effort were not to be permitted to receive any of
the non-titular levels of the British orders of chivalry. In 1952 and 1953 a number of appointments to the Order of St. John were clearly made in recognition of war service that was
rendered outside of the sphere of the work of St. John Ambulance. Once again the Order was
being used to fill the honours vacuum. The end of the Korean War saw the flow of other
honours — aside from long service awards — ceased once again.

Officials of the Order of St. John in Canada, while pleased that Canadian appointments
to the Order were able to continue, were not entirely satisfied with the situation *vis-à-vis* official recognition. Investitures were carried out by the governor general and lieutenant-governors,

but appointments were still not published in the *Canada Gazette*. There were regular questions about this, given that Canadian appointments to other orders were typically published in the *Canada Gazette*, along with the perfunctory inclusion in the *London Gazette*.

In February 1954, the chancellor of the Order approached the secretary of state, who was responsible for honours at the time,[56] to ask if appointments to the Order could be published in the *Canada Gazette*.[57] Cabinet decided, on the secretary of state's recommendation that "only official appointments could be published in the Canada Gazette and that the Order's request would therefore not be met."[58] This decision demonstrated the attitude of senior officials that it was best to just maintain the status quo and not delve into serious questions about honours policy. It is strange that appointments to the Order were not considered "official," even though they are made in the name of the Queen, and investitures were undertaken by the senior-most officials of the Crown in the land.

In 1956 the cabinet passed a directive that instated a more liberal policy towards honours and awards, which had no effect on the Order of St. John.[59] The 1956 policy also allowed for Canadians to accept foreign honours under certain circumstances. This was the first time since the Second World War that Canadian civilians were permitted to accept foreign honours.

The criteria for being appointed to the Order had been further refined by the early 1960s: "generally a member … is admitted or promoted because of the quality of the work he or she has done, is doing or is prepared to do for the Order."[60] There was nevertheless more emphasis on the length of service rendered and on what a nominee was "prepared to do for the Order," than there was on the accomplishment side of the criteria. Nominations continued to be channelled through St. John National Headquarters and the priory secretary, with the National Honours and Awards Committee vetting nominations and putting together the honours list for submission to London. The special centres such as Canadian National Railways, Canadian Pacific Railways, Northern Electric, and Bell Telephone submitted their lists with nominations to St. John headquarters as well.

The manner in which the Department of National Defence dealt with the status of the Order of St. John provides an interesting window into the federal government's policy of tolerance and "intentional unawareness." As one of the earliest special centres, DND developed a standardized method of dealing with nominations. All official honours fit into the order of precedence, which is the sequence in which orders, decorations and medals are properly worn. Until 1967 the Canadian order of precedence was a slightly modified version of the British order of precedence. Although the award of most honours had come to an end in 1946, those who were awarded orders, decorations, and medals were permitted to continue wearing them. From 1916 to 1990 the Order of St. John was incorporated into the Canadian order of precedence immediately before the Albert Medal and Distinguished Conduct Medal, and there it remained.

Members of the Royal Canadian Navy, Canadian Army, and Royal Canadian Air Force continued to be appointed to the Order of St. John after 1946, just as their civilian counterparts were. Indeed, following the Second World War the three services that today comprise the Canadian Forces maintained and enhanced their relationship with St. John Ambulance, primarily through first aid training and in 1962 this was greatly expanded. Within the Department of

National Defence all honours were channelled through the Personnel Members Committee (PMC), which included members from the various services. The PMC would accept nominations from members of the military and these were examined and adjudicated by the Inter-Service Awards Committee, a sub-committee of the PMC. From here a list was drawn up and approved by the surgeon general and then sent to the Priory of Canada for approval and transmission to London. This was the system that was put in place in 1948. In 1957 a short lived change was added to this process: the minister of national defence wanted to be involved in the process as he felt some responsibility for the nominations sent forward to the Priory of Canada.[61] Although Cabinet was unwilling to recognize the Order as "official," a senior minister of the Crown was approving draft appointment lists for the Department of National Defence special centre before they were sent onto the Canadian priory and then on to London. It was a bizarre — although typically Canadian — situation. The authority for members of the military to be appointed to the Order was included in the various service orders issued by the three services.[62] This was further official recognition of the Order as an official Canadian honour. Even if Cabinet was unwilling to deal with the broader question of honours, the Order of St. John was legally bestowed and worn by civilians and members of Canada's military.

Perhaps the principal reason for the Order being accepted as part of the honours system, despite a pervasive government policy against honours, was the role of the sovereign head. A senior official from the Department of National Defence noted "in view of Her Majesty's approval [of the Order] the Minister has agreed that the officers concerned may wear the award."[63] It would have been very difficult for any government to prohibit the award of an honour for which Canadians were nominated by fellow Canadians, for charitable works, that was awarded by and in the name of the Queen. In essence the Order of St. John worked outside the dormant Canadian honours system independently, and was sanctioned by the head of state and supported by senior representatives of the Crown such as the governor general and lieutenant-governors. The Department of National Defence recognized it as an official award, and the Order remained part of the order of precedence for wearing honours in Canada, thus it was official in every way, even if Cabinet chose to ignore these facts.

Canada's centennial year brought a partial resolution to the honours question in Canada. On 17 March 1967, Queen Elizabeth II signed the letters patent establishing the Order of Canada, which initially had parts: Companion of the Order of Canada, the Medal of Courage of the Order of Canada, and the Medal of Service of the Order of Canada. These three awards served as the cornerstone upon which the post-1967 Canadian honours system has developed. In 1972 the Canadian honours system was augmented and expanded; the Order of Canada was restructured into three levels — Companion, Officer, and Member — and the Order of Military Merit was established by the Queen along with the three bravery decorations, the Cross of Valour, Star of Courage, and Medal of Bravery. Although no mention was made of the Order of St. John in 1967 following the creation of the Order of Canada, the 1972 expansion of the Canadian honour system necessitated a restructuring and blending of the many British honours bestowed on Canadians in Right of Canada, along with the newly created Canadian honours.

Predictably, the position of the Order of St. John remained unchanged in the order of precedence, being worn after the Associate Royal Red Cross, but before "Medals for Bravery and Distinguished Conduct, War Medals, Commemorative Medals and Long Service Awards."[64] The federal government continued to take an arms-length approach to the Order of St. John, basically refusing to become involved in its administration. Yet the Order of St. John remained at the end of the Canadian order of precedence for orders and senior gallantry awards ranking after such awards as the Military Cross and Distinguished Flying Cross.[65] The Government's *Manual of Official Procedure* noted "awards in the Order of St. John continue to be made and the decorations conferred at investitures by the Governor General, are worn by members of the Armed Forces, civilians and officials."[66]

Further Changes to the Order of St. John

Since 1972, the Canadian honours system has continued to grow to include a variety of service and long service medals, expanding to become one of the most well-rounded and complete systems in the world. By the 1980s, the position of the Order of St. John was increasingly being questioned. A consistently high number of annual appointments numbering from between 250 to 350 per annum and a lack of government oversight in the nomination and selection process were points of concern. In the eyes of some officials, the Order of St. John remained a British order that Canadians happened to be appointed to, even if the advice for appointments was emanating from a Canadian source and the governor general as prior was investing members, in the name of the Queen. There was, however, the fact that in this case the Queen was acting as the Queen of the United Kingdom and not the Queen of Canada, and the Order was constituted by a Royal Charter issued in Right of the United Kingdom and governed by British orders-in-council.

There was discussion of simply removing the Order from the Canadian order of precedence, which would have had the effect — in theory at least — of preventing subsequent recipients of the Order from wearing its insignia. Such a proposal was fraught with difficulties and would have been an administrative nightmare not only for the Order, but also for the Chancellery of Honours at Rideau Hall. Another issue that concerned government officials was the number of annual appointments and perceived lack of a stringent nomination process.

The consistently high number of appointments could be explained by the fact that Canada was permitted an annual allotment of appointments to the Order and had an overall maximum membership of 6,400 members, out of the worldwide membership of 30,000. Within St. John, there was a fear that if the annual allotment of appointments for Canada was not filled, that the number would be reduced and assigned to another priory. There was also the fact that the Order was being used as much to recognize long service as it was being used to recognize merit of an exemplary nature (The issue of annual allotments will be discussed in the next chapter.) The early 1980s brought little change to the Order and its operation, however, an overall review of Canada's honours system would bring about the most important transformation of the Order since Bennett resumed the appointment of Canadians to the British orders of chivalry.

In 1988 the Chancellery, in cooperation with the Privy Council Office and the Government Honours Policy Committee, undertook a comprehensive review of the Canadian honours system. One of the key goals of this review was to "establish the primacy of Canadian Honours."[67] Up to this point, the Canadian honours system continued to include various British honours that had historically been bestowed on Canadians, although the last of these had been made in 1964.[68] Over the course of their work, discussions arose with the Priory of the Order of St. John in Canada as to its position within the Canadian honours system. The review, which was completed in late 1988, found that "anomalies concerning the Order of St. John were identified. Specifically the Queen of the United Kingdom is the sovereign of the Order, not the Queen of Canada."[69] This was followed by a discussion of the publication of appointments to the Order in the *London Gazette* and not in the *Canada Gazette;* this was another glaring inconsistency.

Canadian honours had not been published in the *London Gazette* since 1964, and after 1904, had always been simultaneously included in the *Canada Gazette.* After discussions with the Priory, two options were devised:

- Maintenance of the Status Quo: Should the Order prefer to maintain its present status, it could no longer be considered in the family of Canadian orders and appointments to the Order would be subject to review in accordance with government regulations as is the case for all requests from foreign powers wishing to honour a Canadian citizen.
- Take steps to have the Order recreated under the Queen of Canada: This option would meet all the conditions for the Order to be part of the Canadian family of honours and the governor general would exercise the powers of the sovereign in matters concerning the Order.

The first option would have had the effect of removing future appointments to the Order of St. John from the Canadian honours system and requiring them to be considered "Commonwealth and Foreign honours," which are worn after all Canadian honours. The second option was by far the most sensible, and Chancellor Frank McEachern took it to the meeting of Priory Chapter on 15 June 1989. Priory Chapter passed a resolution acknowledging that the priory should work "towards becoming a Canadian Order under a Sovereign Head who is the Queen of Canada,"[70] and further discussions ensued between the priory and Rideau Hall. A special committee was struck to review the Royal Charter, statues, and regulations governing the Order in Canada with the view of making them more compatible "with the Canadian reality should Priory Chapter decide to pursue option two."[71] This was a critical moment: Some members of the Order were keen to maintain the historic connection with the Queen in right of the United Kingdom and the constitutional complexity of the Queen of Canada being a separate entity was lost on a number of St. John officials and members of the

Order. In some quarters, the proposed change was viewed as a break with the international dimension of the Order, and there was also a fear that the sense of ownership would be lost, and that control over the Order would be devolved to government officials.

Members of the government Honours Policy Committee along with officials from the Chancellery did discuss the possibility of reducing the six grades of the Order (Bailiff, Knight/Dame, Commander, Officer, Serving Member, and Esquire) to three grades (Commander, Officer, and Member) to bring the Order into conformity with other orders in the Canadian honours system. There was great resistance to this by St. John officials as it would have given Canadians a much different gradation than their counterparts in priories elsewhere in the Commonwealth. The six grades had a long history and given that the top two grades of the Order confer knighthood and the accolade of the Order, and not the accolade of the realm, which includes the title "Sir" or "Dame," such a change was deemed unnecessary.[72] This took a great deal of explaining on the part of priory officials. As late as 2001, the offer was made to St. John that if a three graded system was adopted, the government might consider allowing the use of post-nominals. This offer was never seriously entertained and was viewed more as an attempt to vandalize a historic institution than as a way to elevate the public's perception of the Order.

In August 1990, the special committee met with officials from Rideau Hall to discuss how the Order could be incorporated into the Canadian honours system. It was agreed that a revised nomination and approval process would be put in place, one that augmented the existing process to include oversight by the chancellery. A new standard nomination form was developed and the importance of including an award citation was retained. Nominations would be put forward to a St. John national honours and awards committee (NHAC) that would include officials from the Chancellery.[73] The list approved by the NHAC would be sent to the Grand Priory to be considered by Chapter General, the list would then be submitted to the grand prior for approval and then the list would receive royal approval through the governor general acting in the name of the Queen of Canada. The governor general would then inform the Queen that she had approved the list in her name. The list would then be published in the *Canada Gazette* as the Order was formally incorporated into the national honours system. In this way, the Queen would act as Queen of Canada in relation to all matters relating to the Order of St. John in Canada, and, as sovereign head, would be seen as representing the Order's international dimension.

The incorporation of the Order of St. John into the Canadian honours system and the "Canadianization" of the Order was an important step, well beyond changing the crown worn by the Order's sovereign head when sanctioning appointments to the Order. The practical reality that Canada is an independent country and no longer was a dependent of the United Kingdom made a reality in relation to the Order of St. John in Canada. The historic relationship between the Order and all parts of the Commonwealth — headed by the Queen, as head of the Commonwealth — was also acknowledged, and this heralded a new era of cooperation with all parts of the St. John organization around the globe that were historically linked through the Crown and the old Grand Priory of the Venerable Order of St. John of Jerusalem in the British Realm.

This proposal was reviewed by the Queen and the grand prior and was approved, being viewed as a necessary modernization of the Order's operation in Canada. One senior official noted "Her Majesty thought that the proposal was an ingenious one."[74] For its members, the Canadianization of the Order was virtually invisible. It necessitated a few administrative changes and the Sovereign Head of the Order in Right of Canada was changed from "The Queen of the United Kingdom" to "The Queen of Canada." With this change, all Canadian appointments to the Order have been made by the governor general in the name of the Queen. The governor general is required to notify the Queen of who has been sanctioned for admission to or promotion within the Order in her name as Queen of Canada. The Order moved up in the Canadian order of precedence and was placed immediately after the Member grade of the Royal Victorian Order, precisely the same position the Order had been placed in by King Edward VII in 1905, having been demoted to a lower position in 1916. The new Canadian order of precedence no longer contained any British orders, decorations or medals; only those honours bestowed by the Queen in Right of Canada.[75]

The first investiture carried out under the method of appointment was held on 25 October 1990 when Chancellor Donald Rae invested Governor General Ramon Hnatyshyn as a Knight of Justice of the Order and also installed him as prior. The new prior's first act was to invest Ms. Gerda Hnatyshyn as a Dame of Grace, using the St. John Sword to dub her. For the first time women and men admitted to the Order were dubbed, symbolizing a "new practice of equality," and the Order of St. John was welcomed into the Canadian honours system after more than fifty-five years in a quasi-official position as a Canadian honour.[76]

The inaugural list of Canadian appointments to the Order of St. John was sanctioned by the prior on 6 March 1991 and published in the *Canada Gazette* on 24 August 1991,[77] under the heading "The Governor General, the Right Honourable Ramon John Hnatyshyn, on the recommendation of the Grand Prior, has appointed the following Canadians to the Most Venerable Order of the Hospital of St. John of Jerusalem."

The Order continues to constitute part of the Canadian honours system. With appointments dating from 1931 the Order has the second most continuous record of unbroken appointments in the system, after the Memorial Cross, instituted in 1919. It is older than the RCMP Long Service Medal of 1934.

Australia would follow the Canadian model of having the Queen approve appointments to the Order as Queen of that realm beginning in 1998. In 1999 the Order of St. John was reorganized from The Grand Priory of the Most Venerable Order of the Hospital of St. John of Jerusalem[78] into eight equal priories: Australia, Canada, England, New Zealand, Scotland, South Africa, United States, and Wales. Before 1999 the Grand Priory was the Priory of England and the superior ruling body of the Order, managing the international affairs of the Order, with the other priories being subordinate entities. With this change the Order Secretariat came into existence, in October 1999, based in London but not part of the Priory of England, to serve the Grand Council and assist in the management of the affairs of the Order on a worldwide basis.

At the international level, the grand prior is appointed by the sovereign head of the Order, and is always a senior member of the royal family selected by the Queen. The Grand Council consists of the four "Great Officers" — the lord prior, the prelate, the deputy lord prior, and the sub-prior — and the prior or chancellor of each of the eight priories. There are also thirty-three branches of the Order, St. John associations in various Commonwealth countries, and an associated body in Hong Kong. These changes reflected the equal status of each priory.

Throughout 2006, the Order undertook a comprehensive review of its honours and awards system of the Order of St. John.[79] The review proposed a number of important changes. These included the abolition of the rank of Esquire as a grade of the Order, new criteria for appointment to the Order, the removal of gender differentiations such as Serving Brother/Serving Sister, and other administrative changes. The Order decided on many of these issues in May 2006 when it met in Edinburgh, Scotland. The decisions will be officially confirmed when the statutes of the Order are updated in 2008 or 2009.

The purpose of the Order honours system was defined "to recognize the contribution that a person has made to one or more aspects of the work of the Order; to build the collegiality among members of the Order and those who serve in its foundations and in its other activities, thus helping to reinforce the values of the Order at all levels of its work; and to ensure the long-term sustainability of the Order."[80] There was also a recognition that the honours award system of the Order should be applied without variation, except as "may be required by a national honours authority; or may be appropriate to accord with the practice in relation to the sole or main national order in the relevant country."[81] It was agreed that the grade of Esquire within the Order should be discontinued. It was redesignated as a working appointment within a priory (ie., a priory appointment that has nothing to do with the Order) without reference to being a member of the Order. The designation Serving Brother/Serving Sister will be changed to Member, when the statutes of the Order are modified.

The worldwide compliment of the Order remained unchanged at 35,000 members, although as of June 2007 the Order has 21,752 members. The distribution by grade is as follows:

Table 2

Distribution of the Order of St. John by Grade

Grade	Percent
Bailiff/Dame Grand Cross	0.1 percent (maximum of 21)
Knight/Dame of Grace and Knight/Dame of Justice	4.0 percent
Commander	10.0 percent
Officer	24.9 percent
Serving Brother/Serving Sister (Member)	61.0 percent

Canada's maximum membership in the Order is capped at 6,480. The long standing practice of reviewing the distribution of each grade quinquennially was also retained. Along with this, and perhaps most significantly, a revised set of criteria for admission and promotion for each level within the order was adopted by the Grand Council on 9 May 2006.

Admission to or promotion in the Order is based on merit: A candidate is admitted or promoted because he or she stands out from his or her peers. For candidates to be admitted or promoted to Grade IV (Officer) or above, it must be shown that the merits of the candidate are *over and above* those which might ordinarily be expected of a person in comparable circumstances.[82] The more refined criteria were set along similar lines as that used by other Canadian honours. With the emphasis being placed on the sphere of the contribution — international, national, or regional — and its significance. Much less emphasis is placed on the services that a member is prepared to perform, the overwhelming focus is that of services rendered. Length of service is no longer considered to be one of the principal factors in appointments, but it remains part of the overall honours equation.

Today strict criteria have been developed to guide Priories in determining the most appropriate grade of appointment:

Bailiff/Dame Grand Cross: The nominee shall have demonstrated the utmost integrity, loyalty, and devotion to the Order and over an extended period shall have made a preeminent contribution to the Order or an Establishment by exceptional successful and sustained leadership at either or both a national or international level.

Knight/Dame of Grace and Knight/Dame of Justice: The nominee shall over a sustained period or in circumstances of acute crisis or pressure have made an outstanding contribution to the Order, an Establishment or Foundation by leadership or demonstrable achievement in a position carrying major responsibility, such leadership and achievement being seen as significant and inspirational. This leadership or achievement will usually have been at an international, national, or regional level, but in exceptional cases may have been at a local level. The Justice distinction continues to be given to persons who are armigerous (possessing a coat of arms).

Commander: The nominee shall either have achieved an exceptionally high quality of performance in his or her role at a national, regional or, in exceptional cases, local level, such achievement being demonstrated by, for example proven innovation or effective governance; or have exercised at a national or regional level successful and effective leadership in a prominent role carrying major responsibility.

Officer: The nominee shall either; have achieved over an extended period in a supporting role at a national level a quality of performance over and above that which might ordinarily be expected of a person in his or her role; or have at a regional or local level over an extended period exercised successful and distinguished leadership or made a high level of specialist contribution.

Serving Brother/Serving Sister (Member): The nominee shall have performed notable and committed service at national, regional, or local levels, such service having been to the benefit of the Order, an Establishment, or Foundation through its high quality or persistence.

Nominees are admitted to the Order at the grade justified by their contribution; there is no requirement to graduate through grades of the Order as there had been dating back to the Royal Charter of 1888. This is the same principle used by the Order of Canada and Order of Military Merit, where level of responsibility and contribution are the main considerations in determining the grade to which a person is appointed.

Skipping grades is also permitted where it is justified by the merits of the individual nominee. As a general rule it was decided that promotion within the Order should not occur before the passage of three years,[83] but in special circumstances this can be set aside. In general, no automatic promotions are to be made, and length of time involved with the Order is not considered a sufficient reason for promotion, rather the Service Medal exists for that purpose.

The Orders of St. John

There has long been confusion about the existence of other Orders of St. John. It should be noted that there are only five legitimate and mutually recognized Orders of St. John that continue to carry on the historic work of the Knights Hospitaller. These are the Sovereign Military and Hospitaller Order of St. John of Jerusalem of Rhodes and of Malta (The Order of Malta), Die Balley Brandenburg des Ritterlichen Ordens Sankt Johannis vom Spital zu Jerusalem, commonly known as the Johanniter Orden (Germany), Johanniter Orde in Nederland (Netherlands), Johanniterorden I Sverige (Sweden), and the Most Venerable Order of the Hospital of St. John of Jerusalem (Order of St. John, sometimes referred to as the Most Venerable Order). In 1961 an alliance was formed between the Most Venerable Order, the Johanniter Orden, Johanniter Orde in Nederland, and Johanniterorden I Sverige; these four orders comprise the Alliance of the Orders of St. John.

The agreement set out that "The signatory Order of St. John hereunder mentioned are akin to the older Tongues, respect the ancient rule and its underlying purpose, but are each of them free, independent and autonomous, and they now form an Alliance of Orders of St. John to be known by that description."[84] Two years later in 1963 the Most Venerable Order and the Order of Malta signed a joint declaration. The 1963 declaration dealt with the age old dispute over the legitimacy of the Most Venerable Order:

A dispute, long since relegated to the realms of academic discussion, as to whether the Most Venerable Order was the lineal descendent of the old Grand Priory of the

Sovereign Order, at one time caused division amongst those concerned with such questions. Certain it is that the Most Venerable Order acquired a completely independent existence when it was granted a Royal Charter by Her Majesty Queen Victoria, who became its Sovereign Head.... it is our dearest wish of both Orders, to seek ever more ways in which they can collaborate, to promote God's glory and to alleviate the suffering and miseries of mankind.[85]

In October 1987 the Alliance orders and the Order of Malta signed an agreement clarifying the difference between "those Orders which are recognized as such by the Sovereign authorities of the countries in which they are based and the self-styled 'Orders of Saint John' whose pretension to be Orders of Chivalry are unrecognized by such sovereign authorities."[86] On 23 September 1992 an accord between the Order of Malta, Johanniter Orden, and the Venerable Order was signed in Ottawa pledging mutual cooperation in Canada.

By far the most important development in the relationship between the Orders of St. John came in October 2004; in many ways this was the culmination of a process that began in 1961 when the Alliance of the Orders of St. John was constituted.[87] It was agreed that the Sovereign Military Order of Malta (SMOM) is the original order, and that the four orders of the Alliance, stem "from the same root, are orders of chivalry as well as being Christian confraternities."[88] The agreement also recognized that the five orders share a commitment to the traditions established by The Order of the Hospital of St. John of Jerusalem in the Middle Ages:

Sharing a unique vocation to subject themselves to the lordship of the sick and poor, these five orders are committed to treating the infirm, whatever their religion, as their superiors, rendering to them that respect and quality of treatment which would be due to Christ himself. This, and their centuries-old tradition, distinguishes them from other international or national bodies engaged in similar charitable work.[89]

The British association of the Sovereign Order of Malta was founded in 1875. This was followed by the establishment of the Sub-Priory of the Blessed Adrian Fortescue, which was created in 1972 with Lord Robert Crichton-Stuart as regent. A return to being the Grand Priory of England came in 1993. Friendly relations between the Order of St. John and Order of Malta were resumed in 1946.[90]

The idea behind establishing a Canadian association of the Order of Malta was introduced in 1948, "on the occasion of Quebec's Eucharistic Congress."[91] The Order established a Canadian association in 1952, which was formally incorporated as a non-profit corporation on 27 January 1953. The association elected the Right Honourable Édouard Thibaudeau Rinfret as its first president and Quentin J. Gwyn as its first chancellor. Gwyn would go on to become president of the association in Canada and eventually rise to post of grand chancellor in Rome.

A number of prominent Canadians became involved with the association early after its founding. They included Major General Georges Vanier, who was made a Knight Grand Cross of Magistral Grace with ribband, and his wife Pauline, who was made a Dame Grand Cross of Magistral Grace. Both of these appointments were made in December 1960. In 1975 relations were formally opened between the association and the Priory of Canada of the Order of St. John. The president of the association, Marc Lacoste, held a meeting at St. John House in Ottawa with Brigadier-General Beament, chancellor of the Order of St. John and there have since been many years of cordial relations. In 1995 the headquarters of the association moved from Montreal to Ottawa. The Order of Malta has three classes and various divisions:

The Prince and Grand Master

First Class (Professed):

- Justice: Venerable Bailiff Grand Cross, Commander, Knight in solemn vows, Knight in simple vows, Novice Knight
- Conventual Chaplain: Grand Cross, Chaplain with Commandery, Chaplain

Second Class:

- Obedience: Bailiff Grand Cross, Grand Cross, Commander Jus Patronatus, Knight

Third Class:

- Honour and Devotion: Bailiff Grand Cross, Grand Cross, Commander Jus Patronatus, Knight; Dame Grand Cross, Dame.
- Conventual Chaplain ad honorem: Grand Cross, Chaplain
- Grace and Devotion: Grand Cross, Knight; Dame Grand Cross, Dame
- Magistral Chaplain: Grand Cross, Chaplain
- Magistral Grace: Grand Cross, Knight; Dame Grand Cross, Dame
- Donat: First, Second and Third Classes

The Johanniter has been present in Canada since at least 1925 when it is known that a member of the Dutch association was resident in Alberta. It would not be until the 1980s that the Johanniter would become officially established in Canada; having previously been attached to the Sub-Priory of the United States. The first liaison officer of the Order in Canada was Dr. Joachim O.W. Brabander of Montreal. Brabander was responsible for organizing the Order in Canada. In 1983 the inaugural Johanniter Convocation in Canada was held in Montreal at St. John's Lutheran Church. By 1985 the Johanniter Aid Association in Canada was established, this was followed by the creation of a Canadian sub-commandery in 1986. With this the Canadian members of the Order were formally separated from the sub-commandery of the United States. The first sub-commander of the Order in Canada was Dr. Brabander. The sub-commander is often simply referred to as "The Delegate in Canada." The Johanniter Orden has three classes:

The Herrenmeister
First Class: Commander, Honorary Commander
Second Class: Knight of Justice
Third Class: Knight of Honour

On 22 September 1992 a joint declaration was signed at Ottawa by the Order of Malta, Johanniter, and the Most Venerable Order. The declaration sought to confirm in Canada the friendly relations that had existed between the orders for many years. On 26 June 1999 the three orders of St. John came together in Ottawa's St. Patrick's Basilica to celebrate the 900th Anniversary of the Knights Hospitaller. The event included members of all three orders, including the then prior of the Priory of Canada, Roméo LeBlanc.

The unofficial Orders of St. John, which are often referred to as "self-styled Orders of St. John" carry such grand designations as The Sovereign Order of the Hospitallers of Saint John of Jerusalem — Knights of Malta — Orders of Saint John Incorporated; Association of the Sovereign Order of Saint John of Jerusalem; The Order of St. John of Jerusalem, Knights of Malta; and Sovereign Military and Hospitaller Order of Saint John of Jerusalem Knights of Malta (United States Priory of the Order of St. John) Ecumenical. These are only a sample of a number of organizations that have adopted the name and style "Order of Saint John." None are bestowed by a recognized head of state or have any connection to the Order of Malta or the members of the International Alliance of the Order of St. John of Jerusalem.

As recounted by Sainty, author of *The Orders of Saint John,* many of the self-styled orders claim to be successors of the Russian Grand Priory. A series of court cases in the United States has further discredited a number of them. Nevertheless some of these groups continue to operate in Canada and around the world. Members of the Most Venerable Order of the Hospital of St. John of Jerusalem are prohibited from becoming members of these self-styled orders to further protect the integrity of the legitimate and recognized Orders of St. John. These self-styled orders are little more than private clubs.

TWELVE

LOGISTICAL ASPECTS
OF THE ORDER OF ST. JOHN

Taking into consideration the recommendations which
are being considered for 1947 we will have approximately
two hundred and thirty people awaiting insignia.
W.J. Bennett to Brigadier General W.G.B. Barne,
14 January 1946

As one of Canada's national orders, one that is shared with other Commonwealth countries, the Order of St. John has officials, insignia, investiture ceremonies, and other logistical elements. Many of these traditions are old and are shared with the worldwide Most Venerable Order of the Hospital of St. John of Jerusalem. However, some have been adapted to Canadian circumstances. While the investiture ceremony for the Order is the same as that used in other priories, the appointment certificates in Canada are bilingual, reflecting the linguistic duality of the country. The special position of the lieutenant-governors and commissioners of the Territories also reflect the federal nature of the country and the central role that the Crown plays in the life of the country.

Officials of the Order

Today in Canada there are twenty officials of the Order who hold specific posts. These include the sovereign head, the prior of Canada, the chancellor of the Order, thirteen vice-priors, the dean of the Order,[1] the secretary of the Order, and the registrar of the Order. At present these last two posts are held concurrently. The posts of grand prior and lord prior are specific to the Order of St. John internationally and cannot be considered "purely Canadian" even though the lord prior, Eric Barry, is a Canadian citizen and former chancellor of the Priory of Canada.

It is interesting to examine the development of the relationship between the Order in Canada and the offices of governor general, the lieutenant-governors and the territorial commissioners. Given the close relationship that the Order has with the royal family, it was only natural that this relationship grew to include the senior representatives of the Crown. The first president of the St. John Ambulance Association's Canadian branch was Sir George Airey Kirkpatrick, lieutenant-governor of Ontario. It was not, however, until 1911 that a formal relationship between the Crown and the Order was established in Canada. His Royal Highness Prince Arthur, Duke of Connaught, the youngest son of Queen Victoria and grand prior of the Order, served as Canada's governor general from 1911 to 1916. Being the most senior official of the Order, after his nephew King George V, it was natural that he wanted to help the Canadian branch of St. John Ambulance and the Order of St. John to flourish.

Upon his arrival in Canada "HRH honoured the Canadian Branch by becoming the Patron, and HRH the Patroness."[2] The following year, the lieutenant-governors and the commissioner of the Yukon were made vice-patrons of the Order. When the Canadian branch of the Order of St. John was elevated to a commandery in 1933, the governor general was given the designation Knight Commander of the Order in Canada. This title changed again in 1946 when the commandery was elevated to a priory and the governor general, Lord Alexander, changed from being Knight Commander of the Commandery in Canada to prior of the Priory of the Order of St. John in Canada. The lieutenant-governors and the commissioner of the Yukon were invited to become Knights of Grace of the Order in 1934, and by 1935 all had accepted the appointment. Today, lieutenant-governors and territorial commissioners continue to be appointed as Knights or Dames of the Order upon taking office. The governor general is similarly admitted to the Order after being appointed to that high office.

Levels of the Order

Elias Ashmole, the noted seventeenth century English historian of honours wrote that the Order initially consisted of one level only, that of "Knight." As the influence and revenue of the Order grew following the death of Gerard, the Order elected "out of their own Body another Governor or Head, namely, Raimund de Podio, or Poggio a Florintine, who digested and enlarged their Laws and Institutions, and divided the Body of the Order into three Classes, vis. Knight, Servant and Ecclesiasticks."[3] This is in large part why the term "Serving" was included with the names of certain levels of the Order until recently.

The present five-graded structure used by the Order is a relatively recent development. The first master of the Order, Raymond du Puy, established the original three levels that serve as the foundation for the modern structure of the Order. At the top there was "Knights of Justice," men of noble birth who already held a secular knighthood and were thus armigerous. On rare occasions men whose lineage was not noble and non-armigerous were admitted as "Knights of Grace." The second class was populated by monks and conventual chaplains who discharged ecclesiastical duties of the convent and priories. Lastly there were "Serving Brothers," who composed the largest number of members, being divided into servants of arms, who acted as esquires to knights, and servants of office who performed administrative duties.

The current five-graded (levelled) structure used by the Order follows the general structure on which other major multi-graded orders of chivalry and orders of merit structure themselves.[4] France's *Légion d'honneur* and Britain's Order of the British Empire and Royal Victorian Order are all five-grade orders. From 1926 to 2007 the Order included a sixth grade, that of Esquire, which has been reclassified and is no longer a level of the Order. The earlier structure and criteria for appointment had a rather Byzantine complexity. The 1849 statutes of the Order included four grades:

Grand Cross: This dignity may be conferred by the Chapter General on high and illustrious personages, as well as on distinguished members of the Langue in reward for preeminent services. The Great Officers and also the dignitaries abroad are *virtute officii*, Grand Crosses and a Grand Cross has the privilege of voting by proxy at every assembly of the Langue.

Knights Commander: The Chapter General may for the benefit of the Langue, or to reward services, promote eminent Chevaliers of either class to the rank of Knight Commander; but none except Knights of Justice can offer themselves for this distinction. All Sub-Preceptors and Commissioners are, *virtute officii*, Knights Commander.

Knights: The Knights (Chevaliers) are selected from the Companions at Chapter General by ballot at which two black balls excluded, and must occupy such a position in life as entitles them to attend the Court of their Sovereign. They consist of two classes:

- Those who prove, according to the ancient Statutes of the Order, that they are decedent from four grandparents entitled to coat-armour; and have made a foundation in the Langue of the old established passage dues of £100 sterling; these are designated Knights of Justice
- Those who compensate for the above by certain equivalents, such as marked services to the Langue in the capacity of Companion, near relationship to those who have advanced its interests, together with Knighthood in recognized Orders, high moral worth and social eminence, or other qualifications that may enable them to promote the interest, and add to the lusture of the institution. In their case only one-forth of the foundation of £100 is required, and they are called Knights of Grace.

Companions: Any Knight may nominate as Esquire on becoming his sponsor the following points:

- That he is a Christian of liberal education, eminent for virtue, morals, and good breeding, and in an honourable position in life;
- That he has signed the Declaration prescribed by Chapter X;
- That he has made an oblation to the Treasury of not less than five pounds.[5]

Post-nominals were associated with each of these grades, GCJJ, KCJJ, KJJ, and CJJ. By 1862 the Statues of the Order altered the structure of the Order as follows:

Bailiff or Grand Cross
Commander
Knight of Justice/Knight of Grace
Honorary Knight
Chaplain
Esquire
Donat.

In essence the level of Companion was transformed into that of Esquire and Honorary Knights were added, as were Chaplains and Donats. By 1867, despite the complex hierarchy of the Order, the total membership numbered 101 persons. This included one Donat and one Serving Brother.[6]

The 1872 statutes delineated a structure more akin to that in place today. This was the first time that Serving Sisters were included, and the rank of Honorary Associate was also added at this time:

Bailiff
Chevalier Commander
Chevalier of Justice
Chaplain
Lady of Justice
Chevalier of Grace
Lady of Grace
Esquire
Honorary Associate
Donat
Serving Brother/Serving Sister

The gender differentiation was typical of the Victorians; however, the inclusion of ladies, who were excluded from all the British orders of chivalry save the Order of the Crown of India, was unique and revealed the truly progressive nature of the Order. The term "Chevalier" was used in place of the "Knight" in part so that the Order would not become confused with the existing official orders of chivalry recognized by the Crown in the United Kingdom. Although there is no documentary evidence, this may have also been a tribute to the contribution made by the French tongues of the Order in re-establishing the Order in Britain. From 1871 to 1888, Commanders of the Order were separate from Chevalier Commanders, as they were the managers of commanderies and elected for a five year term from an electorate made up of Chevaliers of Justice, Chevaliers of Grace, Chaplains, and Esquires. It was therefore an office title and not a level of the Order. They ceased to hold the distinction of Commander of the Order upon leaving office.[7] The distinction of Honorary Associate was bestowed on people who were devoted to the objectives of the Order or who were highly distinguished for philanthropic deeds, but who were not involved in St. John Ambulance. This level was discontinued with the Royal Charter of 1926, when Honorary Associates were permitted to become Officers or Serving Brothers/Serving Sisters.

Queen Victoria's granting the Royal Charter to the Order in 1888 required a reclassification of the grades of the Order, and this included the incorporation of several specific offices, which are denoted by an asterix:

Lord Prior*
Sub-Prior*
Grand Bailiff*
Bailiff
Commander
Honorary Commander
Knight of Justice
Lady of Justice
Chaplain
Knight of Grace
Lady of Grace
Esquire
Serving Brother/Serving Sister
Honorary Associate
Associate
Donat (not intended to be worn with official honours)

Associates were persons who, while not members of the Order, had been active in the hospitaller work of the Order.

The Royal Charter granted by King George V in 1926 simplified the grades of the Order into three separate levels, with separate differentiations within each level. This made the structure slightly more confusing that it had been under the 1888 Royal Charter:

Grade I
- Bailiff and Dame Grand Cross
- Knight and Dame of Justice
- Knight and Dame of Grace

Grade II
- Chaplain

Grade III
- Commander Brother and Commander Sister
- Officer Brother and Officer Sister
- Serving Brother and Serving Sister

From the 1926 structure the current levels of the Order can be discerned, and it was in 1936 that the current basic structure was adopted, except the level held by Chaplains:

Grade I
- Bailiff and Dame Grand Cross

Grade II
- Knight and Dame of Justice
- Knight and Dame of Grace

Grade III
- Chaplain

Grade IV
- Commander Brother and Commander Sister

Grade V
- Officer Brother and Officer Sister

Grade VI
- Serving Brother and Serving Sister

Grade VII
- Esquire

When the Order was constituted as a Canadian order and part of the Canadian honours system in 1990, six grades were adopted, that of Chaplain being omitted:

Grade I
- Bailiff and Dame Grand Cross

Grade II
- Knight and Dame of Justice
- Knight and Dame of Grace

Grade III
- Commander

Grade IV
- Officer

Grade V
- Serving Member

Grade VI
- Esquire[8]

As noted, the level of "Esquire" will be phased out by 2008, with the last Canadian appointment to this grade being made to François Payeur in March of 2007. People appointed to this grade of the Order before 2007 are permitted to retain the designation.

There are frequently questions about the top two grades of the Order as conferring knighthood. The "accolade of the Order" confers knighthood upon the recipient, however there is no title associated with this knighthood. The dubbing occurs when the grand prior or his delegate taps the recipient three times on the left shoulder. The act of investiture is the ultimate public award of status as a member of the Order. Appointment to the top two grades of the Order of St. John, unlike other orders, does not require the appointee to attend an investiture.

The "accolade of the Realm" confers the title "Sir or Dame" upon the recipient. The dubbing occurs when the sovereign taps the recipient on each shoulder with a sword. This is the process followed for persons appointed to the Order of the Garter; Order of the Thistle; as Knight Bachelors or to the top two grades of the Order of the Bath; Order of St. Michael and St. George; Royal Victorian Order; or Order of the British Empire. Appointment to these orders is only completed when the appointee is dubbed.

Allotments and Annual Appointments

Following the reactivation of the English tongue of the Order, the overall membership was small, numbering just over 100 in 1867. Appointments of Canadians to the Order of St. John have been made annually without interruption since 1931, although the first Canada specific list was inaugurated in 1991. Earlier Canadian appointments dating from the first in 1842, were sporadic. Indeed until 1931, only a few Canadians were appointed to the Order annually. Even during the height of the First World War when St. John's work reached a peak only twenty-three appointments were made to the Order.

Table 1

The Order of St. John 1914–1919

Grade	Appointments	Total Membership
Knight of Grace	6	31
Honorary Knight of Grace	0	1
Lady of Grace	11	26
Honorary Lady of Grace	0	1
Esquires	6	18
Honorary Serving Brothers	0	2
TOTAL	23	79

Until the reorganization of the Order in 1926, most Canadian appointments were made at the "Knight/Lady of Grace" grade and that of "Esquire." The "Serving Brother/Serving Sister" grade, which would become the workhorse grade of the Order of St. John, did not come into its element until after 1926. The pre-1926 level of "Honorary Serving Brother" was in many ways similar to that of the post-1926 "Serving Brother/Serving Sister." Before 1926, Serving Brothers were full time paid employees of St. John Ambulance in Britain.

While the Order of St. John, like other civilian honours of the period awarded in Canada and throughout the British Empire, was well populated by men of public life, there were a few distinct differences from other honours. Women were admitted to the Order and encouraged to participate. Indeed, during the First World War, the twenty-six ladies of grace undertook some of the most important home-front projects that St. John engaged in. All British orders, save the Order of the British Empire, were restricted to males alone. No distinction was made between military and civilian members of the Order.

With the resumption of Canadian appointments to the Order in 1931, the number of annual appointments grew to better reflect the growth of the St. John Ambulance in Canada. The St. John centennial list saw sixteen Canadian appointments, while in 1933, forty-eight more Canadians were appointed to the Order.[9]

During the Second World War, the numbers grew further to reflect the war work done by St. John Ambulance both in Canada and around the globe. The figures from 1939–1946 reflect the appointments made to the Order during the Second World War. No appointments were made in 1941 on account of war restrictions on the production of insignia for the Order.[10]

Table 2

Appointments to the Order of St. John, 1939–1946

Grade	Appointments
Knight of Grace	10
Lady of Grace	0
Commander Brother	23
Commander Sister	8
Officer Brother	101
Officer Sister	24
Serving Brother	78
Serving Sister	48
TOTAL	292

The number of annual appointments following the Second World War returned to a more limited number, ranging from a high of eighty-three in 1948 to a low of sixteen in 1949. With the new Royal Charter of 1955, there was a fairly rapid expansion of the Order, which was intended to keep pace with the expansion of the organization as a whole and the number of volunteers working with St. John around the world.

The membership of the top three grades of the Order (Bailiff, Knight/Dame, and Commander) was capped with a maximum membership, but today only the top two grades have a maximum membership. The "Officer" and "Serving Brother/Serving Sister" grades were limited only by a maximum number of annual appointments, with no cap on the overall membership. In 1985 the worldwide membership of the Order was capped at 30,000. Before 1985 there was no overall cap on the total membership.

Table 3

Worldwide Membership of the Order

Year	Overall Membership
1867	101
1931	4,268
1936	5,287
1946	9,209
1961	16,502
1965	19,181
1970	22,341
1975	22,000
1980	29,378
1985	30,000
1999	35,000 (fixed as maximum)

As the total membership of the Order increased, so did the number of Canadians appointed annually. On the surface it is difficult not to be critical of the number of Canadian appointments made in the 1960s through to the year 2002. Annual appointments and elevations ranged from 300 to a high of 669 per annum. As Canadian officials had fought hard to obtain a higher annual allotment of appointments, there was rarely a year when the maximum number of appointments was not reached. There was a general fear that if the maximum number of appointments was not filled annually that Canada's share of the Order would be reduced. The Priory of Canada also developed an allotment schedule for each provincial council; this too helped to fuel the large number of appointments, given the fact that provincial councils generally felt they had to fill their allotment with nominations, rather than lose part of their quota. Another reason for the high number of appointments relates to the absence of a fully developed national honours system until recently. From 1946 to 1967, there was no Canadian honours system as we know it today. For civilians performing meritorious acts, there was no official mechanism for recognition. To a small degree, the Order of St. John filled this gap, and people not actively involved in St. John Ambulance were appointed to the Order in recognition of other charitable and meritorious works that may have in some small way touched upon the work of the Order. Indeed, the Order's motto "In the Service of Humanity" allowed for a broad interpretation. A highly critical examination could conclude that the Order was simply trying to buy friends, and indeed this did occur from time to time: how else could one explain the 1951 appointment of Quebec Premier Maurice Duplessis? But these sorts of appointments were not the norm.

In some ways, the large number of appointments and elevations had the effect of devaluing the prestige associated with being a member of the Order. No doubt, most appointees during this period were worthy of some form of recognition for their work with St. John, but it is difficult to justify the wanton distribution of honours that occurred. One explanation is that the Order was seen in part as both a reward for meritorious service and long service, so promotion was in many cases automatic after the perfunctory three to five years. The other reason is related to the fact that St. John Ambulance relies heavily upon volunteers and what is in essence an unpaid workforce, and honours provide an incentive to volunteer and participate.

Canadians' understanding of honours also changed during this period. It was not until the late 1980s that the average citizen became familiar with the Order of Canada and other parts of the Canadian honours system, and it is unfair to make a direct comparison between Canada's senior national order and the Order of St. John. The Order of Canada is the ultimate mark of honour bestowed by the Crown/state in recognition of life long service, and it is greatly limited in the number of annual appointments. Appointments to the Order of St. John are made for exemplary service in the field of serving St. John and its foundations and is used as the primary means of recognizing voluntary contributions — the key point being that the contributions are being made by volunteers. Only 15 percent of appointments to the Order of Canada are made for purely voluntary contributions, the remainder are made in recognition of outstanding contributions made during the course of a person's professional life. A salient parallel can be drawn between the Order of St. John and the Order of Military Merit. Both orders recognize service with a specific organization, in the case of the Order of St. John it is St. John Ambulance, while in the case of the Order of Military Merit it is the Canadian Forces. Even the levels of the two orders are structured according to merit and level of responsibility, which provides for a balanced distribution of appointments to the respective orders.

Even after the Order was incorporated into the Canadian honours system in 1990 the number of annual appointments remained significant. The 1991 list of appointments published in the *Canada Gazette* included 395 appointments and elevations, in 1992, there were 450, and by 2002, it had ballooned to 669. The Chancellery of Honours at Rideau Hall was alarmed by the size of these lists and began to question the nomination process and criteria for appointment used by the Order.[11] Officials at Rideau Hall and in the Privy Council Office made reference to the "inflation of honour" to which the Order of St. John had been subject. St. John officials were not ignorant of this perception, and appropriate changes were made to enhance the integrity of the Order. By 2005, the number of annual appointments had dropped drastically to 225, and a more rigorous nomination and selection process was employed. In 2006 the number of annual appointments had been further reduced to a more conservative 143 appointments and elevations.

One reason for the decline in annual appointments/elevations is related to the tightening of the criteria for admission to the Order. The National Honours and Awards Committee had been much more stringent in its approach to nominations. The review of the honours and awards of St. John undertaken for the Grand Council in 2005 and largely approved in 2006 has also further tightened the criteria for admission to each level of the Order. There is also no longer a feeling that Canada must fill all the vacancies that open up in the Order, which had been the case throughout the 1970s and 1990s.

Insignia of the Order

The insignia is the most visible part of any order; the badge of membership being slightly different depending on the level of membership. The insignia of the Order is of a similar design throughout, being embodied in an eight-pointed cross. The Order consists of five grades with six different sets of insignia: Bailiff or Dame Grand Cross, Knight or Dame of Justice, Knight or Dame of Grace, Commander, Officer, and Member. In the early days following the revival of the Order in England it was deemed so important for members to wear their insignia that the 1872 Statutes of the Order stated that the white cross "must be worn at General Assemblies and Chapter under a penalty of 5s[hillings]."[12] Although wearing the insignia continues to be important there is no longer a penalty associated with failure to do so at St. John events.

This section will focus on the design of modern insignia. Appendix D contains descriptions of the various insignia used throughout the history of the Order. Office-specific insignia, worn by the five senior officials of the Order — the sovereign head, grand prior, lord prior, the prior of Canada, and the chancellor of the Order in Canada — will be examined separately.

Bailiffs and Dames Grand Cross wear a eight-pointed cross breast star, 92 millimetres (mm) wide. The star is gold in colour and enamelled white. The sash badge is worn on the left hip and is an eight-pointed cross with embellishments gold in colour with white enamel. The badge is 85 mm wide for men and 59 mm wide for ladies. The ribbon is black morae and measures 120 mm wide for men and 58 mm wide for women.

Knights and Dames of Justice wear an eight-pointed cross breast star 78 mm wide. Around the neck an eight-pointed cross with embellishments, gold in colour and enamelled white, measuring 58 mm wide, is worn by men. Ladies wear the same neck insignia on a shoulder bow. The ribbon is 38 mm wide and black morae in colour.

The insignia worn by Knights and Dames of Grace is identical to that worn by Knights and Dames of Justice except that the insignia is silver in colour with white enamel and the breast star includes embellishments between the arms of the eight-pointed cross.

Commanders of the Order wear a eight-pointed cross, silver in colour, enamelled white, measuring 58 mm wide. Men wear this around the neck, while ladies wear it on a shoulder bow. The ribbon is 38 mm wide and black morae in colour.

Officers of the Order wear an eight-pointed cross, silver in colour, enamelled white, measuring 38 mm wide. The insignia is hung from a black morae ribbon, 38 mm wide. Serving Members wear an insignia identical to that worn by officers, silver in colour with no enamel.

The insignia of the Order has changed as the Order has grown, and in response to war, shortages, and financial difficulty. The insignia most prone to change has been that of the Serving Brother and Serving Sisters, what is today the Member grade of the Order. The original Serving Brother and Serving Sister insignia was 38 mm wide and consisted of a circular silver medal, enamelled in black, with an embellished eight-pointed cross in silver, with white enamel superimposed on the black background. This insignia was often specially engraved with the recipient's details on the reverse. Given that this insignia was a multi-piece affair it proved to be expensive and time consuming to make. Thus, during the Second World War and until 1947 an "economy issue," sometimes called the "skeleton insignia" was used. These were stamped silver discs with the eight-pointed cross cut out. The entire insignia was plain and not enamelled. Following the end of the war holders of the "skeleton insignia" were permitted to exchange their insignia for a standard pre-war design issue. In 1980 the current design of Serving Member insignia was adopted. Appendix D details the various changes made to the insignia of the Order since 1888.

The 1860 statutes of the Order included a peculiar ordinance related to the insignia: "No member can attend the Chapter-General without the Insignia of the Order, and, with the notification of his election, the secretary-general transmits to each entrant a warrant to the Jeweller of the Langue, to provide him with the same [insignia], according to a fixed price and pattern."[13] There was even a set fine for failure to wear the insignia of the Order at appropriate events. That individuals were required to procure their own insignia was typical of both the period and of continental European custom.[14]

A variety of firms have manufactured the Order both in the United Kingdom, Canada, and New Zealand. The original insignia of the Order were produced by Phillips Brothers and Sons of London from 1867 to 1895. Carringtons of London made the insignia from that time until 1908 when the manufacture was turned over to H.T. Lamb and Company, who were located close to St. John Gate in London. By the end of the Second World War, Toye, Kenning and Spencer Limited were manufacturing the insignia, and have done so ever since. A Canadian manufacturer, Joe Drouin Ltd., has also produced the insignia of all grades. The ribbon of the Order has always been produced by Toye, Kenning and Spencer. As the oldest ribbon weavers in Britain, the company has produced the black morae ribbon for the Order since the re-establishment of the English tongue.

The provision of insignia became a serious problem during the Second World War. Not only did economy issues and recycled insignia had to be used, but in the case of Canada there were no insignia available for bestowal. New members of the Order were simply presented with the undress ribbon of the Order and a letter. By early 1946 Canadian officials of the Order, not fully appreciating the continuing austerity measures in place in Britain, expressed increasing frustration at the lack of insignia. "Taking into consideration the recommendations which are being considered for 1947 we will have approximately two hundred and thirty people awaiting insignia. I find that this goes back to our 1941 list.... Some of our people cannot understand why we cannot give them insignia when medals and insignia are being provided for other Orders."[15] The reality was that production of insignia for the Order of the British Empire and newly created war medals was given precedence over insignia for the Order of St. John. By late 1947 the Canadian backlog was dealt with and insignia was shipped from Britain for bestowal.

Before 1947 all insignia of the Order were made of silver, after this date insignia have been made of plated base metal. In 1947, the effect of war restrictions was still having its effect on the Order and consideration was given to the production of plastic insignia.[16] Thankfully this course was avoided.

Given that the Order is part of a charitable organization the cost of insignia has periodically been a cause of concern, there being a desire to provide decent quality insignia at a reasonable cost. This was especially important because before 1990, recipients of the Order were expected to cover the cost of their insignia, either directly or through a donation to the Order. The governor general and lieutenant-governors were exempted from this practice.

Table 4

Cost of Insignia in Pounds Sterling and Canadian Dollars, 1934–2007

Grade of Insignia	1934	1959	2007 (Canadian Dollars)
Knight of Grace	£6.0.0 ($29.94)	£9.5.0 ($25.55)	$450.00
Knight of Justice	£6.12.6 ($32.68)	£10.5.0 ($28.24)	$425.00
Dame of Grace (shoulder badge alone, not accompanied by star until post-1936)	£2.17.6 ($13.97)	See Knight	See Knight
Commander	£2.17.6 ($13.97)	£2.17.6 ($7.34)	$300.00
Officer	£1.15.0 ($8.11)	£2.6.6 ($7.26)	$150.00
Serving Brother/Serving Sister	£1.15.0 ($8.11)	£0.18.6 ($2.15)	$70.00

As the value of the British pound dropped relative to the Canadian dollar, the cost of insignia dropped for the Canadians. There was the additional problem that because the insignia of the Order was manufactured in the United Kingdom, it was subject to an import duty of 40 percent imposed by the customs department. Canadian officials were not concerned that there was no Canadian firm capable of manufacturing the insignia of the Order.[19] For a number of years the customs duty was cleverly circumvented by having the insignia shipped to the governor general by the diplomatic bag from London to Ottawa.[20] While this saved the Order a good deal of money, it was found to be in violation of the Customs Act, and the practice was promptly discontinued. In 1995, a Canadian firm began producing the Order's insignia, and a mix of Canadian and British manufactured insignia has been used since this time.[21]

Lapel Badge: "The Rosette"

Long before the Order of Canada or other Canadian honours started including a lapel badge for undress wear, the Order of St. John had its own series of lapel badges, known as rosettes or boutonnières. This was a tradition that was common in many European countries dating to the mid-nineteenth century, and was a tradition first adapted and used by the Order of Malta and later the Order of St. John. The first reference to a lapel badge can be found in the 1872 issue of the statues of the Order. The statutes mention that "A button bearing the cross [of the Order] may be used by all members alike."[22] The button was altered to a rosette based upon that used by the Order of Malta, which they began using in the late eighteenth century.

A rosette comprised of a 12 mm piece of black morae ribbon wrapped in a circle, known as a box pattern, defaced in the centre by a 10 mm wide embellished eight-pointed white cross correspondent to the level of Bailiff/Dame Grand Cross or Knight/Dame of Grace/Justice.

In Canada, a slightly altered tradition emerged with relation to the levels of the Order below that of Knight/Dame. Following the lead set by the Order of Canada in 1972 when lapel badges were introduced for all levels of that order, the Order of St. John in Canada adopted lapel badges for members of the Order of St. John in 1985. These are worn on the lapel for everyday use. The lapel badge worn by all members of the Order is 18 mm wide. Bailiffs and Knights/Dames of Justice wear a gold and white enamel representation of the eight-pointed cross with embellishments. Knights/Dames of Grace, Commanders, and Officers wear a silver and white enamel representation of the eight-pointed cross with embellishments. Serving Brothers/Serving Sisters (Members) wear a plain silver representation of the eight-pointed cross with embellishments.

Before 1972 and the introduction of lapel badges for the Order of Canada and other Canadian honours, it was not generally the practice of members of the Order of St. John to wear their lapel badges at non-St. John events. In 1950 a question about when the lapel badge should be worn was brought up with the secretary-general of the Order in London, he replied to the Priory of Canada that "The Lord Prior's view is that it [the lapel badge/rosette] should be worn only when it is desirable that the wearer should be recognizable as a member of the Order. If this is the view taken by the Canadian Priory it would restrict the wearing of the rosette to all functions connection with St. John."[23] Today there are no restrictions on wearing Order of St. John lapel badges, indeed it is encouraged to raise awareness of the work of St. John Ambulance.

Insignia Worn by Officials of the Order

The senior officials of the Order of St. John all wear specific insignia of office to denote the office they hold. The five officials who wear unique insignia are the sovereign head, grand prior, lord prior, prior of Canada, and the chancellor.

The sovereign head of the Order wears a breast star and sash badge. The star is an eight-pointed cross, 8 centimetre (cm) wide, set in gold with enamels. The sash badge is an eight-pointed cross, 8 cm wide, set in gold with embellishments surmounted by an St. Edwards Crown that is not enamelled. The sash badge is hung from a black watered ribbon, 6 cm wide.[24]

The grand prior wears a breast star and sash badge, although on some occasions when a sash is not worn, a sash badge at the neck is permitted. The star is an eight-pointed cross, 8 cm wide, set in gold with white enamel. The sash badge is a eight-pointed cross with embellishments, 8 cm wide, of gold with white enamel, surmounted by a plain imperial crown. The sash ribbon is 12 cm wide.

The lord prior wears a breast star and sash badge, although on some occasions when a sash is not worn, the grand prior is permitted to wear his sash badge at the neck. The star is a eight-pointed cross, 8 cm wide, set in gold with white enamel. The sash badge is an eight-pointed cross with embellishments, 8 cm wide, of gold with white enamel, surmounted by a gold coronet, which is meant to be a representation of the coronet worn by Edward, Prince of Wales, who was the first grand prior under the Royal Charter. The sash ribbon is 10 cm wide.

The latest symbolic additions to the Order of St. John include four chains of office, known as The Chains of Office of the Priory of Canada. These are in many ways modelled on the chancellor's Chain of the Order of Canada and the chains of office worn by officials of the various British orders of chivalry. The chains are "worn on appropriate official occasions such as investitures, both national and otherwise; meetings of Chapter and of Priory Councils; meetings of provincial and territorial councils; meetings of the Grand Council and at other such times as befits the honour of the Priory and of the Order."[25]

The prior of Canada wears a chain of office composed of two separate rows of gold chain, joined in the centre by the shield of Canada, surrounded by the motto of the Order of Canada, and surmounted by a Royal Crown. From this hangs a gold eight-pointed cross in white enamel, defaced with the shield of the Priory of Canada in red and white enamel. On the chain are the thirteen shields of the Canadian provinces and territories in gold with enamels, alternating with gold and white enamel eight-pointed crosses. Each side of the chain bears the shield of the Priory of Canada in gold, with red and white enamels at the point where the chain affixes to the shoulder.

Governor General Michaëlle Jean was the first prior to be presented with the Prior's Chain. It had previously been worn as the chancellor's chain by Chancellor Jeff Gilmour, but in 2006, it was decided that this chain would more appropriately be worn by the governor general as prior, and thus the chain was made by the Prior's Chain of Office and was formally presented to Michaëlle Jean by Lord Prior Eric Barry, at a ceremony held at Government House on 12 April 2006 in Ottawa.

The chancellor of the Priory of the Order of St. John in Canada wears a chain of office composed of two separate rows of gold chain, joined together in the centre by the shield of Canada surrounded by the motto of the Order of Canada and surmounted by a Royal Crown. From this hangs a gold, eight-pointed cross in white enamel, defaced with the shield of the Priory of Canada in red and white enamel. On each side of the shield of Canada are natural gold maple leaves. An immediate past-chancellor's chain of office also exists. It is identical to the chancellor's chain, except that there are no gold maple leaves on each side of the shield of Canada. The past chancellor wears a chain of office in his or her capacity as chair of Priory Chapter. The president of Ontario Council wears a chain similar to that of the chancellor, composed of one row of gold chain, and joined in the centre by the shield of Ontario. From this hangs an eight-pointed cross in white enamel, defaced with the shield of the Priory of Canada in red and white enamel. The concept for the chains was developed by Roger Lindsay and Stephen Connelly of Cleave and Company,[26] which also manufactured them. They are made of sterling silver, gilded where appropriate. Lindsay was responsible for donating the past chancellor's chain. It can be expected that over the next few years that other provincial councils will adopt chains of office for their presidents similar to that worn by the president of Ontario Council.

Robes of the Order

Like other orders of chivalry that were established in Europe over the past thousand years, the Order of St. John possesses robes known as mantles.[27] Mantles are special garb worn at investitures or on specific days commemorating an event important to the order in question. This is usually the day the order was established or the saint's day associated with the order. For the Order of St. John this is June 24th.

In all there are nine different types of robes worn by members of the Order of St. John, four of these are specific to officials of the Order, while five are specific to holders of the various grades of the Order.

The sovereign wears a mantle of black velvet lined with white silk, with a train extending behind. On the left breast is the badge of the Order of St. John, 30 cm in diameter, in white silk with gold wire edging, and the entire badge is surmounted by an imperial crown. The grand prior wears a mantle similar to that of the sovereign but without the crown on the breast badge and no train. The secretary of the Order wears a mantle of black merino faced with black silk, and on the left breast is the badge 15 cm in diameter displaying the badge of the Order behind which are two quills in saltire. According to C.W. Tozer, clerical members of the

Order, "when officiating at functions of the Order may wear over their surplice a tippet of black stuff with red lining and edging and red buttons. On the left breast is the badge of the Order, 3 inches [7.5 cm] in diameter. They may also wear a square black velvet cap with red edging and buttons."[28] This garb has rarely been worn in Canada.

Bailiffs and Dames Grand Cross of the Order wear a black silk mantle, lined with black silk. On the left breast is a 30 cm wide white linen badge of the Order embellished with gold silk. The tongues of the lions and unicorns are red. All other members of the Order, except Serving Brothers and Serving Sisters, may wear mantles of black merino (wool) faced with black silk. Rank is differentiated by the size of the badge of the Order worn on the left breast. Knights and Dames of Justice wear the same 30 cm badge of the Order as Bailiffs and Dames Grand Cross. Knights and Dames of Grace wear a 30 cm wide badge of the Order in white linen embellished with white silk. Commanders and Officers wear a badge similar to that worn by Knights and Dames of Grace but 23 cm and 15 cm in diameter respectively, both in white linen with embellishments of white silk.

Beneath the mantle worn by Bailiffs, Knights, Commanders, and Officers, individuals are permitted to wear a surcoat known as a sopra-vest. This vest is a cassock-like garment that buttons down the side and close round the neck down one side, and falls to the ankles. It is cut so as to entirely cover the tie, shirt, jacket, and trousers. Women do not wear the sopra-vest. Medal ribbons are worn on the sopra-vest in the centre. Bailiffs grand cross have a 30 cm, plain white eight-pointed cross on the chest.[29]

When outdoors, a plain black Tudor flat cap of black velvet can be worn, although this has not been used in Canada for a long time and is not a required part of the ensemble. Since 1974, ladies have been permitted to wear mantles; before that, the only lady to wear a mantle was the Queen. In Canada mantles tend to be worn only at investitures and then only by those holding the rank of Knight/Dame and above.

Post-nominals

The post-nominals assigned to the Order, like other orders and honours correspond to the level of appointment. The 1849 Statutes of the Order included post-nominals, GCJJ (Grand Cross/Bailiff), KCJJ (Knight Commander), CJJ (Companions), however post-nominals were not published with the statutes after 1871. They were, after all, unofficial designations not recognized by the Crown at this point in the Order's history. In 1896, some years after the Order was granted its Royal Charter, the Chapter-General approached the War Office in Britain and suggested that knights of the Order who were serving in the British Army and Royal Navy be permitted to place the letters "K.J." after their names.[30] Members of the Sovereign Military Order of Malta had long used the unofficial post-nominals "K.M.," representing Knight of the Order of Malta, just as "K.G." represented Knight of the Order of the Garter.[31] This petition was refused and subsequent appeals to have post-nominals recognized outside the Order have met with little success.

The post-nominals used by the Order are modelled on those assigned to other honours throughout the Commonwealth:

Bailiff/Dame Grand Cross: G.C.St.J.
Knight/Dame of Grace/Justice: K.St.J. or D.St. J.
Commander: C.St.J.
Officer: O.St.J.
Serving Brother: S.B.St.J., or Serving Sister: S.S.St.J.,
    (what will soon become Serving Member M.St.J.).

Although the designation "M.St.J." was only considered in 2007, it was used unofficially at various times earlier in the twentieth century.[32]

There are no post-nominals associated with the Service Medal of the Order of St. John or the St. John Life Saving Medals. The Order's post-nominials have always been restricted for use within the Order and are not for general usage. Following the formal incorporation of the Order into the Canadian honours system in 1990 there was discussion about the liberalization of this policy, although there has been little movement on this issue. At one point Rideau Hall officials suggested that if the Priory of Canada were to abandon the top two levels of the Order — Bailiff/Dame Grand Cross and Knight/Dame — and reduce the Order to a three-levelled (Commander, Officer, and Member) honour similar to the Order of Canada and Order of Military Merit, consideration would be given to making the post-nominals official for use outside the Order. This offer was refused as it would have handicapped Canadians involved in the Order in relation to other priories.

Order of Precedence

The order of precedence is the sequence in which the insignia of orders, decorations, and medals in the Canadian honours system are worn. All countries that possess an honours system have a formal order in which honours are to be worn. Within the Canadian and British honours systems there are three categories of honours: Orders, which are societies of honours to recognize exemplary service of the highest calibre; decorations, which are awarded for bravery, gallantry or meritorious service; and medals, which are awarded for war/campaign service, commemorative events such as a coronation, long service, and a miscellany of categories for medals such as the Queen's Medal for Champion Shot and Arctic Medals.

Early in the history of the Order, the insignia and undress ribbon were worn immediately after all British orders, but before the senior most decoration, the Albert Medal. This was first set out in "The Memorandum as regards the Wearing of Insignia" issued on 17 June 1889, and subsequently revised in July 1896.[33] This high status was degraded in 1900, though no official reason is known. The 1900 British Army Dress regulations placed all levels of the Order between the Distinguished Conduct Medal and the Meritorious Service Medal; thus, the

Order was worn after decorations but before war and campaign service medals.[34] In 1905, King Edward VII restored the Order to a much more senior position in the order of precedence,[35] ranking it immediately after the "Member" (5th Class)[36] of the Royal Victorian Order, and before all decorations. In 1916, this regulation was again changed and the Order was placed after gallantry crosses (DSC [Distinguished Service Cross], MC [Military Cross], DFC [Distinguished Flying Cross], AFC [Air Force Cross]), and immediately before the Albert Medal and the Distinguished Conduct Medal. There it remained in both the British and Canadian orders of precedence.

With the incorporation of the Order into the Canadian honours system in 1990, the Order reverted to its historic position in the Canadian order of precedence, ranking immediately after the "Member" level of the Royal Victorian Order, but before decorations for bravery, valour, and meritorious service. The Order in Canada has returned to essentially the same position it held from 1905 to 1916 in the order of precedence. All five grades of the Order are in this one place. The reason for this is primarily related to the tradition of combining all five levels of the Order into one position in the order of precedence.

The federal government passed Order-in-Council 1991–841 on 9 May 1991, which incorporated the various provincial orders into the Canadian order of precedence. The provincial orders were placed immediately after the Order of St. John, but before decorations; thus, the Order of St. John was not displaced. There was some discussion at the government Honours Policy Committee about placing provincial honours ahead of the Order of St. John, but this did not go forward for three reasons. First, the Queen is sovereign head of the Order of St. John, while she is not the sovereign of any of the provincial orders, second, the Order is national in scope, and third, it is one of the oldest parts of the honours system and had historically been ranked after national orders in Canada and in the United Kingdom.

Certificate

The original appointment certificates for the Order of St. John were elaborate affairs printed on vellum, often entirely executed by a heraldic artist. These early appointment certificates were signed by the grand prior and issued in his name on behalf of the sovereign head of the Order. These certificates were sealed with a large wax seal contained in a skippit,[37] and attached to the document by a black or red and white silk cord. When the new Royal Charter was granted by King George V in 1926, the appointment certificate was simplified and brought into line with certificates awarded with other British orders of chivalry. The new version measured 28.5 cm x 36 cm, was printed on vellum, and, for an extra fee, the name of the appointee was entered onto the document by a heraldic artist. The seal of the Order was impressed onto a small white seal, which was affixed to the upper left of the document. As with the previous certificate, it was issued in the name of the grand prior, under his signature in the name of the sovereign head.

This version of the certificate was used until 1990, when it was replaced by a Canadian version. This new version was bilingual and issued in the name of the prior of the Order in

Canada. These documents were signed by both the prior and the chancellor of the Order. They were embossed with a gold eight-pointed cross at the top, and sealed with the seal of the Order on a gold disc in the lower left corner.[38] This was perhaps the most attractive appointment certificate awarded since the 1920s.

As a cost saving measure, a plain and unilingual certificate was developed in 1998. This certificate was signed by the chancellor of the Order and contained little text other than the appointee's name, the name of the prior, and the date of appointment. The priory seal was impressed in the lower left usually on a gold seal. In 2007 this certificate was replaced by a bilingual document modelled on the certificate used by the Order of Canada and other Canadian honours.[39] It was also in 2007 that the prior resumed signing the certificates. These were printed on archival quality cotton bond paper, with the seal impressed onto the paper. The new certificate returns to the tradition of a high quality appointment certificate.

Seal of the Order

The seal of the Order used in Canada was adopted in 1985 following alterations made to the Royal Charter. The seal bears the head of St. John the Baptist surrounded by the text SIG : PR : ORD : HOSP : S : JOHIS : HIER : IN CANADA. The seal is impressed on all appointment certificates of the Order, Priory Vote of Thanks Certificates, and other official documents where it is deemed appropriate. The head of St. John the Baptist was displayed on some of the earliest seals of the Order dating back to the fourteenth century. The regulations establishing the commandery of Canada drawn up in 1933 state that the seal "shall be a facsimile of the Seal of the Order with the addition on the face of the name of the Territory where it is to be used."[40]

Investiture Ceremony

Records relating to early investitures are sparse, although we do know that lieutenant-governors often invested appointees into the Order at the various government houses across Canada. As governor general, the Duke of Connaught, who went on to become the longest serving grand prior in the history of the Order, often held investitures at Rideau Hall in Ottawa. As the sovereign's representative in Canada, it was natural for the governor general to act as host for such events. Following the resumption of Canadian appointments to the Order in 1931, the governor general held an investiture in the ballroom at Rideau Hall on 1 March 1932, "We are much indebted to His Excellency for his readiness to hold the Investiture and hope that he will continue to assist the Order in this way,"[41] noted one senior official. The establishment of the Priory of Canada in 1946, and the appointment of Canada's subsequent governors general as priors of the Order further cemented this pattern.

With lieutenant-governors in the provinces acting as vice-priors of the Order after 1946, it became customary for them to hold investitures in their respective provinces once a year. In the early years these were held at a local Anglican church. Since the 1990s locations such as Government House, the provincial legislature, or a government office have been used.

Once a year, a national investiture is held in Ottawa. The tradition had been to conduct these events in the ballroom at Rideau Hall, at Christ Church Cathedral, or at Notre Dame Basilica, but this changed in 1997. That year Governer General Romeo LeBlanc ceased participating in investitures, and this non-participation was continued by Adrienne Clarkson. No official reason has ever given for this, other than it was seen as inconvenient for Rideau Hall staff. In Clarkson's case the lack of involvement may have been related to Clarkson's peculiar attitude towards the Order, which, while warm early in her mandate, became cold. Clarkson was also the first governor general to refuse to wear the mantle of the Order. Governor General Jean has shown a much more genuine interest in the world of the Order, and it is hoped that she will accept to preside over an investiture before the end of her mandate.

With no further national Order of St. John investitures taking place at Rideau Hall, a number of alternative venues have been employed. The National Conference Centre, Notre Dame Basilica, and Christ Church Cathedral in Ottawa were all used for national investiture ceremonies after such events ceased being held at Rideau Hall. In 2006, with the assistance of Senator Marilyn Trenholme Counsell, a former lieutenant-governor of New Brunswick and a Dame of Justice of the Order, the national investiture ceremony was held in the historic Senate Chamber. In this magnificent setting, forty-four Canadians were invested into the Order by Chancellor René Marin on behalf of the prior. The 2007 national investiture ceremony was also held in the Senate Chamber, courtesy of Speaker Noël Kinsella, a long standing Knight of Malta. Members of Canada's Parliament have a historic association with the Order dating back to the establishment of the Canadian branch of the association in 1910. Senate Speaker Hewitt Bostock became involved with St. John Ambulance during the First World War and went on to become president of the Canadian branch from 1928 to 1929.[42] At one time the headquarters of the association were located in the Victoria Building on Wellington Street which today houses Senate offices.

With investitures now taking place in the Senate Chamber, it would appear that a new tradition has been set. Governor General Jeanne Sauvé held a number of Order of Canada investitures in the Senate Chamber, which was an important factor in convincing the Senate that it would be appropriate and fitting for the Order to carry out an investiture there. Following the 2006 and 2007 investitures, a dinner was held in the historic Room 200 of the West Block of the Parliament Buildings, the site of many state dinners and important events in Canadian history.

Chapel of St. John of Jerusalem

In Canada the Chapel of the Order of St. John is located in Montreal at Christ Church Anglican Cathedral. The concept for the Chapel came from the family of Colonel Herbert Molson, former president of the Montreal General Hospital and a Knight Commander of the

Order of St. John. Following his death, his wife made a bequest to Christ Church Cathedral, and on 31 January 1940 the Select Vestry Committee agreed that "the generous gift of Mrs. Molson and her children be accepted and that the Chapel be furnished and beautified as a memorial to the late Colonel Herbert Molson, the work to be carried out by Professor Nobbs under the direction of the Dean and Mr. Jellett as Chairman of the Church Fabric Committee in collaboration with Mr. T.H.P. Molson, representing the donors."[43] The Chapel was designated "The Chapel of St. John of Jerusalem" on 28 May 1940, and it was formally dedicated as part of the Proceedings of the Annual Synod on 23 June 1940 with many members of the Molson family in attendance.

In the floor of the chapel is set a bronze plaque bearing the text "THE CHAPEL OF ST. JOHN OF JERUSALEM — To the glory of God and in loving memory of Lt. Col. Herbert Molson, CMG, MC, VD, 1875–1938."[44] The chapel is located in the north transept of the cathedral and is decorated with several small stained glass windows depicting events from the life of Jesus Christ. Until recently, the cathedral was used for investitures held by the Quebec Provincial Council.

Music

During the Order's centennial year the St. John Centennial March was adopted as the official music for investiture ceremonies. James Gayfer, noted bandmaster and first director of music for the Canadian Forces School of Music, authored the piece, which was completed in 1982. A friend of British composer Ralph Vaughn Williams, Gayfer was a highly accomplished organist, holding a doctorate in music and fellowships in many academic musical societies.

Oblations

Membership in the Order once entailed the payment of annual dues, know as oblations. The amount remitted was directly linked to the level of the Order to which the individual had been appointed. As the Order was both an honour and a working charity, it was seen as fitting to ask and require members to contribute towards the charitable work of the Order annually. There has long been some confusion about the reason for oblations: some viewed them as "payment" to be admitted to the Order, but this is a false conception. Although no other British order of chivalry required the payment of annual dues, "no other order of chivalry does any charitable work and therefore there is no basis of comparison between other Orders and the Order of St. John in this regard."[45] A senior Canadian official of the Order commented "my personal feelings are that I would not want to see any changes [in the payment of oblations] as I feel honoured in being one of those who assists in maintaining the organization."[46] Until the 1980s it had been customary to delete individuals from the membership roll of the

Order if they failed to pay their oblations for three consecutive years. However, explanation notwithstanding, changing times brought an end to this tradition. In 2006 the Priory of Canada decided to abandon oblations. The result has been an increase in annual donations to the Priory of Canada by members of the Order. It is a modern reality that people are often more generous when such giving is not compulsory.

THIRTEEN

SYMBOLS, AWARDS, MEDALS, AND HERALDRY OF THE ORDER OF ST. JOHN

*Gules on a cross Argent a maple leaf Gules, in the first quarter a
representation of the Royal Crest of England.*
Arms of the Priory of Canada
Canadian Heraldic Authority Grant 1999

The broader St. John organization in Canada possesses a number of other honours and awards that do not constitute part of the Order of St. John as an order of chivalry. These include the Service Medal of the Order, two commendations, the Priory Vote of Thanks, the Donat, and the old St. John Ambulance Association first aid medallions and labels. This chapter will examine these awards along with the symbolic elements of St. John and the heraldic grants associated with it.

Service Medal of the Order of St. John

The Service Medal of the Order of St. John was originally approved in 1896 by Chapter-General, although it was not instituted until 1898. The final design was approved by Chapter-General on 31 October 1899. The medal is awarded to members of St. John Ambulance and the Order of St. John who render twelve years of service with a minimum of sixty hours of volunteer service per year. In other parts of the Commonwealth, the medal has been awarded for ten or fifteen years of service.[1] Originally, the medal could also be awarded for meritorious service, although this provision is no longer in effect. The Service Medal of the Order of St. John has been awarded to Canadians since its inception.

The medal itself is a silver-coloured circular medal, 38 mm in diameter. The obverse depicts a veiled effigy of Queen Victoria surrounded by the inscription "VICTORIA : D : G : BRITT : REG : F : D : IND : IMP." The effigy of Victoria was taken from a bust sculpted by her daughter, HRH Princess Louise, consort of Lord Dufferin, governor general of Canada from 1872–78. The reverse of the medal depicts the Royal Arms of the United Kingdom within a garter bearing the motto "*Honi Soit Qui Mal y Pense,*" above the motto is a Tudor crown, and below it is the Prince of Wales's feathers. On either side of the badge of the Order, each bearing a shield — the one on the left charged with the arms of the Order, while the one on the right is charged with the arms of the Prince of Wales. The whole device rests upon a flourish of St. John's wort and is surmounted by the Latin words, *Magnus Prioratus Hospitalis Sancti Johannis Jerusalem in Anglia.*

The ribbon is 38 mm wide, and consists of five equal stripes, three watered black and two white. Bars are awarded for additional periods of service. A thin silver bar with sprigs of St. John's wort and a Maltese cross in the centre is awarded for each five years service period. A maximum of three five-year bars can be awarded. After twenty years of additional service a gilt bar is awarded. Each additional five years of service is recognized with an additional gilt bar.

Table 1

St. John Service Medal Emblems

Years of serving after receiving Service Medal	Emblems worn on the ribbon of the medal	Emblems worn on the undress ribbon
Less than 5	None	None
5	1 silver bar	1 silver cross
10	2 silver bars	2 silver crosses
15	3 silver bars	3 silver crosses
20	1 gilt bar (with the removal of all silver bars)	1 gilt cross (with the removal of all silver crosses)
25	2 gilt bars	2 gilt crosses
30	3 gilt bars	3 gilt crosses
35	4 gilt bars	4 gilt crosses
40	1 gilt laurel leaf (with the removal of all gilt bars)	1 gilt laurel leaf (with the removal of all gilt crosses)

The design of the medal has remained unchanged since 1899, except that between 1899 and 1913 the medal was issued with a ring suspender. This design has been retained as a tribute to the contributions by Queen Victoria, who issued the Royal Charter recognizing the Order, and Edward VII, then the Prince of Wales, who was instrumental in raising the profile of the Order in Britain and throughout the British Empire. This medal remains the most symbolically rich medal in the Canadian honours system. Usually the effigy of the sovereign on medals is changed upon the accession of a new monarch. Queen Victoria remains on the medal, although she has been dead for more than a century. Her granting of a Royal Charter in 1888 remains one of the pivotal events in the Order's history.

The Service Medal was originally struck in sterling silver from 1899 through 1947. From 1948 to 1960, the medal was struck in silver-plated base metal; from 1960 through 1966 in silver-plated cupro-nickel; and since 1966 it has been struck in rhodium-plated base metal.[2] The medal was originally named on the rim, although in Canada this ceased in 1974.[3] A variety of firms have manufactured this medal. Originally it was struck by the noted die engravers J.S. Wyon and Company, H.T. Lamb and Company, and later by the Royal Mint. Most recently the medal has been manufactured by Toye, Kenning and Spencer based in London, England.

Two St. John Service Medals have been awarded in gold, on both occasions to long serving grand priors. The first was awarded to HRH the Prince of Wales, who later became King Edward VII, and the second was awarded to HRH Prince Arthur Duke of Connaught, formerly governor general of Canada, who received his medal in 1935 in honour of the twenty-fifth anniversary of his appointment as grand prior.

In Canada the St. John Service Medal has always been worn after the Queen's/King's Medal for Champion Shot at the end of the order of precedence. Only the Canadian Corps of Commissionaires Medal, created in 1948 and provincial commemorative medals are worn after the St. John Service Medal. The Medal has traditionally been presented by a senior local or national official of the Order of St. John.

Commendations

The Canadian Priory of the Order of St. John possesses two commendations: the Chancellor's Commendation and the Provincial Commendation. Both serve as an intermediate award between the Priory Vote of Thanks and appointment to the Order. The concept behind these commendations is based on the Canadian Forces chief of defence staff and command commendations and the Vice-Regal Commendation.[4] The Chancellor's Commendation is "an exceptional distinction that is personally awarded by the chancellor to recognize a particularly meritorious contribution on the national scene." The Chancellor's Commendation is awarded at the discretion of the chancellor of the Order. The insignia of the Chancellor's Commendation is a gold bar, 3 cm wide, bearing a white enamelled eight-pointed cross in the centre. A circular lapel badge, gold in colour, bearing a white enamelled eight-pointed cross is also included with the bar and award certificate. The first awards of the commendation were made on 23 June 2006, when eight individuals were invested by Chancellor Marin following the Order of St. John investiture dinner held in the West Block of the Parliament Buildings. Unlike the Priory Vote of Thanks, these commendations may be awarded to those who are already members of the Order.

The Provincial Commendation is "an exception distinction that is awarded by the President of a Provincial Council to recognize a particularly meritorious contribution on the provincial scene." The Provincial Commendation is awarded on the recommendation of the local honours and awards committee of St. John. The insignia is a silver bar, 3 cm wide, bearing a white enamelled eight-pointed cross in the centre. A circular lapel badge, silver in colour, bearing a white enamel St. John Cross is also included with the bar and award certificate. The bar insignia for both the Chancellor's and Provincial Commendation are numbered on the reverse. The bar is only worn with medals; it is not worn alone. The lapel badge can be worn on any occasion.

The design concept for the bar and lapel badge were devised with the help of Captain Carl Gauthier from the Department of National Defence. Members of the Canadian Forces and Royal Canadian Mounted Police are permitted to wear the bar on the left pocket of their uniform in the same position as other commendations are worn.

Esquires

Since 2007, persons appointed as Esquires to Knights and Dames of the Order have been considered to hold a specific post, but are not members of the Order. Esquires continue to wear a silver lapel badge, 18 mm in diameter, bearing an eight-pointed embellished white cross. Persons appointed before 2007 have been grandfathered, and can continue to use the post-nominals "Esq.St.J." within the Order.

Other Priory Awards

Aside from the Order, the Priory of Canada possesses a number of other mechanisms to recognize outstanding achievement and service to St. John. These awards include the Priory Vote of Thanks and Honorary Life Membership. Honorary Life Memberships are one of the oldest awards, having been awarded in Canada since the turn of the last century. Honorary Life Membership Certificates are awarded to members of St. John Ambulance upon their retirement from active service. Since 2004, this award has been expanded to include members of Priory Chapter whose term has expired. They are issued with a certificate designating the recipient as an Honorary Life Member of the chapter. Recipients also receive a lapel badge, which is an eight-pointed white cross, 18 mm wide, defaced with the shield of the Order of St. John in red enamel on sterling silver.

The Priory Vote of Thanks (PVOT) is one of the most common awards given by the Order of St. John. In 2007 more than 1,800 PVOT certificates were awarded. These certificates are signed by the prior and bear the name of the recipient. This award began in 1934 as the Commandery Vote of Thanks. The concept behind these awards, considered to be junior to being admitted to the Order, was that a mechanism was required to reward specific service rather than meritorious service over an extended period; it is, in essence, a vote of thanks for good deeds performed. A PVOT cannot be awarded to a person who is already a member of the Order. Beginning in the 1890s, the Grand Priory began awarding Vellum Vote of Thanks, which is described as "The Thanks of the Grand Prior and Chapter General engrossed on Vellum."[5] There was also the Parchment Vote of Thanks, which was described as "Thanks of the Ambulance Committee (St. Johns Gate) on parchment in recognition of distinguished service in furthering the objectives of the Association."[6]

Life Saving Medal of the Order of St. John

This medal was authorized by a statute of the Chapter General in 1871 and instituted on 15 December 1874. The Royal Charter of 1888 refers to it as "The Medal of the Order," which is to be awarded "For Gallantry in Saving Life on Land."[7] Today it is known as the Life Saving Medal of the Order of St. John. It is awarded in three grades, gold, silver, and bronze. The silver and bronze grades have existed since the establishment of the medal, while the gold grade was created in 1907.

That the Order sought to recognize life saving acts is not surprising given that in Victorian Britain there were relatively few rewards for civilian bravery. Other volunteer organizations such as the Royal Humane Society had long possessed bravery awards, which were primarily awarded for saving a person from drowning. Founded in 1774, the Royal Humane Society began to award, and continues to award, medals in gold, silver, and bronze for the saving or attempted saving a human life.[8] There was also the Royal Society for the Protection of Life from Fire, which had its own set of awards for fire related life saving. The annual report of 1874 states clearly that the "medal was issued to fill a gap between the conditions of award of the Royal Humane Society Medal and the Society for the Protection of Life from Fire Medal."[9] It was not until the establishment of the Albert Medal[10] in 1866 that civilians were recognized by the Crown for efforts "in saving or endeavouring to save lives of others."[11] The Albert Medal was rarely awarded and thus the gap in civilian honours for bravery remained until the creation of the George Cross and George Medal in 1940.

The idea for a life saving medal originated with Sir Lechmere in 1869. Lechmere submitted a proposal to Chapter General at St. John's Gate in 1870 and the annual report of that year notes "The want of some system of rewards for acts of bravery upon land, and the supplying of this want, being apparently a work closely connected with the objects of the Order, steps were at once taken to act upon the suggestion."[12] It was noted that awards already existed for saving life at sea and rescue from fire, but that "it appeared that often casualties occur in our mining and colliery districts, and men expose their lives to the greatest risk to rescue their fellow creatures, no recognition from any public body [award] could be obtained, because it was not within the scope of any existing society to reward such merit."[13] It was proposed that "a system of honorary rewards, by means of medals and certificates, should be established on a somewhat similar footing to those granted by the above mentioned societies, but as these latter fully supply the recognition for bravery shown on water, the Order of St. John, desirous not to encroach upon the work of any other public body, has therefore decided to limit its rewards solely to acts of bravery upon land ... especially those which are of so frequent occurrence in our mining and colliery districts."[14]

Indeed, while the Industrial Revolution brought Britain great wealth, it came at a significant cost for labourers and their families: injury and death.[15] By the last half of the nineteenth century the coal mines were perhaps the most deadly, with the annual death toll in the thousands. Thus it was natural for the Order of St. John to desire to establish an award "to those who in their conspicuous act of gallantry have endangered their own lives."[16]

The purpose of the St. John Life Saving Medals retains much of its original purpose. The Life Saving Medal is awarded to a person who:

- has performed a conspicuous act of bravery;
- in performing that act has endangered their own life; and
- has performed that act in saving or attempting to save the life of one or more persons.

The Life Saving Medal can be awarded to any person regardless of their citizenship or where the life saving act was performed, similarly there is no requirement to be involved in St. John Ambulance to receive the medal. The principle of non-duplication is also key: "The Medal or a Bar is not awarded to a person who for the same act has received a national bravery award or an awarded from another body of standing."[17] The medal can be awarded posthumously.

Two different versions of the medal have been awarded and both have been 36 mm in diameter. The first pattern was issued from 1874 to 1888. The obverse depicts the badge of the Order of St. John, without embellishments, and is circumscribed with the text "AWARDED BY THE ORDER OF ST. JOHN OF JERUSALEM IN ENGLAND." The reverse displays a sprig of St. John's Wort and scrolls inscribed with "JERUSALEM, ACRE, CYPRUS, RHODES and MALTA." The entire reverse is circumscribed by the text "FOR THE SERVICE IN THE CAUSE OF HUMANITY." The second pattern, which has been awarded since 1888 contains on the reverse a depiction of the badge of the Order with embellishments, circumscribed by the words "FOR SERVICE IN THE CAUSE OF HUMANITY." The reverse includes a sprig of St. John's Wort and scrolls bearing the words "JERUSALEM and ENGLAND," circumscribed with the text "AWARDED BY THE GRAND PRIORY OF THE ORDER OF THE HOSPITAL OF ST. JOHN OF JERUSALEM IN ENGLAND." Both medals were designed and originally struck by J.S. Wyon and Company. A variety of manufacturers have struck the medal since 1900.

The ribbon from which the medal is hung has changed five times since 1874. From 1874 to 1888 it was plain black, 34 mm, defaced with the badge of the Order without embellishments. From 1888 to 1905, it was plain black and 18 mm wide. In 1905, to allow the medal to be worn with war medals the the ribbon was changed to watered black, 36 mm wide. From 1950 to 1954, the ribbon was watered black, 36 mm wide, edged with 2 mm of scarlet, and two white stripes in the centre, 2 mm wide each. Since 1954, the ribbon has been watered black, 36 mm wide, edged with 2 mm of scarlet and a central 2 mm stripe of white.

From 1874 to 1904, it was worn on the right breast, apart from official honours. This policy was changed in 1905 when the Life Saving Medal was, in essence, incorporated into the British honours system. From 1905 to 1936 the medal was worn on the left breast (the crown side) after decorations but before campaign and war medals, thus holding a place of honour in the order of precedence. In 1936 the Central Chancery of the Orders of Knighthood, the office of the Royal Household responsible for honours, moved the medal to the right breast.[18]

Canada did not, however, follow suit on this matter and the medal continued to be worn on the left breast by Canadians until late 1948. The Department of National Defence failed to incorporate the 1936 change made by the Central Chancery and it was only after an inquiry by W.J. Bennett, commandery secretary, that the change was made "I will have to advise our Department of National Defence of this, as recently we received a copy of orders in which they indicated the Life Saving Medal should be worn on the left breast."[19] Thus, this medal returned to the right breast where it continues to be worn on St. John uniforms. Given the existence of official bravery decorations it is not longer authorized to be worn by members of the Canadian Forces.

Canadians have received all three medals, five gold, forty-six silver, and 116 bronze. The awards of this medal made in the years immediately following its establishment were exclusively to people living in the British Isles. The first Commonwealth award was made in 1888 to E. Smaller of the India Railways Service, who was awarded the medal for saving an Indian lady who had become incapacitated on a railway crossing.[20]

The first Canadian recipient of the Life Saving Medal was Conductor Thomas Reynolds of the Canadian Pacific Railway (CPR).[21] Reynolds was one of the many CPR employees who earned a St. John First Aid Certificate as part of the extensive first aid training program started by the St. John Ambulance Association for railway employees in 1908.

On 21 January 1910 a CPR express train left Sudbury for Minneapolis at noon. On reaching the bridge crossing the Spanish River near Webbwood, Ontario, at a point where the stream is 76 metres wide and 10 metres deep, the first class car and dining car left the track and plunged down the embankment. Reynolds and several passengers were seated in the dining car when it crashed through the ice which was 45-centimetres thick, the first class car quickly settled on the riverbed 3.5 metres below, and it is believed that no one escaped. The dining car was however not completely submerged, although the front of the car rapidly filled with water, all the occupants who were hurled to that end during the collision with the ice were in danger of drowning. Reynolds, in coming to the surface, found the top window some 15 centimetres above the water, he smashed the heavy plate glass with his feet, and dived and pushed himself through, having great difficult in preventing the strong current from washing him away. He succeeded in making his way between the broken ice and the car and gained a foothold in the top of the latter. He wrenched a fanlight from the roof and rescued a lad and another passenger through this small opening. Shortly afterwards in response to his cries, an axe was brought and he was then able to enlarge the opening sufficiently to allow the rescue of other injured passengers. Conductor Reynolds was badly cut and injured, and his recovery took more than a month.

Following his recovery, Reynolds was presented with the St. John's Life Saving Medal in silver at Government House Ottawa on 26 July 1910 by Lord Grey, the governor general, who was acting on behalf of the grand prior, the Duke of Connaught, who would become Canada's governor general less than a year later.

It was not until 1946 that the first Gold Life Saving Medal was awarded to a Canadian,

Leonard Rissanen, "[a] member of the Brigade in Port Arthur, who at great personal risk rendered first aid to several men and removed them to safety at the time of a grain elevator explosion and who continued to search for injured men in the face of imminent danger from new explosions and falling wreckage."[22] A silver lifesaving medal was awarded to Carl Frederick Mellerup for his bravery in the same incident. Sergeant Lawrence Zimmerman of the Toronto Police Force was one of the most recent recipients of the Life Saving Medal, being invested with the medal in silver in June 2006.

Given the existence of three national bravery awards in the Canadian honours system that are open to civilians, the Cross of Valour, Star of Courage, and Medal of Bravery, the awarding of the St. John Life Saving Medal has become much more limited.

Certificates of Honour

In addition to the Life Saving Medal, there is also the Certificate of Honour. Ranked below the Bronze Life Saving Medal, the Certificate of Honour is awarded for lesser yet significant acts of bravery. The Certificate of Honour is awarded to a person who:

- has performed a conspicuous act of bravery;
- has performed that act in saving or attempting to save the life of one or more persons; and
- has performed that act in circumstances which do not merit the award of the Life Saving Medal.

Recipients of this certificate receive a document signed by the chancellor of the Order bearing their name.

Donat

The Order of St. John possesses a unique mechanism to recognize philanthropy and those who make significant donations of funds through the presentation of a Donat insignia. Section 38 of the 1888 Royal Charter makes reference to "Donats" as "persons who, from an appreciation of the works of the Order, have contributed to its funds."[23]

The first mention of Donats appeared in the 1862 statutes of the Order. Originally, Donats did not receive an insignia; they were simply sent a copy of the annual report. The Donat insignia was instituted in 1910, with three levels gold, silver, and bronze. The idea for a Donat insignia was taken directly from the Sovereign Military Order of Malta, which has long possessed such a mechanism to recognize philanthropy directed towards the Order.

Although the Order of St. John Donat is not part of the Canadian honours system — being restricted for wear at Order of St. John functions and then only on the right side, opposite from official honours — it represents an important internal award used by the Order to recognize philanthropy. Recipients of the Donat are not members of the Order of St. John, and if they are subsequently appointed to the Order, they cease to wear the Donat badge.

The insignia is a demi-cross, identical to that of the Order of St. John, 38 mm in width, with white enamel, but the upper arm is replaced by a piece of ornamental metal that is not enamelled. A ring suspension is attached to the top of the insignia and it is hung from ribbon. The ribbon is watered black, 38 mm wide, with a 2 mm white stripe down the centre.

On 23 June 2006, Sidney Sharman of Nanaimo, British Columbia, was presented with a Diamond Donat in recognition of his unprecedented gift of one million dollars to St. John Ambulance. This was the first time in Canada that a Diamond Donat was presented, indeed the use of Donats as a mechanism to recognize philanthropic gifts to the Order has been in decline for the past twenty years.

St. John Ambulance Association Medallions and Labels

An important part of completing a St. John Ambulance first aid course was receiving a first aid certificate. Pupils were encouraged to maintain their first aid proficiency by taking a first aid course every year, to learn about new techniques and improve their skills. If an individual successfully completed a first aid course two years in a row they were awarded what was known as the St. John Ambulance Association First Aid Medallion. Shaped in the form of a cross and defaced with an eight-pointed cross in the centre the Medallion was engraved with the recipients name on the reverse and an issue number. In subsequent years upon successful completion of a first aid course the St. John Ambulance Association issued a label, which was a small bar bearing the year of completion. These bars were attached to the top of the medallion, and it was not uncommon to see some first aiders with upwards of twenty labels attached to their St. John Ambulance Association First Aid Medallion. Each of the labels was engraved with the same issue number as the medallion. These served as "proof" of a person's up-to-date first aid qualifications.

Women tended to wear the medallion around the neck on a thin black ribbon, while men simply kept the medallion and attached labels on their person for presentation. Each medallion recipient was registered with St. John's Gate in London. While most medallions were issued in bronze, special sterling silver and carat gold issues could be purchased for an additional cost.

The first medallions were awarded to a group of sixteen women from Toronto in 1896.[24] In Canada the awarding of medallions and labels ceased in 1959.

• • •

The most recognizable symbol of the Order of St. John is the eight-pointed cross. It has been used by the Order in Canada since its inception, and by the Order worldwide practically since its foundation. Also known as the Amalfi Cross and Maltese cross, it is a highly potent and pervasive symbol of the Order and its good works. The eight-pointed cross has a long history in Canada, dating back to New France and Acadia [25]

Regalia

With the establishment of the Priory of Canada there was a desire to replicate many of the traditions, regalia, and customs of other priories. In typical St. John fashion a special committee was struck to "find out what ceremonial paraphernalia our Priory in Canada requires."[26] Officials at St. John's Gate were keen to help and wrote in some detail about the need for a Sword of Temporal Jurisdiction "which is carried immediately before the Prior, or Presiding Officer in procession to from the meeting of the Priory Chapter and lies before him during their meetings."[27] It was also thought that the new Priory of Canada should possess a banner, something akin to a regimental colour, displaying the "arms of the Order or of the Priory"[28] for use during processions. Another element that was mentioned was a processional cross, which displayed the eight-pointed cross of the Order in white on a background. "This should be carried in front of the clergy in any procession of the Order."[29] The priory took no immediate action on the costly task of acquiring a sword,[30] or Priory Banner

The sword would come in the form of a gift. On 28 February 1952 Sir Otto Lund, commissioner-in-chief of the brigade in the United Kingdom presented the Priory of Canada with an exact replica of a late 15th century weapon commonly known as a hand-and-one-half-sword. The steel hilt of the sword is plated with silver and carries a kite-shaped pommel embossed with the shield of the Order. Swords of similar design had previously been presented to the Grand Priory and the Priory of Australia. The scabbard of the sword is decorated with the embellished eight-pointed white cross. Sir Otto presented the sword to Chancellor C.A. Gray in the presence of several hundred members of the brigade and association. For St. John Ambulance the sword is akin to a mace of authority and continues to be used in all the Order's major ceremonies across the country.

It was not until 1960 that the Priory gained a physical banner. Donated by Donald F. Angus of Montreal, the banner consisted of a white cross on a red field, with a natural maple leaf in the centre and the royal crest in the canton.[31] This particular banner was retired in 1999 when the Priory of Canada was granted arms by the Canadian Heraldic Authority. The current banner is almost identical in design except for two small changes. The maple leaf in the centre is red in colour, not autumnal green, and the royal crest in the canton displays the St. Edwards Crown surmounted by a lion, replacing the Tudor Crown surmounted by a lion.

Colours of the Order and the Eight-pointed Cross

The basic design of all the insignia used by the Order of St. John, along with the colours used by the Order can be traced back to the Order of Malta, and represent part of the Order's shared heritage.

The Order of St. John has three official colours, black, white, and red. The original hospital built in Jerusalem in the eleventh century was affiliated with the Benedictine Church of St. Mary the Latin. As with a number of religious orders, the Benedictines wore black robes. It has been noted that "their habit was the black *cappa clausa* — that is, the long monastic bell-like cloak, with a slit on each side for the arms, and a white cross on the breast, which ultimately took the form of the eight-pointed cross included in the arms of the Republic of Amalfi."[32] According to Elias Ashmole, the 17th century historian of the Most Noble Order of the Garter, "the Knights of this Order [St. John] then took the black habit of Hermitis of St. Augustine, and lived under his rule ... and on the Breast of the habit wore, at first a plain cross of white cloth, since changed to one with eight points [a Maltese cross]."[33] Thus two different accounts exist as to the origins of the colour, black being one of the Order's official colours. Black Robes were subsequently adopted by the Order of Malta, and later the Order of St. John. This is the principal reason why both the robes of the Order of St. John and the ribbon from which the insignia of the Order is hung are black in colour.

Sometime before the thirteenth century, the Order of Malta adopted "a pall of red with a white cross on it."[34] In the middle of the thirteenth century, knights of the Order of Malta were permitted to wear surcoats of plain red superimposed with a white cross. This cross has always appeared as a plain cross of equal proportions. This combination of red and white is the basis for the coat of arms used by the Order of Malta and the various priories of the Order of St. John throughout the world.

The Order of St. John's familiar eight-pointed cross, may also be referred to as the Amalfi Cross, St. John Cross, or Maltese Cross. This historic symbol is shared with the Sovereign and Military Hospitaller Order of St. John of Jerusalem, of Rhodes and of Malta (the Order of Malta), and the Johanniter Orden which is active in a number of European countries. The common historic foundations of these three organizations, and their relatively recent rekindled fellowship make it necessary to recognize that the eight-pointed cross is a shared symbol, one with deep historic roots.

The earliest known statutes of the Order of Malta reveal that members of the Order were required to wear a white cross on their clothing. Initially the white cross was not the eight-pointed variety, but was likely a plain cross. According to Tozer, it was not until the end of the fifteenth century that the eight-pointed cross was formally adopted,[35] and by that point, this had become the custom of the Order.

The eight points of the St. John Cross hold both a religious and secular meaning, reflecting the Order's history as a religious organization, and the secular qualities of a good first aider. The religious meanings are taken from Chapter Five of the Gospel of St. Matthew in the New Testament, the Beatitudes:

- Blessed are the poor in spirit, for theirs is the Kingdom of Heaven.
- Blessed are they that mourn, for they shall be comforted.
- Blessed are the meek, for they shall inherit the earth.
- Blessed are they that hunger and thirst after righteousness.
- Blessed are the merciful, for they shall obtain mercy.
- Blessed are the pure of heart, for they shall see God.
- Blessed are the peacemakers, for they shall be called Sons of God.

- Blessed are they that have been persecuted for righteousness' sake, for theirs is the Kingdom of Heaven.
- Blessed are ye when men shall reproach you, and persecute you, and say all manner of evil against you falsely for My sake.

As the First Aid work of St. John grew, the council of the Order in England assigned each point of the cross a meaning "specially applicable to the essential qualities of a First Aider":[36]

- Observation
- Tact
- Resourcefulness
- Dexterity
- Explicitness
- Discrimination (i.e., being able to treat the most serious injuries first)
- Perseverance
- Sympathy

The eight-pointed cross "embellished" with the lion passant guardant and the unicorn passant in the alternating angles was adopted by the tongue of England when it was re-established in 1831. The lion and unicorn were chosen as they were — and continue to be — used as the supporters of the Royal Arms of the United Kingdom and the Royal Arms of Scotland. These two creatures are also the supporters of the Royal Arms of Canada, which have been in use since 1921. The Order of Malta uses a fleur-de-lys between each arm of the eight-pointed cross, along with the heraldic shield of the Order, and a crown. The tongue of Italy utilized fleurs-de-lys between the angles of the arms, while the Johanniter Orden used a winged eagle between the angles of the arms, thus it was necessary for the English tongue to differentiate its insignia from that of other tongues.

St. John's Wort, known in scientific circles as *Hypercium perforatum*, is a type of shrub that usually blossoms with yellow flowers around St. John's day. This is one of the main reasons that the plant has been adopted as the Order's official floral emblem. In medieval times it was collected and nailed above doors and windows to serve as protection against evil spirits. Thought to have some medicinal qualities, it was often used to help ease nerve pain. The plant was also ground into a paste with water and used as a salve for open wounds. In recent years it has been used as a natural treatment for mild depression.[37]

Motto

Unlike other Canadian and British orders, the Order of St. John possesses two mottoes. Given that the Order is the only Canadian order that is both a charitable organization involved in humanitarian works and an honour — that is, part of the national honours system — it is fitting that the Order be embodied in two phrases. The mottoes are used in tandem and usually only appear with the priory coat of arms.

The two mottoes of the Order: "*Pro Fide*" and "*Pro Utilitate Hominum*," are best described in the context of the purpose and objects of the Order. The encouragement of all that makes for the moral and spiritual strengthening of mankind in accordance with the first great principle of the Order, embodied in its motto "'*Pro Fide*,' (For the Faith)."[38] "The encouragement and promotion of all works of humanity and charity for the relief of persons in sickness, distress, suffering, danger, without distinction of race, class or creed, and the extension of the second great principle of the Order, embodied in its motto '*Pro Utilitate Hominum*' (For the Service of Humanity)."[39]

Heraldry

Many of the heraldic elements of the Order of St. John can be traced to the founding of the Order in 1099. The plain white cross on a red field is used by the Order of Malta, the Order of St. John, and the Johanniter Orden. From 1888 to 1926, the Order of St. John used the same shield as the Order of Malta but with lions and unicorns in the alternating angles. The embellishments were removed from the shield in 1926 after Prince Arthur, Duke of Connaught, petitioned King George V to permit the Order to use the "Royal Crest" (a lion guardant atop a royal crown) in the first quarter of the shield, heraldically described as a "Cross in the first quarter a representation of Our Royal Crest."[40] On the occasion of the impending reorganization of the Order and the granting of a new Royal Charter in 1926, King George V granted this honour.

Until 1946, the St. John Ambulance Association's Canadian branch, and later the Commandery in Canada, simply used an embellished eight-pointed white cross on a black disc on documents and as its principal symbol. When the Priory of Canada was established, a new coat of arms and banner were adopted. Identical in design to that used in England, the centre of the white cross was defaced by a natural maple leaf (originally green, it is now red). Largely through the efforts of Chancellor Ted Beament and Yvette Loiselle, the Canadian Heraldic Authority granted these arms 16 September 1999 along with the banner of the priory. The arms and banner of the priory are based on the arms and banners used in other priories, where the central device indicates the specific priory. Thus for Canada the device is a maple leaf, while for England uses a rose, and New Zealand uses a fern leaf. The St. John Ambulance Badge, which dates from 1982, comprises a red maple leaf, defaced with a black disc containing an eight-pointed white cross. This was formally adopted as the badge of St. John Ambulance in Canada and is generally treated as the "logo" of the organization. It was granted as a badge by the Canadian Heraldic Authority in 1999 with the addition of white edging around the disc.

The practice of displaying the insignia of honours with coats of arms can be traced back to the early fifteenth century, shortly after the establishment of the Order of the Garter. Knights of the Garter would often encircle the shields of their arms with the motto of the order, a practice that became commonplace by the reign of Henry VII (1485–1509).

It was only in the early nineteenth century that it became common for the actual insignia of orders to be hung from the shield of a person's coat of arms. In more recent times, it has been customary for the holders of the higher ranks of the British orders of chivalry (knights and dames, companions, and commanders) to surround their shield with the circlet bearing the motto of the Order to which they belong.

In Canada, the general rule related to the inclusion of the insignia of orders and decorations in heraldic grants is that such insignia must be an official honour from the Crown. In the case of Commonwealth and foreign orders and decorations, the award must have been approved by the government Honours Policy Sub-Committee, which acts on behalf of the Queen. Although members of the Order of Canada, Order of Military Merit, and Order of Merit of the Police Forces are all entitled to surround their shields with the motto circlet of their senior most order, the Order of St. John follows a different and more ancient practice.

The heraldic practice of including some symbolic element signifying membership in the Order is very old. Knights of the Order of Malta and later of the "the Hospital of St. John in England display above their personal arms a chief of the order."[41]

The Royal Charter sets out that Bailiffs Grand Cross and Dames Grand Cross may add supporters to their arms. In addition, they may bear their arms on the badge of the Order, and include the arms of the Order in their arms in the chief position. Knights and Dames of the Order, whether they are of Justice or of Grace, are permitted to bear their arms over the badge of the Order, and suspend insignia from their shields. Commanders, Officers, and Members are simply permitted to hang the ribbon and insignia of their particular grade from their shield of arms.

Only a person who is armigerous can accede to the "Knight/Dame of Justice" grade of the Order. The confirmation whether or not a person is eligible to become a Knight/Dame of Justice is made by the priory genealogist. Both the College of Arms (England) and the Court of the Lord Lyon (Scotland) have "Officers of Arms" (heralds) appointed as priory genealogists in the respective priories. While the Priory of Canada does possess a genealogist, this post is not, and has never been held by a serving officer of arms employed by the Canadian Heraldic Authority (CHA). A working relationship has been developed between the Priory of Canada and the CHA. Before any reclassification of a Knight/Dame of Grace to a Knight/Dame of Justice, the CHA is consulted to confirm whether or not the candidate is armigerous. Since 1992, reclassification of Knights/Dames has been published in the *Canada Gazette*.

One honours historian has noted that this process of informal consultation, and absence of a herald who is concurrently priory genealogist, is not a literal implementation of the Royal Charter with regard to the practice of reclassification.[42] The same expert also commented "the Chancellery does not appreciate the importance of supporting the installation of a Herald as Priory Genealogist."[43] No doubt the Priory of Canada would welcome the appointment of a member of the Canadian Heraldic Authority to serve as genealogist. Indeed, given the regulations associated with the other Canadian orders, it would be appropriate for CHA heralds to be appointed heralds to each of Canada's national orders.

The first grant of arms from the Canadian Heraldic Authority to include the insignia of the Order was to James R. Breithaupt, CStJ, who was granted arms on 10 October 1990. Subsequently grants have been made depicting the insignia of every grade of the Order to both men and women. Three of Canada's eight grand crosses have been granted arms, Yvette Loiselle, Cy Laurin, and Eric Barry.

Depicted in the photo section are representations of the arms of four members of the Order. Eric Barry's grant includes the sash insignia of Bailiff Grand Cross. His shield is superimposed upon an eight-pointed white cross, which is a further indication of his appointment to the Bailiff or Knight/Dame grades of the Order. Dr. Marie des Agnes Loyer's grant of arms depicts the insignia of a Dame of Grace. In the year following the presentation of Dr. Loyer's arms her appointment to the Order was reclassified and she is now a Dame of Justice. The grant of Owen William Lockyer includes three insignia, Officer of the Order of Military Merit, Officer of the Order of St. John, and the Canadian Forces Decoration. Lastly Bruce Patterson's grant includes the insignia of a Serving Brother.

CONCLUSION

From the labours of the Blessed Gerard to the modern day hospitaller work of St. John Ambulance, the motto of *pro utilitate hominum* — for the service of humanity — remains the driving principle and purpose behind the Order of St. John. The modern day hospitaller work continues through the provision of first aid training and first aid services, to people throughout Canada and in the broader context of the Most Venerable Order, around the globe.

The Order has made a significant contribution to Canada over the past century and a quarter. During the two world wars and in times of disaster St. John Ambulance has been present, taking a leading role in the relief efforts. St. John Ambulance was present following the Halifax Explosion, Influenza Epidemic, S.S. *Noronic* fire, Westray mining disaster, and the 1998 Ontario–Quebec Ice Storm, providing important aid and assistance to victims of circumstance. Countless lives have been saved through St. John first aid training, and its full influence can never be known, simply because of its ubiquity: One life saved can have an immeasurable impact.

The historic relationship with the Department of National Defence, Royal Canadian Mounted Police, Canadian National Railway, and Canadian Pacific Railway has seen St. John Ambulance through periods of difficulty and success. Through the 1920s without the patronage of these entities, the fate of St. John Ambulance first aid training in Canada would have been uncertain. That the impetus for first aid training came from workers and employers alike is further evidence of the mutually beneficial effect of such training has right to the present time.

The bit of silver tinsel hung from a black ribbon would have little meaning without the work of St. John Ambulance. Our ceremonies and history give us a context of who we are, and the first aid work of the Order gives us a modern identity and purpose. The Order holds a privileged place in Canada in that we are the only volunteer organization to comprise part of the national honours system. Our special relationship with the Crown, through the Queen, governor general, and lieutenant-governors is an important asset; we honour them and the history of the Order through our service to humanity. Losing sight of the importance of first aid work would reduce the Order to little more than it was in England during the 1830s — a society of honour for honours sake, void of any meaningful purpose.

Members of St. John Ambulance have always been innovators, much as the original Knights Hospitaller were during the Crusades with their tent hospital and treatment methods.

In times of peace and war, St. John Ambulance has continued this tradition of innovation. Shining examples include the VAD movement of which St. John Ambulance became the principal part, the first ski patrols set up in the late 1920s, through to the therapy dogs of today. Other less obvious innovations have included the publication of the first widely available French language first aid manual in Canada, and the provision of bilingual subtitles for training films released in the early 1920s. An open and accepting order that pioneered the involvement of women, we must continue to welcome Canadians from all walks of life, religions, genders, and cultural groups into our family.

Through the alliance with other orders of St. John, we are linked both to our past and our common hospitaller tradition. These relationships enrich our experience as a charity and can offer valuable lessons.

Throughout our history in times of great crisis, St. John Ambulance has worked closely with other organizations, most notably the Canadian Red Cross. The remarkable achievements of these organizations during the two world wars of the last century were unprecedented. Looking towards the future, it can be hoped that points of contention once held can be put aside. It is time for these noble organizations to enter a new period of increasing cooperation. Both the Red Cross and St. John Ambulance have a common founder in this country, George Sterling Ryerson. Our common founder and history of cooperation is much more potent than the conflicts that have hampered relations.

What is the future of St. John Ambulance? A hagiographical response to this would be one of glowing promise and hope. Such platitudes should be tempered with reality. In the past decade, at the national level, and in some provinces, St. John Ambulance came precariously close to going bankrupt. Although this would not have necessarily resulted in the end to our work, it would have severely impaired the effectiveness of the overall organization as a provider of first aid services and training. We have a bright future ahead; with sound stewardship, prudent planning, and by maintaining our innovative spirit the work of the Order can become an even greater force for good.

Appendix A

Canadian Honours Post-Nominals
1867–2008

Senior Canadian Valour Decorations

VC   Victoria Cross

CV   Cross of Valour

Canadian Orders

CC	Companion of the Order of Canada
OC	Officer of the Order of Canada
CM*	Member of the Order of Canada
SM	Medal of Service of the Order of Canada (became Officer of the Order of Canada in 1972)
CMM	Commander of the Order of Military Merit
OMM	Officer of the Order of Military Merit
MMM	Member of the Order of Military Merit
COM	Commander of the Order of Merit of the Police Forces
OOM	Officer of the Order of Merit of the Police Forces
MOM	Member of the Order of Merit of the Police Forces
CVO	Commander of the Royal Victorian Order
LVO	Lieutenant of the Royal Victorian Order
MVO	Member of the Royal Victorian Order
RVM	Royal Victorian Medal
GCStJ	Bailiff/Dame Grand Cross of the Most Venerable Order of the Hospital of St. John of Jerusalem
DStJ	Dame Commander of the Most Venerable Order of the Hospital of St. John of Jerusalem
KStJ	Knight Commander of the Most Venerable Order of the Hospital of St. John of Jerusalem

CStJ   Commander of the Most Venerable Order of the Hospital of St. John of Jerusalem

OStJ   Officer of the of the Most Venerable Order of the Hospital of St. John of Jerusalem

SBStJ   Serving Brother of the Most Venerable Order of the Hospital of St. John of Jerusalem

SSStJ   Serving Sister of the Most Venerable Order of the Hospital of St. John of Jerusalem

MStJ   Member of the Most Venerable Order of the Hospital of St. John of Jerusalem

EsqStJ   Esquire of the Most Venerable Order of the Hospital of St. John of Jerusalem

Canadian Military Valour Decorations

SMV   Star of Military Valour

MMV   Medal of Military Valour

Canadian Bravery Decorations

SC   Star of Courage

MB   Medal of Bravery

Canadian Meritorious Service Decorations

MSC   Meritorious Service Cross

MSM   Meritorious Service Medal

Canadian Long Service Decoration

CD   Canadian Forces Decoration

Other

PC   Privy Councillor

Senior British Valour Decorations

VC   Victoria Cross

GC   George Cross

British Orders of Chivalry and Knighthood

KG/LG   Knight of the Garter/Lady of the Order of the Garter

KT/LT   Knight of the Thistle/Lady of the Order of the Thistle

KP   Knight of the Order of St. Patrick

OM   Order of Merit

CH   Companions of Honour

GCB   Knight Grand Cross of the Order of the Bath

KCB	Knight Commander of the Order of the Bath
CB	Commander of the Order of the Bath
GCMG	Knight Grand Cross of the Order of St. Michael and St. George
KCMG	Knight Commander of the Order of St. Michael and St. George
CMG	Commander of the Order of St. Michael and St. George
GCSI	Knight Grand Commander of the Order of the Star of India
KCSI	Knight Commander of the Order of the Star of India
CSI	Commander of the Order of the Star of India
GCVO	Knight Grand Cross of the Royal Victorian Order
KCVO	Knight Commander of the Royal Victorian Order
CVO	Commander of the Royal Victorian Order
LVO	Lieutenant of the Royal Victorian Order
MVO	Member of the Royal Victorian Order
GCIE	Grand Commander of the Order of the Indian Empire
KCIE	Knight Commander of the Order of the Indian Empire
CIE	Commander of the Order of the Indian Empire
GBE	Knight/Dame Grand Cross of the Order of the British Empire
DBE	Dame of the Order of the British Empire
KBE	Knight Commander of the Order of the British Empire
CBE	Commander of the Order of the British Empire
OBE	Officer of the Order of the British Empire
MBE	Member of the Order of the British Empire
BEM	British Empire Medal
ISO	Imperial Service Order
CI	Companion of the Order of the Crown of India
Bt	Baronet of the United Kingdom
Kt	Knight Bachelor (also sometimes listed as KB)

British Bravery Decorations

AM	Albert Medal
GM	George Medal
DSO	Distinguished Service Order
DSC	Distinguished Service Cross
MC	Military Cross
DFC	Distinguished Flying Cross
AFC	Air Force Cross
DCM	Distinguished Conduct Medal
DSM	Distinguished Service Medal
MM	Military Medal

DFM	Distinguished Flying Medal
AFM	Air Force Medal
EGM	Empire Gallantry Medal

British Long Service Decorations

ED	Efficiency Decoration
TD	Territorial Decoration
RD	Reserve Decoration
VD	Volunteer Decoration

APPENDIX B

CANADIAN GRAND CROSSES

Being appointed a Bailiff Grand Cross of Dame Grand Cross of the Most Venerable Order of the Hospital of St. John of Jerusalem is the most significant honour that can be bestowed upon any person involved with St. John Ambulance. At any given time the total number of grand crosses is limited to twenty-one for the entire Order worldwide. It is a rare honour.

The first Canadian Bailiff Grand Cross was appointed before Queen Victoria's Royal Charter of 1888 and thus, he is not included in the list below. Sir Alan Napier MacNab was the first Canadian to be appointed to Order of St. John after its revival in 1831. As a long serving member of the Legislative Assembly of Canada, aide-de-camp to Queen Victoria and premier of the Province of Canada[1] from 1854 to 1855, MacNab was appointed as a Knight of Justice in 1842 during a visit to London. He was subsequently appointed a Bailiff Grand Cross on 20 August 1855.[2] MacNab also served as the preceptor of the Order of Canada and was, in theory at least, its principal promoter.

Aside from MacNab, there have been only eight Canadian Grand Crosses, five Bailiffs and three Dames. These are the leaders who built and lead St. John Ambulance in Canada, and around the world:

The Right Honourable Vincent Massey, PC, CH, CC, GCStJ, CD
Massey remains the most prominent Canadian to have been appointed a Grand Cross. His involvement with the Order began in the late days of the First World War and he would go on to become involved with the work of the association through the 1930s. In many ways Massey was Canada's first diplomat, serving first as Canada's minister plenipotentiary to Washington from 1927 to 1930 and later as the Canadian high commissioner to the United Kingdom from 1935 until 1946. King George VI appointed Massey as Canada's first native born governor general in 1952. Massey was appointed a Commander of the Order in 1934, and subsequently was made a Knight of Grace while serving as Canadian high commissioner. In 1955, while serving as prior, Massey was made a Bailiff Grand Cross. He remained a proud supporter and member of the Order until his death in 1967.

Margaret MacLaren, GCStJ
Canada's first Dame Grand Cross served as superintendent-in-chief from 1946 until 1963. MacLaren played an important part in the development of the nursing divisions throughout

Canada and also in the drafting of the 1951 agreement between St. John Ambulance and the Red Cross. Throughout her time as superintendent-in-chief she encouraged the expansion of female involvement in the work of the brigade and association. Suffice to say her contributions permeated every aspect of St. John Ambulance throughout the country. In 1960 she headed a delegation that visited the Eye Hospital in Jerusalem. MacLaren was invested as a Dame Grand Cross by the prior, Major General Vanier just months before her death in 1963.

Commissioner Leonard Nicholson, OC, MBE, GCStJ

A graduate of the Royal Military College of Canada, Nicholson would serve in the New Brunswick Provincial Police and later the Nova Scotia Provincial Police before joining the RCMP. During the Second World War he served as provost marshal of the Canadian Provost Corps (Military Police) and would be appointed commissioner of the RCMP in 1951. He oversaw a massive expansion of the RCMP throughout Canada. In 1960 following his resignation from the RCMP he served as chief commissioner of the brigade in Canada and would later serve as chancellor of the Order from 1969 to 1972. His chancellorship was marked by new efforts to modernize the operations and outreach of St. John Ambulance. He was appointed a Bailiff Grand Cross in 1971, a dignity he enjoyed until his death in 1983.

Kathleen Gilmour, MBE, GCStJ

Throughout her entire adult life "Kay" Gilmour was active in the work of St. John Ambulance and played an important role in building the organization. During the Second World War she was responsible for the recruitment of VADs from across Canada and would travel to London to set up the brigade's VAD headquarters in London. For this extraordinary contribution she was awarded the Service Medal with Palms by Lord Alexander in 1946. Gilmour served as lady superintendent-in-chief from 1943 to 1946. After her retirement she remained active in the work of the brigade, even organizing a 1975 reunion of VADs who had served in the First and Second World Wars. Canada's second Dame Grand Cross was appointed in 1975. Five years later, in 1980 one of the most public faces of St. John Ambulance and the most persistent reminder of the war service rendered by St. John Ambulance passed away.

Brigadier-General Cyrille J. Laurin, OBE, GCStJ

A veteran of the Second World War, at the age of thirty-three, Laurin became one of the youngest brigadier-generals in Canadian history. A highly effective administrator he went on to work as publisher for MacLean-Hunter. As director of the association he worked on meeting the demands of the early 1970s, when an increasing number of public servants were required to take first aid training. He was active in the preparations for the 1976 Olympics and the part that the brigade played in it. Laurin served as chancellor of the Order from 1978 to 1981, and oversaw a significant increase in the number of Canadians taking first aid from St. John Ambulance and further growth in the size of the brigade. He was appointed a Bailiff Grand Cross of the Order in 1980 and died in 1999.

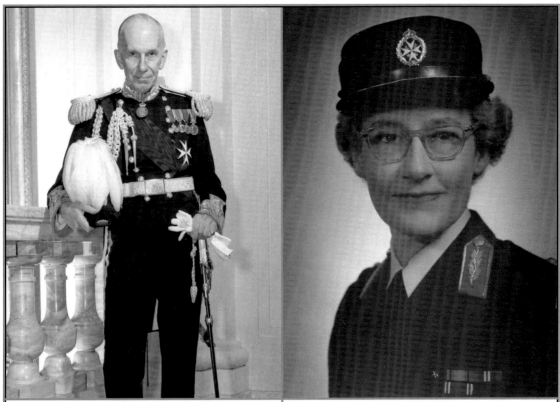

The Right Honourable Vincent Massey, PC, CH, CC, GCStJ, CD

Margaret MacLaren, GCStJ

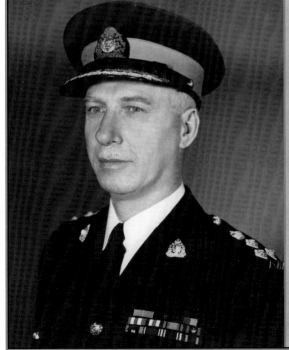

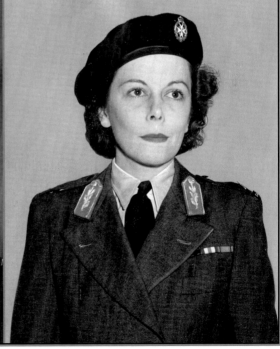

Commissioner Leonard Nicholson, OC, MBE, GCStJ

Kathleen Gilmour, MBE, GCStJ

Plate 18   Canadian Bailiffs and Dames Grand Cross

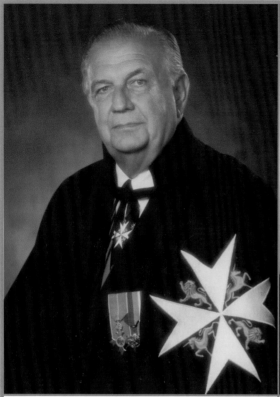

Brigadier General Cyrille J. Laurin,
OBE, GCStJ

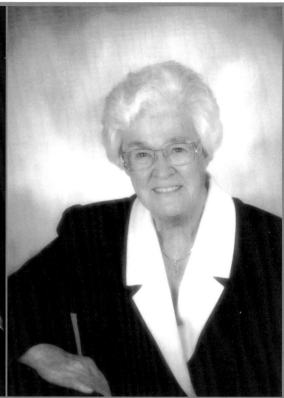

Yvette Loiselle, CM, GCStJ

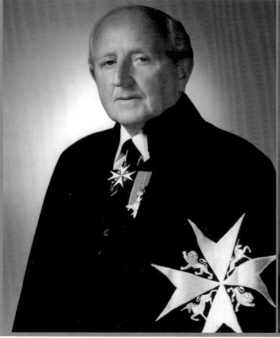

Brigadier General George Edwin Beament,
OBE, CM, GCStJ, ED, CD, QC

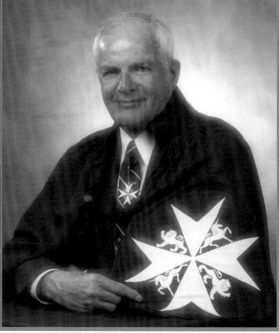

Lieutenant Colonel Eric L. Barry, GCStJ, CD

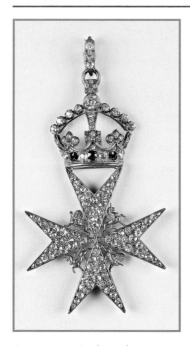

Sovereign's Sash Badge.

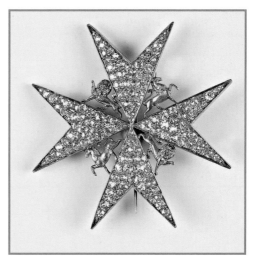

Sovereign's Breast Star.

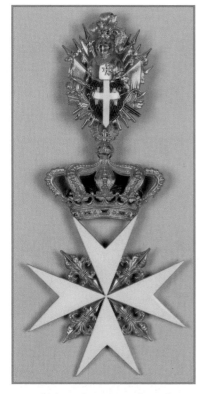

King Edward VII's Order of
Malta Insignia.

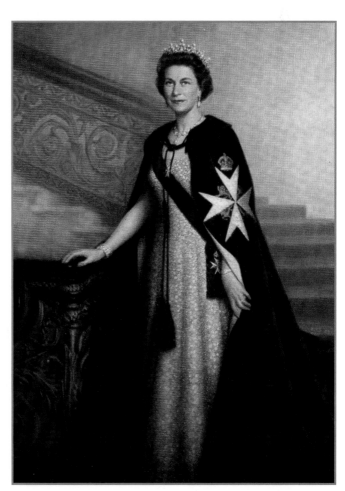

Queen Elizabeth II wearing the Sovereign's Insignia.

Plate 20
Chains of Office of the Priory of Canada

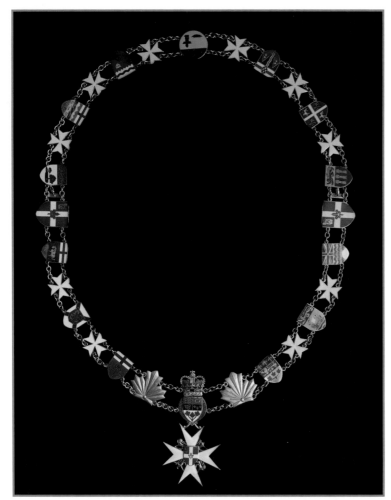

Chain of Office of the Prior of the Priory of Canada.

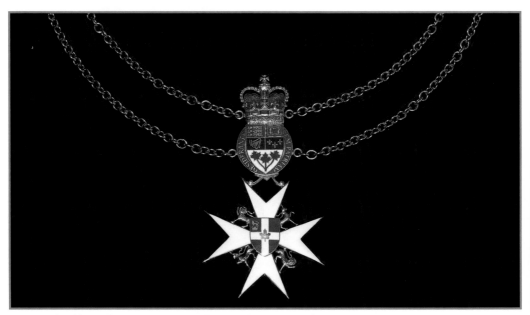

Chain of Office of the Past Chancellor of the Priory of Canada.

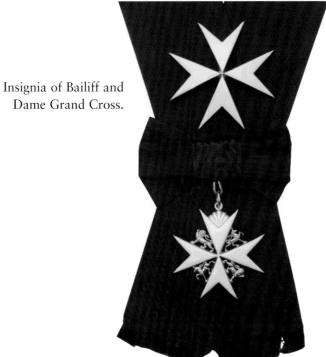

Insignia of Bailiff and
Dame Grand Cross.

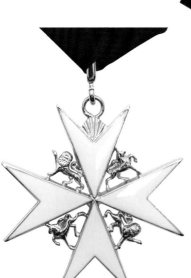

Insignia of Knight
and Dame of Justice.

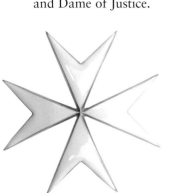

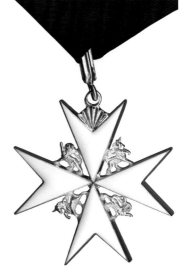

Insignia of a Knight
or Dame of Grace.

Plate 22   Modern Insignia of the Order of St. John

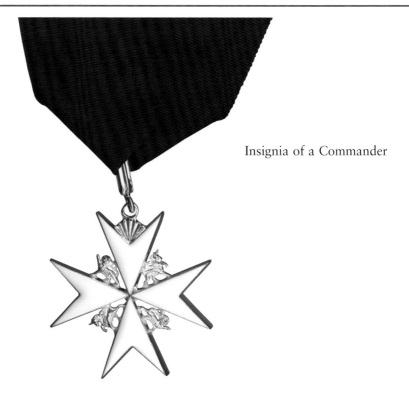

Insignia of a Commander

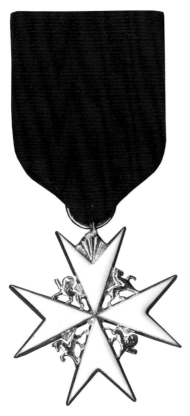

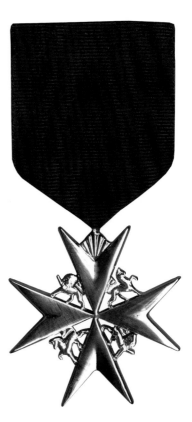

Insignia of an Officer.

Insignia of a Serving Brother or Serving Sister.
(Member)

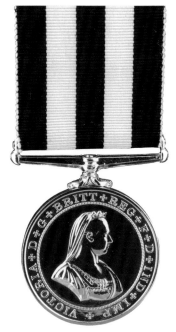

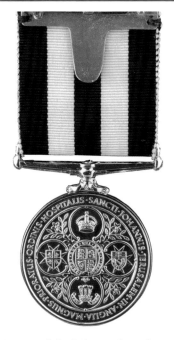

Service Medal of the Order of St. John, Obverse.

Service Medal of the Order of St. John, Reverse.

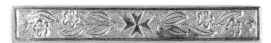

Silver Bar for 5 years of additional service.

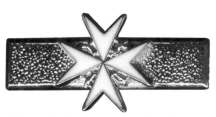

Chancellor's Commendation Bar.

Chancellor's Commendation Lapel Badge.

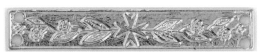

Gold Bar for 20 years of additional service.

Provincial Commendation Bar.

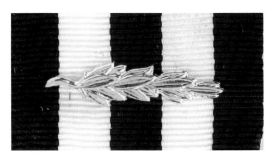

Gold Oakleaf for 50 years service.

Provincial Commendation Lapel Badge.

Plate 24   Obsolete Insignia of the Order and Donat Awards

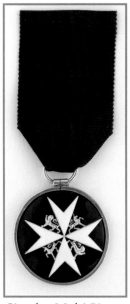

Circular Multi-Piece
Issue of the Serving
Brother's Insignia.

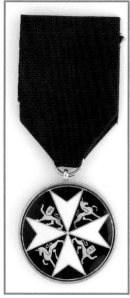

Circular Serving
Brother's Insignia.

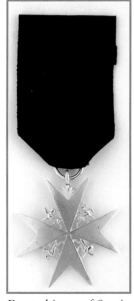

Frosted issue of Serving
Brother's Insignia.

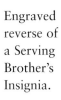

Engraved
reverse of
a Serving
Brother's
Insignia.

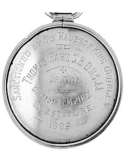

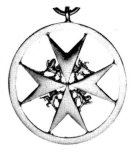

First Issue five-year
service bar for
Service Medal of
the Order.

Skeleton
Issue of the
Serving
Brother's
Insignia.
Known as
the "War
Economy"
Issue.

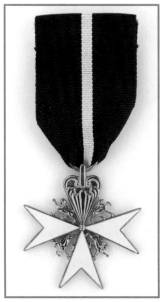

Bronze Donat Insignia.

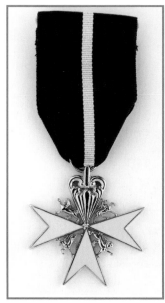

Silver Donat Insignia.

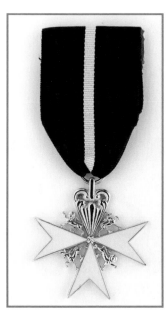

Gold Donat Insignia.

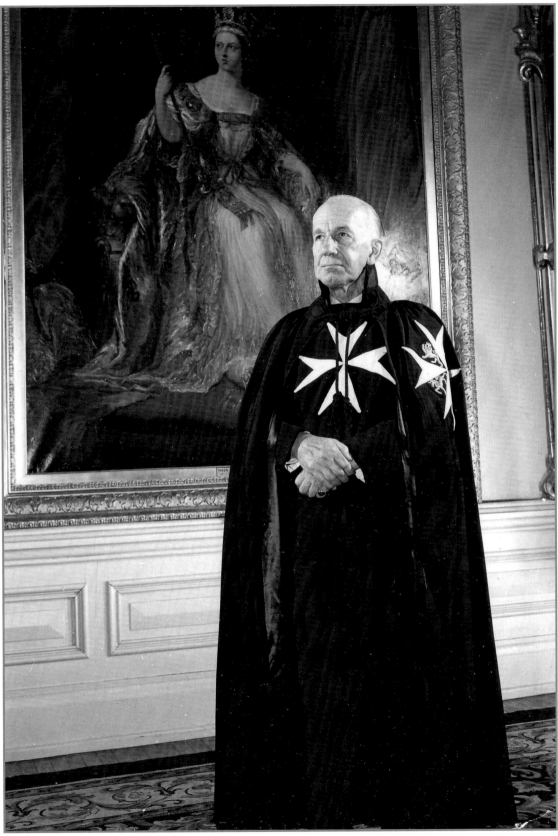

Vincent Massey wearing the Robes of the Order, including the Sopra Vest.

Henry Duke of Gloucester

Knight of the Most Noble Order of the Garter, Grand Prior in the British Realm of the Venerable Order of the Hospital of St John of Jerusalem, to

Herman John Ferrier, Esquire, M.D.

Greeting.

Whereas Her Majesty the Queen, the Sovereign Head in the British Realm of the Venerable Order of the Hospital of St John of Jerusalem, has thought fit to sanction your appointment, as an Officer in the said Venerable Order.

Now therefore I, by these presents, in the name, and by the authority of Her Majesty, do grant unto you the Dignity of an Officer in the said Venerable Order, and I do hereby authorize you to have, hold and enjoy the said Dignity, as an Officer of the aforesaid Order, together with all and singular the privileges thereunto belonging or appertaining.

Given at St John's Gate, under the Signature of His Royal Highness The Grand Prior and the Seal of the said Venerable Order this Twenty-fourth day of July One thousand, Nine hundred and Fifty-two in the First year of Her Majesty's Reign.

By the Grand Prior's Command

Henry R. Pownall
Chancellor.

Grant of the Dignity of an Officer of the Venerable Order of the Hospital of St John of Jerusalem to Herman John Ferrier, Esquire, M.D.

Reg No. 21576.

Older Appointment Scroll.

The Governor General of Canada
Prior of the Priory of Canada of the
Most Venerable Order of the Hospital
of St. John of Jerusalem

La Gouverneure générale du Canada
Prieur du Prieuré du Canada de
l'Ordre très vénérable de l'Hôpital de
Saint-Jean de Jérusalem

Gwendolyn Point

to   à

Greeting!

Salut !

Whereas, with the approval of Her Majesty Queen Elizabeth the Second,
Queen of Canada, Sovereign Head of the Most Venerable Order of the
Hospital of St. John of Jerusalem. We have been pleased to appoint you an
Officer in the said Order.

We do by these Presents appoint you to be an Officer in the said Order and
authorize you to hold and enjoy the dignity of such appointment together with
membership in the said Order and all privileges thereunto appertaining.

Given at Rideau Hall in the City of Ottawa under the Seal of the Priory of
Canada of the Most Venerable Order of the Hospital of St. John of Jerusalem
this 21st day of December in the year Two Thousand and Seven, in the 56th
year of Her Majesty's Reign.

By the Prior's Command

Attendu que, avec l'assentiment de sa Majesté la Reine Elizabeth Deux,
Reine du Canada, Chef souveraine de l'Ordre très vénérable de l'Hôpital
de Saint-Jean de Jérusalem, il Nous a plu de vous nommer Officier dudit
Ordre.

Nous vous nommons par les présentes Officier dudit Ordre et Nous vous
autorisons à bénéficier et à jouir de la dignité d'une telle nomination ainsi que du titre
de Membre dudit Ordre et de tous les privilèges y afférents.

Fait à Rideau Hall dans la ville d'Ottawa, sous le Sceau du Prieuré du
Canada de l'Ordre très vénérable de l'Hôpital de Saint-Jean de Jérusalem ce
21ème jour de décembre de l'an deux mille sept, 56ème année du règne de
Sa Majesté.

Par Ordre du Prieur

The Chancellor

Le chancelier

Current Appointment Scroll.

Plate 28

Order of St. John Investitures in Canada; Past and Present

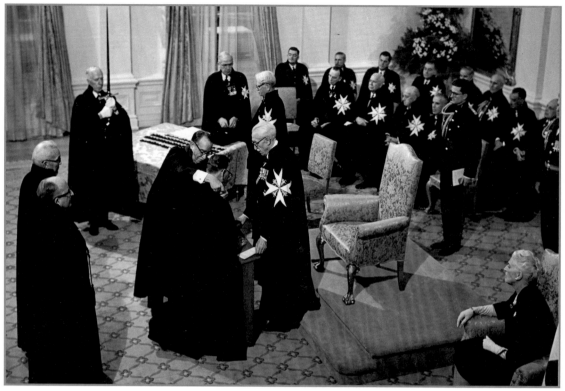

Major General Georges Vanier presiding over an Investiture Ceremony at Rideau Hall, 1961.

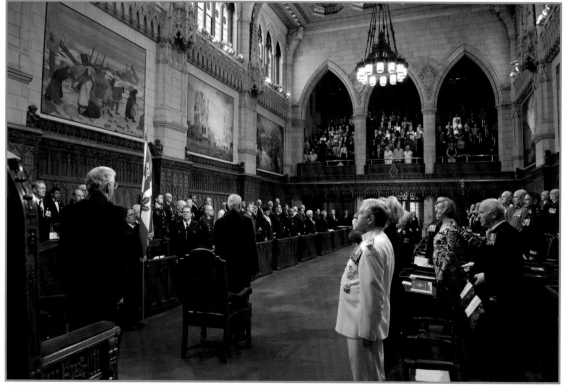

2006 National Investiture Ceremony held at Parliament in the Senate Chamber.

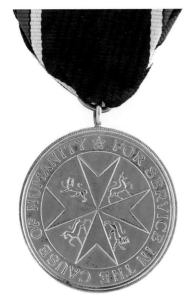

Life-saving Medal of the Order of St. John in Gold, Obverse.

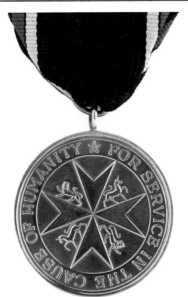

Life-saving Medal of the Order of St. John in Silver, Obverse.

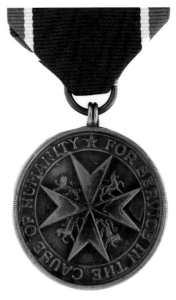

Life-saving Medal of the Order of St. John in Bronze, Obverse.

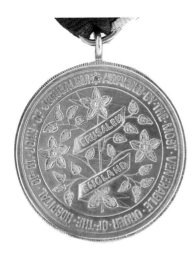

Life-saving Medal of the Order of St. John in Silver, Reverse.

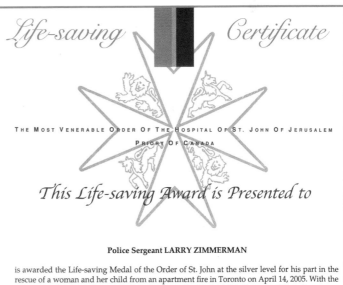

Life-saving *Certificate*

THE MOST VENERABLE ORDER OF THE HOSPITAL OF ST. JOHN OF JERUSALEM

PRIORY OF CANADA

This Life-saving Award is Presented to

Police Sergeant LARRY ZIMMERMAN

is awarded the Life-saving Medal of the Order of St. John at the silver level for his part in the rescue of a woman and her child from an apartment fire in Toronto on April 14, 2005. With the apartment already fully engulfed in flames and with thick black smoke filling the rooms, Police Sergeant Zimmerman immediately assisted with the rescue of a woman from the burning apartment. He was then informed that a young child was still inside. Without hesitation or thought for his own safety, Sergeant Zimmerman re-entered the burning apartment in search of the child. Crawling on his stomach through thick smoke, he continued searching until fire-fighters arrived and were able to rescue the child. Regretfully and despite their best efforts, the woman succumbed to her injuries days later in hospital, but was survived by her child. Police Sergeant Larry Zimmerman is to be commended for his courageous act of gallantry, quick actions, teamwork and for his knowledge and use of first aid in saving and attempting to save lives.

Recorded in the
Official Records of the
Priory of Canada

April 2006

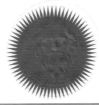

Chancellor

Life-saving Certificate.

Plate 30   Historic First Aid Medallions and Certificates

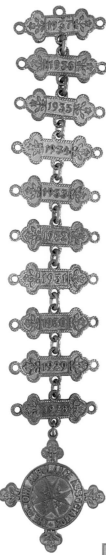

St. John Ambulance Association Medallion with Labels.

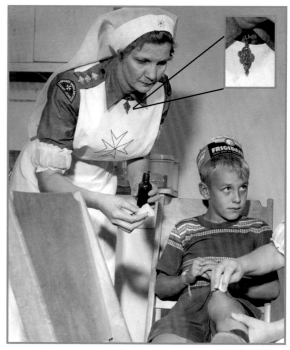

Nursing Division member wearing her St. John Ambulance Association Medallion around the neck, 1958.

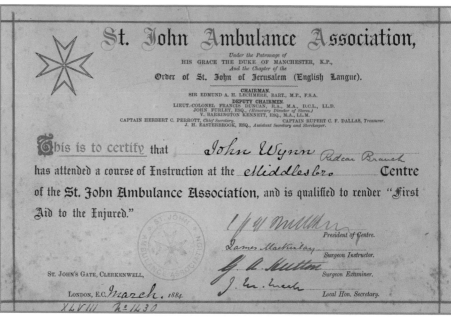

Early St. John Ambulance Association Medallion in silver.

St. John Ambulance Association First Aid Qualification Certificate, c. 1884. This is the same pattern of certificate that was issued to the first Canadians to successfully complete their first aid training in Quebec City and Kingston in 1883 and 1884.

St. John Ambulance Association,

Under the Patronage of
HIS GRACE THE DUKE OF MANCHESTER, K.P.,
And the Chapter of the
Order of St. John of Jerusalem (English Langue).

CHAIRMAN.
SIR EDMUND A. H. LECHMERE, BART., M.P., F.S.A.
DEPUTY CHAIRMEN.
LIEUT.-COLONEL FRANCIS DUNCAN, R.A., M.A., D.C.L., LL.D.
JOHN FURLEY, ESQ., (Honorary Director of Stores.)
V. BARRINGTON KENNETT, ESQ., M.A., LL.M.
CAPTAIN HERBERT C. PERROTT, Chief Secretary.   CAPTAIN RUPERT C. F. DALLAS, Treasurer.
J. H. EASTERBROOK, ESQ., Assistant Secretary and Storekeeper.

This is to certify that _John Wynn_ Redcar Branch has attended a course of Instruction at the _Middlesbro_ Centre of the St. John Ambulance Association, and is qualified to render "First Aid to the Injured."

President of Centre.

James Mackinlay
Surgeon Instructor.

Surgeon Examiner.

ST. JOHN'S GATE, CLERKENWELL,   Local Hon. Secretary.

LONDON, E.C. _March_. 1884.

XLVIII   N° 1630

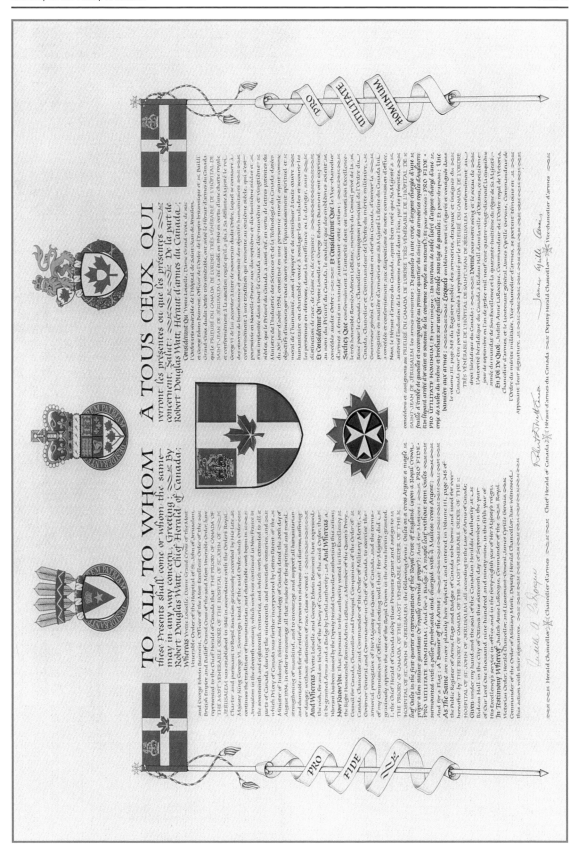

Grant of Arms to the Priory of Canada.

Plate 32   The Order of St. John in Canadian Heraldry

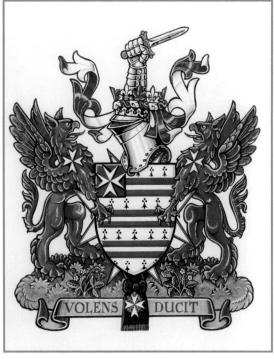

Grant of Arms to Lieutenant Colonel Eric Barry, GCStJ, CD

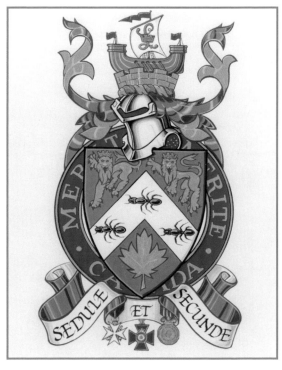

Grant of Arms to Brigadier General Owen William Lockyer, OMM, OStJ, CD.

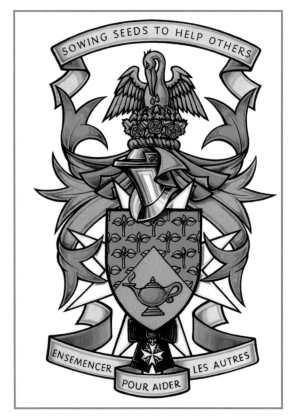

Grant of Arms to Dr. Marie Loyer, DStJ.

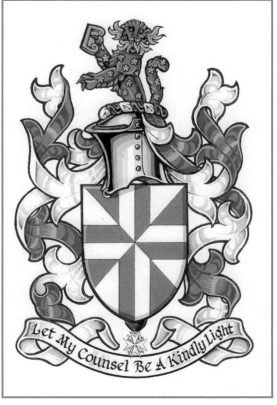

Grant of Arms to Bruce Patterson, SBStJ.

Yvette Loiselle, CM, GCStJ

As a young lady, Loiselle became a VAD in 1944, she would rise through the ranks of the brigade, eventually taking up its senior most office in Canada. In 1972 Loiselle became superintendent-in-chief of the brigade and this was followed by her appointment as chief commissioner of the brigade from 1978 to 1981. She became the first woman in the Commonwealth to fill such a senior position within the brigade. During her time as chief commissioner the membership of the brigade reached new levels and the problem of attrition that had begun in the early 1970s was halted. Like the other Dames Grand Cross she played a significant role in ensuring that the role of women within the organization was made a priority. Loiselle was appointed a Dame Grand Cross in 1982, being invested by the grand prior at St. Bartholomew's Church in Ottawa during the 1983 St. John Ambulance Centennial Celebrations. Loiselle died in 2003.

Brigadier-General George Edwin (Ted) Beament, OBE, CM, GCStJ, ED, CD, QC

A lawyer and soldier, Beament attended the Royal Military College of Canada and would continue his military service throughout his life. After being called to the Ontario Bar, Beament commenced a successful law practice in Ottawa. He served an artillery officer during the Second World War being decorated with the *Croix de Guerre* and Czechoslovakia's Order of the White Lion. In peacetime he returned to the legal profession and devoted much of his time to charitable causes. Foremost among his charitable works was St. John Ambulance, which he served as legal advisor, vice-chancellor, and, finally, as chancellor from 1975 to 1978. He oversaw the successful joint project with the Red Cross and the revitalization of the brigade. He was made a Bailiff Grand Cross of the Order in 1995, becoming the oldest recipient of the honour. Brigadier-General Beament died in 2005 after a life full of devotion to the service of humanity.

Lieutenant-Colonel Eric Lawrence Barry, GCStJ, CD

Canada's most recent Bailiff Grand Cross has worked in a variety of capacities; as a longtime military officer he rose to become commanding officer of the Royal Canadian Hussars. In the field of business he would serve for many years as the president of the Canadian Textile Institute and work with a number of other textile-related industry groups. Barry was appointed a Serving Brother in 1971 and would eventually progress through all the grades of the Order. During his time as director of association, St. John Ambulance received a $1.5 million grant from the McConnell Foundation. As chancellor from 1993 to 1996 Barry oversaw the operations of St. John Ambulance in a time of financial restraint and growing participation in St. John first aid training. In 1999 Barry was appointed a Bailiff Grand Cross and in 2002 he became lord prior of the Order.

Appendix C

Officials of the Order of St. John in Canada

Sovereign Head

Queen Victoria	1888–1901
King Edward VII	1901–1910
King George V	1910–1936
King Edward VIII	1936
King George VI	1936–1952
Queen Elizabeth II	1952–

Grand Priors Following Revival of 1831

The Reverend Robert Peat	1831–1837
Sir Henry Dymoke, Bt	1838–1847
Sir Charles Lamb, Bt	1847–1860
Sir Alexander Arbuthnot	1860–1861
William, Duke of Manchester, KP	1861–1888

Grand Priors Following Queen Victoria's Royal Charter of 1888

HRH Edward, Prince of Wales (Edward VII)	1888–1901
HRH George, Prince of Wales (George V)	1901–1910
HRH Arthur, Duke of Connaught and Stratheran	1910–1939
HRH Henry, Duke of Gloucester	1939–1974
HRH Richard, Duke of Gloucester	1974–

Sub Priors*

HRH Albert Victor, Duke of Clarence	1888–1892
HRH George, Duke of Cornwall and York (GeorgeV)	1893–1901
John Adrian Louis Hope, 1st Marquess Linlithgow, KT, GCMG, GCStJ	1906–1907
Vacant	1908–1910
Henry Thurstan Holland, 1st Viscount Knutsford, GCMG, GCStJ	1910–1914
Robert George Windsor-Clive, 1st Earl of Plymouth, GBE, CB, GCStJ	1915–1923

Alfred Frederick Lumley, 10th Earl of Scarborough, KG, GBE, KCB, GCStJ   1923–1943

Priors*
Ivor Miles Windsor-Clive, 2nd Earl of Plymouth, GCStJ   1943
George Herbert Hyde Villiers, 6th Earl of Clarendon, KG, PC, GCStJ   1943–1946
John de Vere Loder, 2nd Baron Wakehurst, KG, KCMG, GCStJ   1947–1950

Lord Priors*
John de Vere Loder, 2nd Baron Wakehurst, KG, KCMG, GCStJ   1950–1969
Harold Anthony Caccia, Lord Caccia, GCMG, GCVO, GCStJ   1969–1981
Sir Maurice Dorman, GCMG, GCVO, GCStJ, DL   1982–1985
Major General Alan Cathcart, 6th Earl Cathcart, CB, GCStJ, MC   1986–1987
Ralph Francis Alnwick Grey, Lord Grey of Naunton, GCMG, GCVO,   1988–1990
    OBE, GCStJ
Samuel George Armstrong Vestey, 3rd Lord Vestey, GCStJ, DL   1991–2001
Eric L. Barry, GCStJ, CD   2002–

Patrons of the Canadian Branch
Earl Grey, PC, GCB, GCMG, GCVO   1910–1911
HRH Prince Arthur, Duke of Connaught, KG, KT, KP, PC, GCB, GCSI,   1911–1916
    GCMG, GCIE, GBE, GStJ, VD, TD
Duke of Devonshire, KG, PC, GCVO, GCMG, KStJ   1916–1921
Field Marshal Viscount Byng of Vimy, GCB, GCMG, MVO   1921–1926
Viscount Willingdon, PC, GCMG, GCSI, GCIE, GBE   1926–1931
Earl of Bessborough, PC, GCMG, KStJ   1931–1933

Patronesses of the Canadian Branch
Alice, Countess Grey, DStJ   1910–1911
HRH Princess Louise, Duchess of Connaught, CI, VA, DStJ, RRC   1911–1916
Evelyn, Duchess of Devonshire, GCVO, DStJ   1916–1921
Marie Evelyn, Viscountess Byng, DStJ   1921–1926
Marie Adelaide, Countess of Willingdon, CI, CBE   1926–1931
Roberta, Lady Bessborough, GCStJ   1931–1933

Knights Commander of the Commandery of Canada
Earl of Bessborough, PC, GCMG, KStJ   1933–1935
Lord Tweedsmuir, PC, GCMG, CH   1935–1940
Earl of Athlone, KG, PC, GCB, GCMG, GCVO, KStJ, DSO   1940–1946
Field Marshal the Right Honourable Viscount Alexander of Tunis,   1946
    KG, OM, PC, GCB, GCMG, CSI, KStJ, DSO, MC, CD

Priors of Canada

Field Marshal the Right Honourable Viscount Alexander of Tunis, KG, OM, PC, GCB, GCMG, GCVO, CSI, KStJ, DSO, MC, CD	1946–1952
The Right Honourable Vincent Massey, PC, CH, CC, GCStJ, CD	1952–1959
Major General The Right Honourable Georges Vanier, PC, DSO, KStJ, CD	1959–1967
The Right Honourable Roland Michener, PC, CC, CMM, KStJ, CD, QC	1967–1974
The Right Honourable Jules Léger, PC, CC, CMM, KStJ, CD	1974–1980
The Right Honourable Edward Schreyer, PC, CC, CMM, KStJ, CD	1980–1985
The Right Honourable Jeanne Sauve, PC, CC, CMM, DStJ, CD	1985–1990
The Right Honoruable Ramon Hnatyshyn, PC, CC, CMM, KStJ, CD, QC	1990–1995
The Right Honourable Romeo LeBlanc, PC, CC, CMM, KStJ, CD	1995–2000
The Right Honourable Adrienne Clarkson, PC, CC, CMM, COM, DStJ, CD	2000–2006
The Right Honourable Michaëlle Jean, CC, CMM, COM, DStJ, CD	2006–

Presidents

F. Montizambert, CMG, ISO	1910–1913
The Right Honourable, Sir L.H. Davies, PC, KCMG	1914–1915
J.M. Courtney, CMG, ISO, KStJ	1916–1917
Fred Cook	1918–1919
The Honourable Mr. Justice J.F. Orde, KStJ	1920–1921
The Honourable D.T. Irwin, CMG	1922–1923
The Honourable Murray MacLaren, CMG	1924–1925
Sir Percy Sherwood, KCMG, MVO, KStJ, VD	1926–1927
The Honourable H. Bostock, KStJ	1928–1929
The Honourable J.J. King, PC, KStJ	1930–1931
C.G. Cowan, KStJ	1932–1936
R.E. Woodhouse, OBE, KStJ	1937–1942
Allan T. Lewis, CBE, KStJ, QC	1943–1946
Charles A. Gray, KStJ	1946–1960
John H. Molson, OC, MBE, ED	1960–1963
Arthur A. Crawley	1963–1966
N.I.M. MacLaren, MC, KStJ	1966–1969

Lieutenants of the Commandery in Canada

C.G. Cowan, KStJ	1933–1936
R.E. Woodhouse, OBE, KStJ	1937–1942
The Hon. H.A. Bruce, KStJ	1942–1943
Allan T. Lewis, CBE, KStJ, QC	1943–1946

Chancellors**

Charles Gray, KStJ	1946–1960
J.H. Molson, MBE, KStJ, VD	1960–1963
A.A. Crawley, KStJ	1963–1966
Ian Maclaren, MC, KStJ	1966–1969
L.H. Nicholson, OC, MBE, GCStJ	1969–1972
J.R. Roche, OBE, KStJ, ED, QC	1972–1975
G.E. Beament, OBE, CM, GCStJ, ED, CD, QC	1975–1978
C.J. Laurin, OBE, GCStJ	1978–1981
J.C. Dubuc, KStJ, CD	1981–1984
Frank Brown, KStJ	1984–1987
Frank McEachren, CVO, CM, KStJ, ED, CD	1987–1990
Donald W. Rae, OC, KStJ, CD	1990–1993
Eric Barry GCStJ, CD	1993–1996
David Johnston KStJ, CD	1996–1999
Robert Langdon KStJ	1999–2002
Jeffrey Gilmour, KStJ, CD	2002–2005
The Honourable René Marin, CM, OMM, OOnt, KStJ, CD, QC	2005–2007
John Mah, KStJ, CD, QC	2007–

Priory Secretary

William Bennett, KStJ	1946–1957
A.G. Cherrier, OBE, KStJ, CD	1957–1961
Teryl A. Johnston, OBE, KStJ, ED, CD	1961–1972
Douglas W. Cunnington, KStJ, GM, CD	1972–1982
James A. Cowan, OStJ, CD	1982–1989 (also CEO)
Duncan J. Phillips, MMM, CStJ, CD	1989–1999 (also CEO)
André Denis Lagassé, CStJ	1999–2001
Mark W. Tinlin, OStJ	2002–2005 (also Registrar)
Dawn Roach	2005– (also Registrar)

Registrars

Brigadier General C.H. Maclaren, CMG, DSO, CStJ, VD	1950–1957
Colonel G.W. Cavey, OBE, MC, KStJ, MM	1958–1965
John R. Matheson, OC, KStJ, CD	1966–1969
J.K.Tambling	1970–1973
Vacant	1974–1975
Marguerite F.E. Wylie, DStJ	1976–1977

Vacant	1978
Major L.M. Bloomfield	1979–1982
M.H. Rayner	1983–1992
Colonel D.V. Reynolds	1993-1994
Jeffrey Gilmour	1994-1997
Reg Brown	1998-2002
Mark W. Tinlin (also Priory Secretary)	2002–2005
Dawn Roach (also Priory Secretary)	2005–

Hospitaller and Almoner

Robert E. Wodehouse, OBE, , KStJ	1934–1935
Brig Gen R.M. Gorssline, DSO, OStJ, MB	1936–1942
Senator The Honourable Norman Paterson, CStJ	1943–1948

Hospitallers

Colonel Henry Willis O'Conner, CVO, CBE, DSO, KStJ	1949
Briagdier General W.P. Warner, CBE, DSC, MB	1950–1955
J.N.B. Crawford, MBE, CStJ, ED, MD	1956–1963
Brigadier General G.R.D. Farmer	1964–1970
A.M. Davidson	1971–1973
Bryan St. Liddy, KStJ, CD	1974–1991
Brian C. Leonard	1992–1997
Harold W. Climenhaga	1998–2003
George Beiko, OStJ	2004–

Almoners

Thomas Guerin, OBE, KStJ, PhD	1949–1954
Colonel C.P. Gaboury, OBE, KStJ, ED, MD	1955–1963
H.W. Adams	1965–1971
J.C. McKinnon	1972–1976
Colonel J.C. Dubuc	1977
A.H. Harrop	1978–1980
Yvette Loiselle, CM, GStJ	1981–1989
E. Edmonds, KStJ	1990–1995
J.H. Antonio Tremblay, OMM, KStJ, CD	1996–2001
Cyril Woods, KStJ	2001–2005
Vacant	2006
Sandra Wilson, CM, SSStJ	2007–

Genealogists

G.H. Craig, CStJ	1950–1954
C.L. Burton, CBE, CStJ	1955–1958
Colonel Fraser, CStJ, VD	1959–1966
Paul Bienvenu	1967–1969
John R. Matheson, OC, CStJ, CD	1970–1992
Gordon Macpherson, KStJ	1993–2003
David Tysowski	2003–2004
Charles Maier, CStJ, CD	2005–

* This changed to prior from 1947–1949, and became lord prior in 1950

**The post of chancellor was know as sub-prior between the establishment of the Priory of Canada in 1952.

Appendix D

The Royal Charters, 1955 and 1974

Royal Charter, 1955

ELIZABETH THE SECOND by the Grace of God of the United Kingdom of Great Britain and Northern Ireland and of Our other Realms and Territories Queen, Head of the Commonwealth, Defender of the Faith. To all to whom these Presents shall come, Greeting!

WHEREAS by a Royal Charter under the Great Seal, bearing date at Westminster the fourteenth day of May in the fifty-first year of the Reign of Her Majesty Queen Victoria and in the year of our Lord One thousand eight hundred and eighty-eight (hereinafter referred to as the Original Charter) "The Grand Priory of the Order of the Hospital of Saint John of Jerusalem in England," was incorporated for the objects and purposes declared in the original Charter and in the Statutes set forth in the Schedule thereto:

AND WHEREAS by a Supplemental Charter bearing date at Westminster the twenty-second day of May in the seventh year of the Reign of His Majesty King Edward the Seventh and in the year of our Lord One thousand nine hundred and seven certain alterations were made in the provisions of the original Charter:

AND WHEREAS by a further Royal Charter under the Great Seal bearing date at Westminster the twelfth day of June in the seventeenth year of the Reign of His Majesty King George the Fifth and in the year of our Lord One thousand nine hundred and twenty-six (hereinafter referred to as "the Charter of 1926") the provisions of the Original Charter and the said Supplemental Charter were amended, consolidated and superseded and in particular it was declared and ordained that the name, designation and title of the said Order should from the date of issue of the Charter of 1926 be "the Grand Priory in the British Realm of the Venerable Order of the Hospital of St. John of Jerusalem":

AND WHEREAS by a further Royal Charter under the Great Seal bearing date at Westminster the first day of August in the first year of the reign of His Majesty King Edward the Eighth and in the year of our Lord One thousand nine hundred and thirty-six (hereinafter referred to as "the Charter of 1936") the Charter of 1926 was amended and superseded and it was ordained that the Charter of 1936 was and should be the sole Charter of the Grand Priory aforesaid:

AND WHEREAS it has been represented to Us by Our most dear and entirely beloved Uncle and most faithful Counsellor Henry, Duke of Gloucester, Knight of Our Most Noble Order of the Garter, who is now the Grand Prior of the Grand Priory aforesaid, that the Charter of 1936 should be amended and superseded by a further Charter granted by Us AND WHEREAS it is considered expedient to amend and supersede the Charter of 1936 by the grant of a further Charter being these Presents:

NOW KNOW YE that We, having taken the premises into our consideration, by Our special Grace Certain Knowledge and Mere Motion for Us Our Heirs and Successors, by this further Charter, under the power by the Charter of 1936 reserved to Us Our Heirs and Successors and every other power Us hereunto enabling, do DECLARE AND ORDAIN as follows:

Clause 1.—Amendment—and Supersession of the Charter of 1936 —
We do hereby amend and supersede the Charter of 1936 and grant to the Grand Priory aforesaid this further Royal Charter superseding the Charter of 1936 and We Ordain that this Our Royal Charter is and shall be the sole Charter of the Grand Priory aforesaid.

Clause 2.—Title —
We do hereby further ordain that the name, designation and title of the Grand Priory aforesaid is and shall continue to be "the Grand Priory in the British Realm of the Most Venerable Order of the Hospital of St. John of Jerusalem," and we further Declare that the same usually shall be styled and designated for brevity "The Order of St. John" and shall in this Charter be referred to as "the Order."

Clause 3.—Rights and Privileges —
We do hereby further ordain that the Order shall have a Common Seal and have perpetual succession, and that it may by and in the said name and style, sue, implead and answer, and be sued, impleaded and answered in all Courts whatsoever, whether of Law or Equity, and be competent to do all other acts, matters and things incidental or appertaining to a body politic and corporate and to enjoy all rights and privileges lawfully appertaining to bodies politic and corporate.

(Clauses 4, 5, and 6 were revoked by the provisions of the Supplemental Royal Charter of 1974.)

IN WITNESS WHEREOF We have caused these Our letter to be made Patent.

WITNESS Our self at Westminster the fifteenth day of March in the fourth year of Our Reign.

BY WARRANT under the Queen's Sign Manual.

Supplemental Royal Charter, 1974

ELIZABETH THE SECOND by the Grace of God of the United Kingdom of Great Britain and Northern Ireland and of Our other Realms and Territories Queen, Head of the Commonwealth, Defender of the Faith. To all to whom these Presents shall come, Greeting!

WHEREAS by a Royal Charter dated the fourteenth day of May in the fifty-first year of the Reign of Her Majesty Queen Victoria and in the year of our Lord One thousand eight hundred and eighty-eight (hereinafter referred to as "the Original Charter") all the Members (excluding Associates) for the time being of the Order created by the Original Charter were incorporated under the name and style of "The Grand Priory of the Order of the Hospital of Saint John of Jerusalem in England" for the objects and purposes declared in the Original Charter and in the Statutes set forth in the Schedule thereto:

AND WHEREAS by a Supplemental Charter dated the twenty-second day of May in the seventh year of the Reign of His Majesty King Edward the Seventh and in the year of our Lord One thousand nine hundred and seven certain alterations were made in the provisions of the Original Charter:

AND WHEREAS by a further Royal Charter dated the twelfth day of June in the seventeenth year of the Reign of His Majesty King George the Fifth and in the year of our Lord One thousand nine hundred and twenty-six (hereinafter referred to as "the Charter of 1926") the provisions of the Original Charter and the said Supplemental Charter were amended, consolidated and superseded and in particular it was declared and ordained that the name, designation and the title of the said Order should from the date of issue of the Charter of 1926 be "the Grand Priory in the British Realm of the Venerable Order of the Hospital of St. John of Jerusalem":

AND WHEREAS by a further Royal Charter dated the first day of August in the first year of the Reign of His Majesty King Edward the Eighth and in the year of our Lord One thousand nine hundred and thirty-six (hereinafter referred to as "the Charter of 1936") the Charter of 1926 was amended and superseded and it was ordained that the Charter of 1936 was and should be the sole Charter of the Grand Priory aforesaid:

AND WHEREAS by a further Royal Charter dated the fifteenth day of March in the fourth year of Our Reign and in the year of our Lord One thousand nine hundred and fifty-five (hereinafter referred to as "the Charter of 1955") the Charter of 1936 was amended and superseded and it was ordained that the Charter of 1955 was and should be the sole Charter of the Grand Priory aforesaid:

AND WHEREAS the Charter of 1955 was subsequently amended by two Supplemental Charters dated respectively the fourteenth day of November in the seventh year of Our Reign and the year of our Lord One thousand nine hundred and fifty-eight and the twenty eighth day of February in the nineteenth year of Our Reign and the year of our Lord One thousand nine hundred and seventy (hereinafter referred to collectively as "the Supplemental Charters of 1958 and 1970"):

AND WHEREAS it has been represented unto Us by Our most dear and entirely beloved Uncle and most faithful Counsellor Henry, Duke of Gloucester, Knight of the Most Noble Order of the Garter, who is now the Grand Prior of the Grand Priory aforesaid, that the Supplemental Charters of 1958 and 1970 should be revoked and that the Charter of 1955 should be amended by a further Supplemental Charter granted by US providing among other things that the name, designation and title of the Order should again be amended and that the Statutes set forth in the Schedule to the Charter of 1955 which regulate the internal adminis-tration and organisation of the Order should be replaced in revised form so that the objects and purposes of the Order may be better attained:

NOW KNOW YE that We, having taken the premises into Our Royal Consideration, of Our especial grace, certain knowledge and mere motion have declared and ordained and by these Presents do for Us, Our Heirs and Successors DECLARE AND ORDAIN as follows:

Clause 1.—Interpretation —
This Our Royal Charter shall supersede the Charter of 1955 except in so far as any provisions of the said Charter are not hereby revoked.

Clause 2.—Amendment of Charter of 1955 —
The provisions of the Charter of 1955, except so far as they incorporate the said Grand Priory and confer on it perpetual succession and authorise it to have a Common Seal, to sue and be sued and to enjoy all the rights and privileges lawfully appertaining to bodies politic and corporate, are hereby revoked.

Clause 3.— Revocation of Supplemental Charters —
The Supplemental Charters of 1958 and 1970 are also revoked.

Clause 4.—Saving —
The revocation in part of the Charter of 1955 and the revocation of the aforesaid Supple-mental Charters shall not affect the validity or legality of any thing done or executed or of any dealing with property or of any investment made under any of the revoked provisions of the said Charters or of any of the Statutes of the Order annexed thereto.

Clause 5.—Change of Name of the Corporate Body —
All persons who are at the date of this Our Supplemental Charter enrolled as Members of the Order in the roll of members thereof in the custody of the Secretary-General of the Order and are of any of the grades of Members hereinafter specified and all persons who shall for the time being in pursuance of and in accordance with these Presents be Members of the Order shall continue to be one body politic and corporate by the name and style of "The Most Venerable Order of the Hospital of Saint John of Jerusalem" which as heretofore may be styled and designated for brevity "The Order of St. John" and shall herein and in the Statutes be referred to as "the Order."

Clause 6.—Property —

The Order shall have power to purchase, acquire, take and hold in perpetuity or otherwise any property, lands, tenements and hereditaments.

Clause 6A—Gifts to the Priory of England and the Islands —

With effect from 24 October 1999 unless a contrary intention shall be manifest, all gifts, legacies, and payments under covenant or Gift Aid to the Order made by a donor, testator or payor resident within the territory of the Priory of England and the Islands shall be deemed to vest in the Priory of England and the Islands.

Clause 7.—Powers of Investment —

The powers of the Order to invest moneys and funds of the Order not immediately required to be expended shall be such as shall be specified in the Statutes of the Order.

Clause 7A—Indemnity—Insurance —

The Order shall have power to provide indemnity insurance to such extent and subject to such conditions as shall be specified in the Statutes of the Order.

Clause 8.—Statutes—of the Order —

The Statutes contained in the Schedule to this Our Supplemental Charter are hereby declared to be the sole Statutes of the Order until they shall be altered in the manner hereinafter appearing.

Clause 9.—Saving—for Establishments, etc., Overseas —

Notwithstanding the provisions of the Charter of 1955 and of this Our Supplemental Charter, it is hereby declared that any Establishment or other subordinate body of the Order shall have and shall be deemed always to have had power to incorporate or register itself under any local law.

Clause 10.—Amendment—of Charter and Statues —

The Order may revoke, amend or add to any of the provisions of the Charter of 1955 or this Our Supplemental Charter or the Statutes of the Order by a Resolution passed by not less than three-quarters of the members present and entitled to vote at a meeting of the Grand Council of the Order specially summoned for the purpose, and of which at least three months' notice has been given, and any such revocation, amendment or addition shall when allowed by Us, Our Heirs or Successors in Council become effective so that the Charter of 1955 or this Our Supplemental Charter or the Statutes of the Order shall thenceforth continue and operate as though they had been originally granted and made accordingly. This provision shall apply to the Charter of 1955 or to this Our Supplemental Charter or the Statutes of the Order as revoked, amended or added to in the manner aforesaid.

IN WITNESS WHEREOF We have caused these Our letters to be made Patent.

WITNESS Ourself at Westminster the twenty-ninth day of April in the twenty-third year of Our Reign.

BY WARRANT under the Queen's Sign Manual.

Note: The headings to clauses are not included in the charter documents and are inserted here for information only.

APPENDIX E

STATUTES OF THE MOST VENERABLE ORDER OF THE HOSPITAL OF ST. JOHN OF JERUSALEM

PART ONE: INTRODUCTORY

1. Short title

These Statutes may be cited as "the St. John Statutes 1974 to 2003."

2. Interpretation

(1) In these Statutes, unless the context otherwise requires:

(a) "Appointed Day" means (except in Part Five) 1 January 2004;

(b) "Associate Member" means a person who on or prior to St. John's Day 1999 was attached to the Order in pursuance of the provisions of the statute which immediately before that date was numbered Statute 26(2) and who has not ceased for any reason to be attached thereto;

(c) "Establishment" means a Priory, Independent Commandery, Dependent Commandery or St. John Association;

(d) "the Lord Prior" means the Lord Prior of St. John whose Great Office is referred to in Statute 8;

(e) "Member" or "Member of the Order" means a person possessing the qualifications set out in Statute 33 who, having been duly admitted to the Order, has not ceased for any reason to be a Member;

(f) "the Order" or "The Order of St. John" means all the Members of the Order for the time being comprising the corporate body referred to in the Royal Charter;

(g) "Regulations" means Regulations made by the Grand Prior in pursuance of Statute 7(3);

(h) "Royal Charter" means the Royal Charter of 1955 and the Supplemental Royal Charter of 1974;

(i) "Rules" means Rules made in pursuance of Statutes 19(2), 20(3), 22(3) or 24(5);

(j) "Specified Body" has the meaning ascribed to it by Statute 34A;

(k) "St. John Ambulance" means the Foundation of that name and formerly known as the "St. John Ambulance Association and Brigade";

(l) "St. John's Day" means the Feast of the Nativity of St. John the Baptist save that in relation to the year 1999 it shall mean 24 October 1999.

(2) In these Statutes, unless the context otherwise requires, words importing the masculine shall include the feminine, words in the singular shall include the plural and words in the plural shall include the singular.

(3) If at any time the Grand Prior in the exercise of powers conferred on him shall ordain that any office or body constituted by or under these Statutes shall have its title changed to a new title, any reference to such office or body in these Statutes or in any Regulations or Rules made thereunder shall be read and construed as a reference to such office or body by such new title.

(4) If any question arises as to the interpretation of these Statutes, the matter shall be referred to the Grand Prior whose decision shall be final.

3. Mottoes of the Order

The Mottoes of the Order shall be "Pro Fide" and "Pro Utilitate Hominum."

4. Objects and Purposes of the Order

The Order is an ancient Christian brotherhood and its objects and purposes shall be:

(a) The encouragement of all that makes for the spiritual and moral strengthening of mankind in accordance with the first great principle of the Order embodied in the Motto "Pro Fide";

(b) The encouragement and promotion of all work of humanity and charity for the relief of persons in sickness, distress, suffering, or danger, without distinction of race, class, or creed and the extension of the second great principle of the Order embodied in the Motto "Pro Utilitate Hominum";

(c) The rendering of aid to the sick, wounded, disabled or suffering and the promotion of such permanent organisation during times of peace as may be at once available in times of civil emergencies or war, including the training and provision of technical reserves for the medical services of the Armed Forces or any Civil Defence Organisations;

(d) The award of medals, badges or certificates of honour for special services in the cause of humanity, especially for saving life at imminent personal risk;

(e) The maintenance and development of the St. John Eye Hospital in Jerusalem and the clinics and research projects connected therewith;

(f) The maintenance and development of the St. John Ambulance, the objects and purposes of which are:

(i) The instruction of members of the public in the principles and practice of First Aid, Nursing, Hygiene and other allied or ancillary subjects;

(ii) The preparation, publication and distribution of text-books and other training aids to facilitate such instruction and the organisation of examinations and tests for the purpose of issuing certificates of proficiency in such subjects;

(iii)The organisation, training and equipment of men, women and youngpersons to undertake, on a voluntary basis either as individuals or as organised groups, First Aid, Nursing and allied activities, in the streets, public places, hospitals, homes, places of work or elsewhere as occasion may require for the relief, transport, comfort or welfare of those in need;

(iv)The instruction of boys and girls in First Aid, Nursing and other subjects conducive to the education of good citizens;

(v) The provision of trained personnel to give assistance to Central or Local Government Departments or to the Armed Forces at times of emergency in peace or in war;

(g) The formation of ambulance and medical comforts depots and the organisation and administration of transport by ambulance;

(h) The formation and administration of establishments, councils, associations, centres or other subordinate bodies to facilitate the work of the Order in local geographical areas;

(i) The maintenance of contact and the development of collaboration with kindred Orders and bodies;

(j) The manufacture and distribution by sale or presentation of publications, equipment or materials useful for or connected with furthering the objects and purposes of the Order;

(k) The receipt and acceptance of donations, endowments and gifts of money, lands, hereditaments, stocks, funds, shares, securities or other assets whatsoever, and the borrowing, investing or raising of money with or without security for any objects or purposes of the Order and either subject to or free from any special trusts or conditions;

(l) The maintenance, administration or development of all real and personal property vested in or under the control of the Order, and the sale, lease, mortgage, loan, exchange, gift, or any other disposition of the same as circumstances may arise or permit; and

(m)The establishment and maintenance of libraries and museums and the collection of works of art and objects of historical interest relating to the Order.

PART TWO: THE ORGANISATION OF THE ORDER

5. The Sovereign Head

(1) Her Majesty the Queen, Her Heirs and Successors shall be the Sovereign Head of the Order.

(2) The Sovereign Head shall make such appointments to and within the Order as She in her absolute discretion shall think fit.

6. The Grand Prior

There shall be a Grand Prior of the Order who shall be appointed by the Sovereign Head after consultation with the Grand Council and who shall hold office during the pleasure of the Sovereign Head or until resignation.

7. Powers of the Grand Prior

(1) Subject to any directions he may receive from the Sovereign Head, the Grand Prior shall exercise supreme direction and administrative and executive control over the Order, its Establishments, its other subordinate organisations, and its Members and shall make all appointments other than those made by the Sovereign Head. The Grand Prior shall have the right to veto any recommendation, resolution, decision or proceeding of the Grand Council, or of any Establishment or other subordinate organisation of the Order.

(2) The Grand Prior shall submit to the Sovereign Head for approval or direction any matter which he deems to be of important principle and, in particular, shall submit for the sanction of the Sovereign Head all proposals for admission to or promotion in the Order as shall have been recommended by the Grand Council and approved by him.

(3) The Grand Prior, on the recommendation of the Grand Council, shall have power by Instrument under his hand and the Seal of the Order to make, amend, revoke or suspend (in whole or in part and either generally or in relation to any specified area) Regulations or Rules (not being repugnant to the Royal Charter or any law) for any purpose expressed in the Royal Charter or Statutes or otherwise as he may deem necessary or expedient for the conduct, control or management of the affairs or work of the Order and, when published in such manner as the Grand Prior may direct, such Regulations or Rules shall be binding on the organisations or persons to which they are applicable.

(4) To facilitate the conduct of the affairs and work of the Order, the Grand Prior may, in his discretion and subject to such limitations as he may impose, delegate in such manner as he deems fit any of his powers or authority to any other Great Officer or other officer of the Order as he may specify: Provided always that he shall not delegate his power of veto or his authority to make Regulations or Rules or to approve and submit to the Sovereign Head recommendations for admission to or promotion in the Order except when he is unable to exercise such power or authority owing to absence abroad or ill-health in which circumstances such power or authority may be exercised by the Lord Prior on his behalf.

(5) The Grand Prior, on the recommendation of the Grand Council, may appoint Standing or other Committees of such membership and with such terms of reference as he may specify or as may be prescribed by Regulations. Unless the Grand Prior otherwise directs, all such Committees shall report to and exercise their functions under the general supervision of the Grand Council.

8. The Great Officers of the Order

(1) The Grand Prior and those holding the four offices hereinafter mentioned shall be the Great Officers of the Order and *ex officio* shall be Bailiffs Grand Cross or Dames Grand Cross of the Order, that is to say:

(a) *The Lord Prior of St. John* who shall be the Lieutenant and Deputy of the Grand Prior.

(b) *The Prelate* shall be a Member of the Order of episcopal rank in the Church of England as by law established. The Prelate shall be the adviser to the Grand Prior in all matters of an ecclesiastical nature and shall determine the form of religious service and prayers to be used on such occasions as are not provided for by the Statutes or Regulations; save that in Scotland the Grand Prior shall be advised in these matters by the appropriate Executive Officer of the Priory of Scotland.

(c) *The Deputy Lord Prior* or if for the time being the Grand Prior shall think fit two Deputy Lord Priors. A Deputy Lord Prior shall be the Deputy of the Lord Prior. If the Lord Prior is unable to perform the functions of his office by reason of absence or ill-health, a Deputy Lord Prior shall act as Lieutenant and Deputy of the Grand Prior.

(d) *The Sub-Prior* who shall have special interest in Independent Commanderies and St. John Associations.

(2) The Grand Prior, on the recommendation of the Grand Council, may change the title of, or abolish, any Great Office or may create any new Great Office:
Provided always that any such change, abolition or creation shall forthwith be notified by the Secretary-General in writing to the Clerk of Her Majesty's Most Honourable Privy Council.

(3) The Great Officers (other than the Grand Prior)   shall be appointed by the Grand Prior following consultation with the Grand Council.

(4) The duties of the Great Officers (other than the Grand Prior) may be prescribed by Regulations.

(5) The Prelate shall hold office during the pleasure of the Grand Prior or until resignation.

(6) A Great Officer (other than the Grand Prior and the Prelate) shall be appointed to hold office for such period not exceeding three years as the Grand Prior may determine but shall be eligible for re-appointment on one occasion only for a further period not exceeding three years: Provided that if the holder of one Great Office is appointed to another then the period for which he may be appointed to that subsequent office shall not be restricted by the time which he served in the former office.

(7) A Great Officer

(a) who is a member of a Priory shall remain on the Roll of that Priory;

(b) shall be eligible to be or to continue to be a member of the Priory Chapter of his Priory; but

(c) shall not hold concurrent office within any Priory.

(8) Before being appointed to any Great Office the postulant Great Officer shall in such

form as the Prelate shall prescribe make a declaration that he or she personally professes the Christian faith.

9. The Principal Officers of the Order

(1) The Secretary-General and the holders of any other Principal Offices that may hereafter be created by the Grand Prior on the recommendation of the Grand Council shall be the Principal Officers of the Order.

(2) The Grand Prior, on the recommendation of the Grand Council, may change the title of, or abolish, any Principal Office or may create any new Principal Office: Provided always that any such change, abolition or creation shall forthwith be notified by the Secretary-General in writing to the Clerk of Her Majesty's Most Honourable Privy Council.

(3) The Principal Officers shall be Members of Grade I or Grade II of the Order. They shall be appointed by the Grand Prior to hold office for such period not exceeding three years as he may determine and they shall be eligible for re-appointment save that the Secretary-General shall hold office during the pleasure of the Grand Prior or until resignation.

(4) The duties and responsibilities of the Principal Officers may be prescribed by Regulations.

(5) A Principal Officer other than the Secretary-General

(a) who is a member of a Priory shall remain on the Roll of that Priory;

(b) shall be eligible to be or to continue to be a member of the Priory Chapter of his Priory; but

(c) shall not hold concurrent office within any Priory.

10. The Hospitaller

(1) There shall be a Hospitaller of the Order who shall be appointed by the Grand Prior on the recommendation of the Grand Council.

(2) The provisions of Statute 9 shall *mutatis mutandis* apply to the Hospitaller save that the Hospitaller shall be entitled to hold concurrent office within a Priory.

11. Honorary Officers of The Order

(1) There shall be a Genealogist of the Order who shall be appointed by the Grand Prior on the recommendation of the Grand Council. The Genealogist shall be an Honorary Officer of the Order.

(2) There shall be such other Honorary Officers of the Order as the Grand Council may deem expedient from time to time.

(3) The Honorary Officers shall be Members of the Order in any Grade and shall be appointed to hold office for such period not exceeding three years as the Grand Council may determine and shall be eligible for re-appointment.

12. Secretary of the Order

The Grand Prior may appoint a Member of the Order in any Grade to be Secretary of the Order who shall hold office during the pleasure of the Grand Prior or until resignation and shall perform such duties as may be prescribed by Regulations.

13. The Grand Council

(1) There shall be a Grand Council of the Order which, subject to the authority and the powers of the Sovereign Head and the Grand Prior, shall be the governing body of the Order and may deliberate upon and make recommendations to the Grand Prior regarding all matters which appertain to the affairs or work of the Order and may exercise any of the powers or authority expressly conferred upon the Grand Council by the Royal Charter, these Statutes, and any Regulations, or Rules.

(2) Without prejudice to the generality of the foregoing the Grand Council shall:

(a) ensure the observance of provisions of the Statutes which are designed to safeguard the Christian nature of the Order;

(b) promote the furtherance of the objects of the Order as laid down in Statute 4;

(c) be responsible for the strategic planning of measures for strengthening or expanding the Order's objectives;

(d) consider and, if thought fit, recommend the establishment, suspension or dissolution of Priories, Independent Commanderies, and St. John Associations and, subject to the provisions of Statute 20, recommend the establishment, suspension or dissolution of Dependent Commanderies;

(e) consider and, if thought fit, propose to the Grand Prior and the Sovereign Head any changes to the Statutes;

(f) consider proposed changes to Regulations and to the Rules of Priories, Commanderies and St. John Associations and advise the Grand Prior thereon, provided that before advising the Grand Prior to approve such changes the Grand Council shall be satisfied that the proposed Regulations and Rules accord with the Statutes of the Order;

(g) co-ordinate and encourage the activities and the development of Independent Commanderies and St. John Associations;

(h) be responsible, through an Honours and Awards Committee, for the policy on appointments to and promotions in the Order;

(i) consider any proposals from the Honours and Awards Committee for changes to the complements of Grades in the Order and the allocation between Establishments;

(j) adopt a budget for the Secretariat and central services of the Order;

(k) determine the basis of financial contributions by Establishments;

(l) exercise the powers of investment conferred on the Order by Statute 31;

(m) endeavour to co-ordinate and harmonise the use and exploitation by the Order or by any Establishment or other subordinate body of intellectual property rights held by any or by any other Establishment or other subordinate body;

(n) liaise with Priories on matters of common concern;

(o) liaise with Independent Commanderies and St. John Associations;

(p) recommend to the Grand Prior the appointment of the Secretary-General, any other Principal Officers, the Hospitaller of the Order and Honorary Officers of the Order;

(q) through the Secretariat, co-ordinate activities involving more than one Priory or more than one Independent Commandery or St. John Association (without having power to direct the activities of any such body);

(r) direct the work of the Secretariat;

(s) liaise with other bodies on matters affecting the Order as a whole; and

(t) appoint representatives of the Order (but not representatives of Priories) on such other bodies.

14. Membership of the Grand Council

(1) The Grand Council shall consist of *ex officio* and appointed members as follows:

    (a) The *ex officio* members shall be:

        (i) The Great Officers; and

        (ii) The Prior or (if he so appoints) the Chancellor of each Priory; and

    (b) there shall be such number (if any) of appointed members as the Grand Prior having regard to the advice of the Grand Council shall from time to time determine.

(2) The appointed members shall be Members of the Order selected by the Grand Prior. An appointed member shall be appointed to hold office for such period not exceeding three years as the Grand Prior may determine but shall be eligible for re-appointment on one occasion only for a further period not exceeding three years.

(3) The Grand Prior may on a recommendation of not less than three-quarters of all members of the Grand Council make changes in the composition of the Grand Council.

(4) The Hospitaller of the Order shall have the right to attend any meeting of the Grand Council when any matter affecting his office is on the agenda. He shall be entitled to speak but not vote upon such matter.

15. Procedure in the Grand Council

(1) The Grand Council shall be convened by authority of the Grand Prior not less than once in each year upon not less than twenty-eight days' previous notice at such place as the Grand Prior may from time to time appoint.

(2) Meetings of the Grand Council shall always be opened and closed with prayer, provided nevertheless that no Form of Prayer shall be used which is inconsistent with the forms of worship of the Church of England or of the Church of Scotland as by law established.

(3) The Grand Prior, on the recommendation of the Grand Council and subject to the provisions of paragraph (2) of this Statute, may make Regulations as to the manner in which the Grand Council shall conduct its business and, without prejudice to the generality of the foregoing, such Regulations may prescribe who shall preside in the absence of the Grand Prior, the number of members forming a quorum, the method of voting and the circumstances in which persons who are not members of the Grand Council may be admitted to and be heard at any meeting.

16. The Honours and Awards Committee

(1) There shall be an Honours and Awards Committee which shall be a standing committee of the Grand Council.

(2) The Honours and Awards Committee shall advise the Grand Council on all matters relating to appointments to and promotions in the Order and relating to the eligibility for the award of The Life-Saving Medal and The Service Medal.

(3) Without prejudice to the generality of Statute 16(2) the Honours and Awards Committee shall:

    (a) consider all recommendations for appointment as or promotion to the grade of Bailiff or Dame Grand Cross of the Order;

    (b) consider all recommendations for the appointment to or promotion in the Order in any grade of any person who is not resident within the territory of any Priory;

    (c) keep under review and advise the Grand Council with regard to complements for the purposes of Statute 37;

    (d) keep under review and where it thinks fit make recommendations to the Grand Council in respect of the criteria for the award of The Life-Saving Medal; and

    (e) keep under review and where it thinks fit make recommendations to the Grand Council in respect of the criteria for the award of The Service Medal.

(4) The Honours and Awards Committee shall consist of the Lord Prior as President, the Prelate, the Deputy Lord Prior or Deputy Lord Priors and the Sub-Prior and the Secretary-General shall be the secretary of the committee.

(5) The Honours and Awards Committee shall meet whenever the Grand Prior or the Lord Prior may see fit to convene it.

(6) Subject to the approval of the Grand Prior, the Honours and Awards Committee may make By-laws to regulate its own procedures.

17. Delegation to Priories in respect of Honours and Awards

The Grand Council shall have the power to delegate to Priories in all cases subject to such conditions as it may from time to time prescribe:

    (a) the power to make recommendations to the Grand Prior in respect of appointments to or promotions in the Order other than appointments or promotions to Grade I in the Order;

(b) the award of The Life-Saving Medal;

(c) the award of The Service Medal; and

(d) the appointment of Donats.

18. Establishments of the Order

(1) Distinct Establishments of the Order, designated Priories, Commanderies or St. John Associations, may be constituted within the Order in accordance with the provisions of Statutes 19, 20 and 22 in any area where the work of the Order is being carried on, subject to the Grand Prior being satisfied, in the case of Priories and Commanderies, that the number of Members of the Order resident in that area, and in all cases that the importance and value of the work being carried on therein, make it desirable to do so.

(2) A Priory shall be governed by a Prior and a Priory Chapter; a Commandery shall be governed by a Knight or Dame Commander and a Commandery Chapter.

(3) A St. John Association shall be governed in accordance with Rules made under Statute 22(3).

(4) Each Priory, Commandery and St. John Association shall have the immediate general control and supervision of the affairs and work of the Order and the Members of the Order resident within its geographical area of authority.

(5) Each Establishment shall be subject to the provisions of the Royal Charter and these Statutes as are in force from time to time.

19. Priories

(1) A Priory may properly be constituted with the widest practicable degree of autonomy in any country or group of countries.

(2) Where in any case, having regard to the foregoing provisions and to Statute 18, the Grand Council so recommends, the Grand Prior with the sanction of the Sovereign Head may by Instrument under his hand and the seal of the Order constitute a Priory and declare its style and title, its area of authority and its membership. In addition the Grand Prior, on the same recommendations, shall make Rules for the government of the Priory including its powers and functions and the composition of its Priory Chapter and thereafter such Rules shall be capable of addition, amendment or revocation from time to time (as shall be stated therein) by the Grand Prior on the recommendation of the Prior of the Priory and his Priory Chapter and having regard to the advice of the Grand Council. The provisions of the Priory Rules for the time being in force shall in all respects be consistent with local law.

(3) The Grand Prior shall have power to suspend temporarily all or any part of the operations of a Priory and all or any of the Rules applicable thereto and, on the recommendation of the Grand Council, may vary the constitution of the Priory, or dissolve it or any of its dependent Establishments.

(4) All Priories shall rank *pari passu*:

Provided that the Grand Council shall be entitled to prescribe differential rates of financial contribution to the central work of the Order and provided also that Priories which are in existence on St. John's Day 1999 shall be listed in the order set forth in Statute 57 and any Priories which are created after that date shall be listed in the order of the dates on which they are created.

20. Commanderies

(1) A Commandery may properly be constituted in any country or part of a country or group of countries.

(2) A Commandery shall be either:

(a) an Independent Commandery, that is an Establishment the territory of which is wholly outside the territory of a Priory; or

(b) a Dependent Commandery, that is an Establishment the territory of which is wholly or partly within the territory of a Priory and which is dependent on that Priory.

(3) Where in any case, having regard to the foregoing provisions and to the provisions of Statute 18, the Grand Council so recommends and in the case of a Commandery dependent on a Priory, the Priory Chapter also recommends, the Grand Prior with the sanction of the Sovereign Head may by Instrument under his hand and the seal of the Order constitute a Commandery and declare its style and title, its membership, its area of authority and in the case of a Dependent Commandery its dependence on a stated Priory. In addition, the Grand Prior, on the same recommendations, shall make Rules for the government of the Commandery including its powers and functions and the composition of the Commandery Chapter and thereafter such Rules shall be capable of addition, amendment or revocation from time to time (as shall be stated therein)

by the Grand Prior on the recommendation of the Grand Council together with, in the case of a Dependent Commandery, the recommendation of the Prior concerned and his Priory Chapter.

(4) The Grand Prior, or the Prior of a Priory on which a Commandery is dependent, shall have power to suspend temporarily all or any part of the operations of a Commandery and all or any of the Rules applicable thereto and on the recommendation of the Grand Council, coupled with that of the Priory Chapter where appropriate, the Grand Prior may vary the constitution of a Commandery or dissolve it or vary its dependence.

21. Grand Prior's Advisory Council

(1) There shall be a Grand Prior's Advisory Council to which the Grand Prior may refer any matter concerning the Order in regard to which he may desire its advice.

(2) The Grand Prior's Advisory Council shall consist of *ex officio* and appointed members as follows:

(a) the *ex officio* members shall be the members for the time being of the Grand Council; and

(b) the appointed members, who shall be styled Grand Prior's Councillors, shall be not more than fifty in number and shall be appointed by the Grand Prior on the recommendation of Priors of Priories in the manner prescribed by Regulations.

(3) The Secretary-General shall be the secretary of the Grand Prior's Advisory Council.

(4) The Grand Prior's Advisory Council shall meet if and whenever the Grand Prior shall see fit to convene it.

(5) Not less than ten per centum of the Grand Prior's Councillors for the time being in office may require the Grand Council to consider any matter concerning the Order of which they give notice in writing to the Secretary-General.

(6) This Statute and all appointments of Grand Prior's Councillors shall cease to have effect on St. John's Day 2010 unless before that day the Grand Council shall resolve that this Statute shall continue in force.

(7) Subject to the approval of the Grand Prior, the Grand Prior's Advisory Council may make By-laws to regulate its own procedure.

22. St. John Associations

(1) A St. John Association may properly be constituted in any country or group of countries (but not being within the territory of another Establishment).

(2) Within the territory for which it is constituted, the general objects and purposes of a St. John Association shall be to further any one or more of the objects of the Order as prescribed by Statute 4 and without prejudice to the generality of the foregoing:

(a) To encourage and promote all work of humanity and charity for the relief of persons in sickness, distress, suffering, or danger without distinction of race, class, colour or creed; and

(b) To render aid to the sick, wounded, disabled, or suffering and to promote such permanent organisation during times of peace as may be at once available in times of civil emergencies or war, including the training and provision of technical reserves for the medical services of the Armed Forces or Civil Defence Organisations, and in particular a St. John Association shall have within its area the control and management of St. John Ambulance.

(3) Where in any case, having regard to the foregoing provisions, the Grand Council so recommends the Grand Prior may by Instrument under his hand and the seal of the Order constitute a St. John Association and declare its style and title together with its area of authority. In addition, on the same recommendation, the Grand Prior shall make Rules for the government of the St. John Association extending to all such matters as he shall deem appropriate including the powers, functions, organisation and membership thereof.

(4) The Rules of a St. John Association shall be capable of addition, amendment or revocation from time to time by a Resolution passed in such manner as the Rules may from time to time prescribe at a duly convened meeting of the Association and, subject to the provisions of its constitution and of any relevant provisions of local law, as the Grand Prior having regard to the advice of the Grand Council shall approve.

(5) Whenever possible, Members of the Order and members of the St. John Ambulance shall together form the majority of the members of the governing body of any St. John Association.

(6) The Grand Prior may call upon any St. John Association to suspend temporarily or to abandon all or any part of its operations. In addition, the Grand Prior may, on the recommendation of the Grand Council, by Instrument under his hand and the seal of the Order, deprive any specified St. John Association of its powers, authority and functions under this Statute and declare that it is no longer recognised by the Order as being lawfully constituted under the Royal Charter and Statutes of the Order.

(7) All National St. John Councils in existence immediately prior to the Appointed Day shall become St. John Associations on the Appointed Day.

(8) All Special Regulations or Rules applicable to a National St. John Council made under the powers previously vested in the Grand Prior as subsequently lawfully added to, amended or revoked shall be the Rules for that St. John Association within the meaning of paragraph (3) of this Statute.

23. Rules of Incorporated Establishments

(1) Where a Priory, Independent Commandery, Dependent Commandery or St. John Association is incorporated under local law, the instrument of incorporation of that Establishment and any amendment thereto for the time being in force shall be capable of constituting the Rules of that body.

(2) Nothing in Statute 23(1) shall modify the requirement for such approvals as are specified in Statutes 19, 20 and 22: Provided that where the Grand Prior has approved instruments of incorporation which are intended to operate as Rules he shall for the purposes of those Statutes be deemed to have made such Rules.

24. Foundations

(1) A Foundation shall be an institution or an organised body constituted for the furtherance of any of the objects or purposes of the Order and may be either a Foundation of the Order or a Priory Foundation as hereinafter provided.

(2) The Grand Prior may, on the recommendation of the Grand Council, constitute any Foundation of the Order in any part of the world in such manner as may be requisite by law and he may on the like recommendation, in the same manner alter, abolish, extend or restrict the objects or purposes of any Foundation of the Order as he may deem desirable in the interests of the Order.

(3) Foundations of the Order shall be under the entire control of the Grand Prior and the Grand Council. Nevertheless the Grand Prior may, on the recommendation of the Grand Council, assign the control and management of any specified Foundation insofar as it concerns its operation within the territorial limits of a Priory, of an Independent Commandery or of a St. John Association, to the Prior and the Priory Chapter or the Knight or Dame Commander and the Commandery Chapter or the St. John Association as the case may be of that territory. In like manner and after such recommendation, the Grand Prior may revoke or modify any such assignment.

(4) The Grand Prior may, at the request of any Prior and on the recommendation of the Priory Chapter, constitute a Priory Foundation for the territory of that Priory in such manner as may be requisite by law and he may, on the like request and recommendation, in the same manner alter, abolish, extend or restrict the objects or purposes of any such Foundation. A Priory Foundation shall be under the joint control of the Grand Prior and the Prior and Priory Chapter concerned.

(5) The Grand Prior may, on the recommendation of the Grand Council in the case of a Foundation of the Order, or, on the recommendation of the Prior and Priory Chapter concerned in the case of a Priory Foundation, make Rules under his hand and the seal of the Order for governing the activities of any Foundation and may on the like recommendation, suspend, revoke or amend such Rules from time to time.

(6) A Foundation of the Order may be incorporated in any part of the world or may be unincorporated.

25. Visitations

(1) For the maintenance of discipline, sound administration and uniform policy throughout the Order all Establishments and other subordinate bodies shall be subject to visitation by the Grand Prior or his representative, whenever the Grand Prior thinks fit. Similarly all Establishments and other subordinate bodies dependent on a Priory shall be subject to visitation by the Prior of that Priory or his representative.

(2) On the completion of the visitation, the visitor shall render a report in writing to the Grand Prior through the Secretary-General, or, in the case of a visitor appointed by a Prior, to that Prior. In the latter case, the Prior concerned shall consider the report without undue delay and shall forward it to the Grand Prior through the Secretary-General stating what action has been taken or is proposed to be taken thereon.

(3) All such reports reaching the Grand Prior shall also be presented at the next meeting of the Grand Council and in the case of a report prepared by a visitor appointed by a Prior to that Priory Chapter, unless the Grand Prior in his discretion decides to treat the whole report or any part of such report as confidential.

(4) The Grand Prior shall take such action as he thinks desirable in the interests of the Order upon any visitation conducted by him or any report of a visitation submitted to him.

26. Allocation of Property

(1) Property held by or for the purposes of the Order in any part of the world may be allocated by the Grand Prior either for a particular purpose or for the general purposes whether of the Order or of any Establishment and property not allocated expressly under this Statute shall be deemed to be held for the general purposes of the Order (when not impressed with any special trust at the time of acquisition).

(2) Every such allocation under this Statute shall be made on the recommendation of the Grand Council and if it is in favour of a Commandery dependent on a Priory also on the recommendation of the Priory Chapter of that Priory.

(3) Every such allocation shall be by instrument in writing under the hand of the Grand Prior and the seal of the Order and any such Instrument of Allocation may be revoked or varied by the Grand Prior on the like recommendation.

(4) Where property has been allocated to an Establishment under the foregoing provisions of this Statute, such Establishment shall have and may exercise on behalf of the Order all such powers of control and disposition over such property as are vested in the Order. Such allocated property shall be held in the name of the Order or, in case of land, buildings or money to be invested, shall if the Establishment or the Grand Prior so directs be vested in a trust holding company or corporation or in some individual person or persons holding as trustees under a trust created by the Establishment or by its superior Establishment, if any.

(5) Nothing herein contained shall restrict the rights or powers of the Order in respect of property not allocated to an Establishment.

27. Transfers of Property to Establishments

(1) In addition to the power of allocation conferred by Statute 26 property held by or for the purposes of the Order in any part of the world may be transferred by the Grand Prior to any Establishment (the transfer being subject to any special trust which was impressed on such property at the time of acquisition).

(2) Every such transfer under this Statute shall be made on the recommendation of the Grand Council and if it is in favour of a Commandery dependent on a Priory also on the recommendation of the Priory Chapter of that Priory.

(3) Every such transfer shall be by instrument in writing under the hand of the Grand Prior and the seal of the Order.

28. Liabilities

(1) All liability in contract or otherwise arising out of (a) the operations of an Establishment, or (b) the operations of any Foundation which are carried on in the territory of an Establishment, shall be discharged out of the property owned by or allocated to that Establishment.

(2) Every Establishment shall so far as may be practicable in any contract relating to such operations as are specified in Statute 28(1) arrange that liability under such contract shall only be met out of the property owned by or allocated to that Establishment.

29. Indemnity Insurance

(1) Subject to the provisions of Statute 29(2) the Order may at its expense procure the provision of indemnity insurance to cover the liability of members of the Grand Council which by virtue of any rule of law would otherwise attach to them in respect of any negligence, default, breach of trust or breach of duty of which they may be guilty in relation to the Order.

(2) Any such insurance shall not extend to:

(a) any claim arising from any act or omission which the members of the Grand Council knew to be a breach of trust or breach of duty or which was committed by the members of the Grand Council in reckless disregard of whether it was a breach of trust or breach of duty or not; or

(b) the costs of an unsuccessful defence to a criminal prosecution brought against the members of the Grand Council in their capacity as trustees of the Order.

30. Financial Contributions by Establishments

The Grand Council shall have power to require Priories, Independent Commanderies and St. John Associations to make financial contributions to the central administration and work of the Order.

31. The Order's Powers of Investment

(1) Moneys and funds of the Order not immediately required to be expended may be invested in or upon any of the investments following that is to say:

(a) in any investments authorised by the law for the time being in force for the investment of trust funds;

(b) upon the security of freehold or leasehold property in the United Kingdom (such leasehold property being held for a term of which at least sixty years remain unexpired at the date of investment);

(c) in the purchase and subsequent development of freehold or leasehold land in the United Kingdom (such leasehold property being held for a term of which at least sixty years remain unexpired at the date of investment);

(d) in any of the securities of the government of any country within the Commonwealth or of any province or constituent part of any such country that has a separate legislature;

(e) in or upon the mortgages or other securities of any municipal, county or other local or public authority incorporated in any country within the Commonwealth;

(f) in or upon the debentures or debenture stock or bonds, or loan stock or notes of any kind, or guaranteed, or preference, or preferred stock or shares of any company incorporated under any general or special Act of the United Kingdom Parliament or any general or special enactment of the legislature of any other country within the Commonwealth;

(g) in or upon any debentures, or debenture stock or bonds, or loan stock or notes of any kind, or guaranteed or preference, or preferred stock or shares, or ordinary, or deferred stock or shares normally dealt in on any investment Exchange recognised for the purpose of the Financial Services Act 1986 or on one of the Stock Exchanges authorised from time to time in Regulations;

(h) in or upon any debentures, or debenture stock or bonds, or loan stock or notes of any kind, or guaranteed, or preference, or preferred stock or shares, or ordinary, or deferred stock or shares, of any Investment, Financial or Unit Trust which is at the time of making the investment quoted on a recognised Stock Exchange in the United Kingdom;

(i) in the shares of or on loan to or deposit with any Building Society incorporated or registered in the United Kingdom;

(j) on deposit at any Bank: Provided nevertheless that the powers hereby conferred shall be subject to the following stipulations and conditions:

   (i) No investment shall be made which would transgress the powers (if any) contained in the instrument of gift (if any) governing the moneys or funds to be invested;

   (ii) No investments shall be made in any company having an issued and paid-up share capital of less than £750,000 or its equivalent at the current rates of exchange. In the case of a company having shares of no par value such paidup capital shall be deemed to include the capital sum (other than capital surplus) appearing in the company's accounts in respect of such shares;

   (iii) The Order may accept and hold for such period as is thought fit any investment or property transferred or to be transferred to the Order by any person or corporation and whether within the range of investments hereinbefore prescribed or not, subject always to the limitations for the time being imposed by the Charter of 1955 or any Supplemental Charter relating to the holding of land;

   (iv) The Order shall not invest money in or retain any securities in respect whereof any liability exists unless the liability is of limited amount and is to be discharged or is capable of being discharged within a fixed period from the date of investment provided that this sub-paragraph shall not apply to investments in the stock or shares of banks and insurance companies the price whereof is normally quoted on a recognised Stock Exchange in the United Kingdom;

(v) Money awaiting investment may be advanced on the security of stocks, funds or securities the purchase of which would be authorised by the powers conferred by this Statute.

(2) Any investments belonging to the Order may at any time be varied and transposed for or into any other investment or investments of any kind authorised by this Statute and subject to the provisions hereof.

(3) Where any moneys or funds of the Order have been allocated under Statute 26 or have otherwise accrued to an Establishment or other subordinate body situate in a country outside the United Kingdom, the foregoing provisions may be construed in relation to the investment of such moneys or funds in such country as if references to such country were substituted for the United Kingdom and such provisions shall then apply only to the extent that so construed they do not conflict with any law of such country or the terms of any subsisting trust applicable to the investment of such moneys or funds.

(4) In the following provisions of this Statute 31:

(a) the expression "the 1986 Act" means the Financial Services Act 1986 and any statutory modification or re-enactment thereof; and

(b) the expression "Investment Manager" means a person appointed as such pursuant to Statute 31(5).

(5) The Grand Council may appoint as the Investment Manager a person whom it is satisfied after inquiry is a proper and competent person to act in that capacity and who is either:

(a) an individual of repute with at least 15 years' experience of investment management and who is an authorised person within the meaning of the 1986 Act; or

(b) a company or firm of repute which is an authorised or exempted person within the meaning of that Act otherwise than by virtue of section 45(1) (j) of that Act.

(6) The Grand Council may delegate to the Investment Manager power at his discretion to buy and sell investments for the Order in accordance with the investment policy laid down by the Grand Council. The Grand Council may only effect such delegation on terms consistent with this Statute 31.

(7) Where the Grand Council makes any delegation under this Statute 31 it shall:

(a) inform the Investment Manager in writing of the extent of the Order's investment powers;

(b) lay down a detailed investment policy for the Order and immediately inform the Investment Manager in writing of that policy and of any changes to it;

(c) ensure that the terms of the delegated authority are clearly set out in writing and notified to the Investment Manager;

(d) ensure that the Grand Council is kept informed of and reviews on a regular basis the performance of its investment portfolio managed by the Investment Manager and the exercise by him of his delegated authority;

(e) take all reasonable care to ensure that the Investment Manager complies with the terms of his delegated authority;

(f) review the appointment of the Investment Manager at such intervals not exceeding 24 months as it thinks fit; and

(g) pay such reasonable and proper remuneration to the Investment Manager and agree such proper terms as to notice and other matters as the Grand Council shall decide and as are consistent with this Statute 31: Provided that such remuneration may include any or all of commission and fees earned and reimbursement of expenses incurred by the Investment Manager if and only to the extent that such commission fees and expenses are disclosed to the Grand Council.

(8) Where the Grand Council makes any delegation under this Statute 31 it shall do so on terms that:

(a) the Investment Manager shall comply with the terms of his delegated authority;

(b) the Investment Manager shall not do anything which the Order does not have power to do;

(c) the Grand Council may with reasonable notice revoke the delegation or vary any of its terms in a way which is consistent with the terms of this Statute 31; and

(d) the Grand Council shall give directions to the Investment Manager as to the manner in which he is to report to it all sales and purchases of investments made on its behalf.

(9) Where the Grand Council makes any delegation under this Statute 31 it may also delegate to the Investment Manager power to exercise the voting rights attaching to investments in accordance with the policy on such voting for the time being laid down by the Order.

(10) The Grand Council may:

(a) make such arrangements as it thinks fit for any investments of the Order or income from those investments to be held by a corporate body as custodian trustee or as the Order's nominee; and

(b) pay reasonable and proper remuneration to any corporate body acting as custodian trustee of the Order's nominee in pursuance of this provision.

PART THREE: MEMBERS

32. Grades of the Order

(1) The Order shall be divided into the following Grades:
- Grade I Bailiffs or Dames Grand Cross (G.C.St.J.)
- Grade II Knights or Dames of Justice or Grace (K.St.J. or D.St.J.)
- Grade III Commanders (Brothers or Sisters) (C.St.J.)
- Grade IV Officers (Brothers or Sisters) (O.St.J.)

- Grade V Serving Brothers or Serving Sisters (S.B.St.J. or S.S.St.J.)
- Grade VI Esquires (Esq.St.J.)

(2) The letters specified above after each Grade may be used by those to whom they apply to such extent as may be prescribed in the case of those borne on a Roll of a Priory by the Priory Rules of that Priory and in the case of those borne on the Roll of the Order by Order Rules but admission or promotion to any Grade of the Order or the privileges derived therefrom of wearing the insignia appertaining or belonging thereto shall not confer any rank, style, title, dignity, appellation or social precedence whatsoever.

32A. Clerical Brethren

(1) Save as hereinafter provided in this Statute, clerical Grades in the Order shall cease to exist on the day immediately before the Appointed Day and ministers of the Christian religion who are then or who are thereafter admitted to be members of the Order shall be placed in the appropriate Grade specified in Statute 32(1).

(2) (a) A minister of the Christian religion placed in the Grade of Chaplain prior to the Appointed Day shall unless and until he or she shall be promoted be entitled to style himself or herself "Chaplain" and to use in accordance with Statute 32(2) the postnominal letters "Ch.St.J."

(b) Subject to paragraph (a) a minister of the Christian religion placed in the Grade of Chaplain prior to the Appointed Day shall be re-classsified as a "Commander" with seniority according to the date on which he or she was placed in the Grade of Chaplain.

(3) (a) A minister of the Christian religion who is a Member in Grade IV or V of the Order who prior to the Appointed Day desired to be termed a Sub-Chaplain or an Assistant Chaplain shall unless and until he or she shall be promoted continue to be entitled to be so termed and to use in accordance with Statute 32(2)the postnominal letters Sub-Ch.St.J. and Asst.Ch.St.J. respectively.

32B. Sub-Prelates

(1) The Senior Ecclesiastical Officer (or Officers) of each Priory shall for as long as he holds that office be concurrently a Sub-Prelate of the Order but in relation to his duties as such he shall be accountable to the Prior of the Priory and not to the Prelate of the Order.

(2) A Member of Episcopal rank or other eminent status in the Christian Church appointed prior to 24 October 1999 by the Grand Prior to be a Sub-Prelate of the Order shall from the Appointed Day be styled an "Honorary Sub-Prelate."

33. Qualifications for Membership of the Order

(1) No person shall be qualified for membership in any Grade of the Order unless he or she:

    (a) makes a declaration in the terms specified in Statute 34;

    (b) furnishes a certificate in accordance with Statute 34A;

    (c) either:

        (i) has performed or is prepared to perform good service for the Order and its objects and purposes in accordance with the Mottoes of the Order; or

        (ii) has acted conspicuously in a manner which furthers such objects and purposes; and

    (d) has undertaken to comply with the provisions of the Royal Charter, the Statutes, and the Regulations and Rules of the Order.

(2) No person shall be admitted to the Order in Grade VI unless he has attained the age of 16 or in any other Grade unless he has attained the age of 18.

(3) Persons who were Associate Members of the Order on St. John's Day 1999 shall be re-classified as Members of the Order retaining the same Grade.

(4) An Associate Member who is re-classified as a Member of the Order shall rank for seniority according to the date of his or her attachment in the Grade which is applicable at the date of reclassification.

34. Declaration before Admission to the Order

Subject to the provisions of Statute 35, before initial admission to the Order, a Declaration in the following terms shall be signed by prospective Members: "I do solemnly declare that I will be faithful and obedient to The Order of St. John and its Sovereign Head as far as it is consistent with my duty [to my Sovereign/President and] (*) to my country; that I will do everything in my power to uphold its dignity and support its charitable works; and that I will endeavour always to uphold the aims of this Christian Order and to conduct myself as a person of honour."

* The words in brackets to be adapted according to the circumstances of the declarant.

34A. Specified Bodies

(1) No person shall be admitted to the Order if he or she shall also be a member of a Specified Body.

(2) Before initial admission to the Order and before any promotion in the Order the Member or prospective Member shall furnish a certificate in such form as the Grand Prior on the recommendation of the Grand Council shall prescribe that he or she is not a member of a Specified Body and that he or she will not become a member of a Specified Body for so long as he or she is a Member of the Order.

(3) (a) A Specified Body is any body of persons (whether or not incorporated and whether or not a legal entity) which:

(i) holds itself out or represents itself or styles itself to be an order which is:

    (aa) an order of St. John; or

    (bb) derived from an order of St. John; or

    (cc) associated with an order of St. John;

(ii) is not one of the Mutually Recognised Orders of St. John (as defined in paragraph (3)(c) of this Statute); and

(iii) either or both:

    (aa) uses the words "St. John" or any translation or variant thereof in its title (irrespective of any other words used in the title); or

    (bb) uses:

        i. the Emblem (as defined in paragraph (3)(d) of this Statute) with or without any other device or motif; or

        ii. any other device or motif sufficiently similar to the Emblem as to be likely to cause confusion therewith.

(b) For the purposes of sub-paragraph (i) of this paragraph a body shall be capable of being an order of St. John whether or not it is one of the Mutually Recognised Orders.

(c) The Mutually Recognised Orders of St. John are:

(i) the Order;

(ii) the three other Orders which comprise the Alliance of the Orders of St. John, namely:

    (aa) Die Balley Brandenburg des Ritterlichen Ordens Sankt Johannis vom Spital zu Jerusalem (commonly referred to as "the Johanniter Orden");

    (bb) Johanniter Orde in Nederland; and

    (cc) Johanniterorden I Sverige; and

(iii) the Sovereign Military and Hospitaller Order of St. John of Jerusalem, called of Rhodes, called of Malta (commonly referred to as "the Sovereign Military Order of Malta" or "the Order of Malta").

(d) The Emblem is a white equidistant eight-pointed cross (commonly referred to as "the Maltese Cross" or "the Amalfi Cross") with or without embellishments in the angles on a background of any colour or colours and of any shape.

(4) A decision of the Grand Council as to whether any body is or is not a Specified Body shall be final and binding on all persons interested under these Statutes.

35. Modified Declarations

(1) Notwithstanding and in priority to the provisions of Statute 34 a Priory shall be entitled to prescribe a modified form of declaration to be signed before initial admission to the Order of a person who will be borne on the Roll of that Priory. Such declaration, which shall be in such terms as the Grand Prior may approve, shall require the declarant to declare that he personally professes the Christian faith and subject thereto shall as nearly as the circumstances permit be in the form set forth in Statute 34.

(2) Before initial admission to the Order of a person who will be borne on the Roll of a Priory which has not prescribed a modified form of declaration under Statute 35(1), that person may, if he so wishes, in the Declaration to be made by him under Statute 34 include a statement that he personally professes the Christian faith. Such statement shall be in such form as the Prelate may approve.

(3) Where a Member wishes to transfer to the Roll of a Priory which has prescribed a modified form of declaration for the purposes of Statute 35(1), he may be required by that Priory to make a declaration in such modified form before such transfer is effected.

36. Concurrent Membership

(1) A Member of the Order who is resident within the territory of a Priory shall be concurrently a member of that Priory.

(2) A Member of the Order who is resident within the territory of a St. John Association shall, if the constitution of that Council so provides, be concurrently a member of that Council.

37. Complements of the various Grades

(1) The aggregate maximum complement for Members in all Grades shall be 35,000 or such other number as the Grand Prior on the recommendation of the Grand Council shall from time to time prescribe.

(2) (a) The maximum complement for Grade I of the Order shall be:
    (i) the Great Officers; and
    (ii) twenty-one other Bailiffs or Dames Grand Cross.

(b) When a Great Officer shall cease to hold such office he shall continue in the Grade of Bailiff or Dame Grand Cross but shall not count against the complement thereof. This shall be so whether or not such Member was a Bailiff or Dame Grand Cross before being appointed to be a Great Officer.

(c) A Member in Grade I on the Appointed Day who is a Head of State or a member of a Commonwealth or Foreign Royal Family and a person who after the Appointed Day is admitted to the Order in Grade I in accordance with Statute 38(1) shall not count against the complement of Grade I.

(3) The maximum complement for each of the other Grades in the Order and the method of allocation between those to be borne on the Roll of the Order and those to be borne on the rolls of Priories shall be prescribed by Regulations.

38. Appointments to and Promotions in the Order

(1) The Grand Prior on the recommendation of the Grand Council and with the sanction of the Sovereign Head may invite any Head of State or any member of the British Royal Family or of any other Commonwealth or of any Foreign Royal Family to become a Member of Grade I or Grade II of the Order as the Sovereign Head shall approve and upon acceptance he or she shall thereupon be admitted as such and be supernumerary to the Grade without the payment of any Foundation Due or Annual Oblation.

(2) All other admissions to and promotions in the Order shall be sanctioned by and be made in the name of and by the authority of the Sovereign Head after recommendation by the Grand Council and approval by the Grand Prior. The names of those approved by the Sovereign Head shall be published in the *London Gazette* or such other official Gazette as the Grand Prior shall specify. The procedure relating to the selection of suitable persons and verification of their qualifications under these Statutes before submission of their names to the Sovereign Head may be prescribed by Regulations.

(3) Unless in any particular case the Grand Council otherwise recommends or it is otherwise provided by these Statutes or any Regulation, admissions to the Order shall normally be in Grade V and promotions from a lower to a higher Grade shall be dependent upon the rendering of good service in the lower Grade.

(4) On appointment, each Prior of a Priory shall become a Knight or Dame of Justice if he or she does not already hold that rank and if he or she is not a Bailiff or Dame Grand Cross. Further the Grand Prior may at his discretion sanction the reclassification, for good cause *motu proprio*, of a Knight or Dame of Grace as a Knight or Dame of Justice. No other person shall be qualified to be classified as "of Justice" on promotion or appointment to Grade II of the Order unless at such time he or she is entitled to bear Arms. A Knight or Dame of Grace may elect at any time to be re-classified as a Knight or Dame of Justice, as the case may be, without any change in seniority in the Order if he or she is able to satisfy the Genealogist of the Order, or if domiciled in Scotland, the Genealogist of the Priory of Scotland, or in the case of other Priories, the Genealogist of the Priory, provided the latter is an Officer of Arms in Ordinary to the Sovereign Head of the Order, that he or she is entitled to bear Arms.

(5) There shall be a Homage Roll for Members which shall be signed by Members as soon as possible after first admission to the Order in token of their voluntary submission to the supreme authority of the Sovereign Head and of the Grand Prior.

(6) Each Priory shall maintain a Roll of all Members of the Order within that Priory.

(7) Subject to the provisions of Statute 35(3), a Member may be transferred from the Roll of one Priory to the Roll of another Priory in such manner as may be prescribed by Regulations.

(8) The Secretary-General shall maintain a Roll of all Members of the Order who are not borne on the Roll of a Priory in such manner as may be prescribed by Regulations.

39. Personal Esquires

Each Member of the Order in the Grade of Bailiff or Dame Grand Cross or Knight or Dame of Justice shall have the right to nominate two Personal Esquires and each Member of the Order in the Grade of Knight or Dame of Grace shall have the right to nominate one Personal Esquire. Each nominee shall possess the qualifications prescribed by Statute 33.

(1) and subject to the recommendations of the Grand Council and the approval of the Grand Prior the name of the person shall be submitted in the usual manner for admission to the Order in Grade VI and appointment as a Personal Esquire. Such person shall hold his appointment during the pleasure of his nominator and, unless he is subsequently promoted to a higher Grade, his admission to Grade VI shall lapse should his nominator revoke the appointment or cease for any reason to be a Member of the Order.

40. Donats

(1) Any person not being a Member of the Order who from an appreciation of the objects or work of the Order makes a worthy contribution to its funds or to the funds of a Priory may be appointed:

    (a) by the Grand Prior, on the recommendation of the Grand Council, a Donat of the Order; or

    (b) by the Prior of a Priory, on the recommendation of his Priory Chapter, to be a Donat of the Priory and thereafter his name shall be recorded in the List of Donats of the Order which shall be maintained by the Secretary-General or as the case may be in the List of Donats of the Priory which shall be maintained by the proper officer of the Priory.

(2) The rights and privileges of a Donat of a Priory shall in all respects be the same as those of a Donat of the Order.

(3) The appointment of a Donat shall lapse and his name shall be deleted from the List of Donats if he shall subsequently be admitted as a Member of the Order in any Grade.

41. Precedence within the Order

(1) Precedence within the Order shall be as follows:

- The Sovereign Head
- The Grand Prior
- The Lord Prior of St. John
- The Prior of a Priory or the Knight or Dame Commander of a Commandery when within the territory of the Establishment
- The Prelate of the Order

- The Deputy Lord Prior or the Deputy Lord Priors, if more than one in the order of seniority in their Grades
- The Sub-Prior of the Order
- Former Great Officers
- Bailiffs and Dames Grand Cross
- The Prior of a Priory outside the territory of the Priory
- The Members of the Grand Council not included above in the order of seniority in their Grades
- The Principal Officers in the order of their offices as laid down in Statute 9
- The Sub-Prelates and the Honorary Sub-Prelates
- The Hospitaller of the Order
- Knights and Dames
- Chaplains
- Commanders
- Officers
- Serving Brothers and Serving Sisters
- Esquires

(2) Precedence in any Grade is determined by the date of appointment within the Grade, subject to the observance of the following special provisions:

(a) Members of the British Royal Family shall take precedence in their respective Grades, followed immediately by the undermentioned in the order stated:

(i) Commonwealth Heads of State;

(ii) Foreign Heads of State;

(iii) Members of Commonwealth Royal Families;

(iv) Members of Foreign Royal Families.

(b) The precedence of a Knight or Dame Commander of a Commandery outside the territorial limits of his or her Commandery shall be determined by his or her seniority within his or her Grade.

(c) A Knight or Dame of Grace who is re-classified as a Knight or Dame of Justice shall rank for seniority according to his or her date of original appointment as a Knight or Dame.

42. Foundation Dues and Oblations

The Order is devoted to works of Charity and Humanity and it is a fundamental rule that those who belong to the Order should contribute to its Charities such Foundation Dues and Oblations according to their position in the Order as may from time to time be prescribed by Regulations made under Statute 7(3) or subject thereto, by Rules made in that behalf by the Grand Prior or, as the case may be, by a Prior in respect of his Priory or by a Knight or Dame Commander in respect of his or her Commandery.

43. Termination of Membership

(1) (a) A Member who is borne on the Roll of a Priory and who is desirous of resigning from the Order shall give written notice of such desire to the Priory Secretary or other proper officer of the Priory.

(b) A Member who is borne on the Roll of the Order maintained under Statute 38(8) and who is desirous of resigning from the Order shall give written notice of such desire to the Secretary-General.

(c) Upon receipt of a notice given under paragraphs (a) or (b) the Member shall cease to be a member of the Order.

(2) (a) If any Member shall for three years or more be in arrears with his or her Foundation Due or Annual Oblation any Great Officer in the case of a Member borne on the Roll of the Order or the Prior in the case of a Member borne on the Roll of a Priory shall be entitled to terminate the membership of the Order of that person.

(b) If such membership is terminated but all arrears are subsequently paid such person may be re-admitted if the Grand Prior thinks fit.

(3) Without prejudice to the generality of Statute 43(4), if a member shall also be a member of a Specified Body any Great Officer in the case of a Member borne on the Roll of the Order (acting under specific or general authority of the Grand Council) or the Prior in the case of a Member borne on the Roll of a Priory (acting on a recommendation of his Priory Chapter) may terminate the membership of such person; provided that if such person shall thereafter cease to be a member of a Specified Body he may be considered for readmission to the Order as if he had never been a Member.

(4) The Grand Prior on the recommendation of the Grand Council and with the sanction of the Sovereign Head may terminate the membership of any person and on the like recommendation and with the like sanction may re-admit such person.

(5) If the Grand Council shall recommend to the Grand Prior the dissolution or derecognition of a Priory or Commandery or a St. John Association then the Grand Prior on the recommendation of the Grand Council and with the sanction of the Sovereign Head may terminate the membership of the Order of some or all of those who are borne on the Roll of that Priory or Commandery or as the case may be of the section of the Roll of the Order relating to that St. John Association.

(6) Where any person who is borne on the Roll of a Priory ceases in accordance with any of the provision of this Statute to be a Member of the Order he shall thereupon automatically also cease to be a member of the Priory.

(7) As from the date on which any person ceases to be a Member of the Order, he or she shall cease to be liable to pay any future Annual Oblations and shall lose any right to wear or use the Insignia, Augmentation of Arms and any other distinction or privilege of the Order or of membership thereof.

PART FOUR: ARMS, INSIGNIA, ETC.

44. Arms of the Order

The Arms of the Order shall be: Gules a cross argent, in the first quarter a representation of the Sovereign's Crest and they shall be depicted and used in conformity with such provision as may from time to time be made by Regulations.

45. Badge of the Order

The Badge of the Order shall be a white eight-pointed cross embellished in argent in the four principal angles alternately with a lion passant guardant and a unicorn passant, and it shall be designed and used in conformity with such provision as may from time to time be made by Regulations.

46. Great Banner of the Order

The Great Banner of the Order shall bear the Arms of the Order as defined in Statute 44 and it shall be designed and flown in conformity with such provision as may from time to time be made by Regulations.

47. Seal of the Order

(1) The Seal of the Order shall have engraved thereon the Badge of the Order, as laid down in Statute 45, surmounted by an Escutcheon of the Arms of the Order, as laid down in Statute 44, the whole surrounded by the legend: "SIGILLUM MAGNI PRIORATUS ORDINIS HOSPITALIS SANCTI IOHANNIS HIERUSALEM." This may be abbreviated to "SIG:MAG:PR:ORD:HOSP:S.IOHIS:HIER."

(2) The Grand Prior shall make Regulations providing for the custody and use of the Seal of the Order.

48. Seals of Priories and Commanderies

(1) The seal of a Priory, Commandery or St. John Association shall bear the head of St. John Baptist surrounded by the same words similarly abbreviated as appear on the seal of the Order with the substitution of the name of the Establishment in place of the words "MAGNI PRIORATUS." Provided that nothing in these Statutes shall affect the right of the Priory of Scotland to bear on its seal and otherwise the Arms of the Priory of Scotland as recorded under the Law of Arms of Scotland.

(2) The Prior of each Priory and the Knight or Dame Commander of each Commandery, on the recommendation of his or her Priory or Commandery Chapter and the Council or other governing body of a St. John Association, shall provide for the custody and use of the Priory, Commandery or St. John Association Seal, as the case may be.

49. Armorial Bearings

Members of the Order in the following Grades shall be permitted to display their Arms, and to bear the Augmentations of Arms, as hereinafter laid down, provided that their right to Arms is duly established and recorded in the Offices of Arms in England or Scotland or as otherwise authorised by Statute 38(4):

(a) Bailiffs Grand Cross and Dames Grand Cross may bear and use supporters to their Arms, and Garter Principal King of Arms for the time being is hereby authorised to grant supporters to such Bailiffs Grand Cross and Dames Grand Cross as shall not otherwise be entitled thereto; the Lord Lyon King of Arms for the time being is likewise authorised to grant supporters to those of them whose arms are Scottish, and Officers of Arms in other Priories are similarly authorised to grant supporters.

(b) Bailiffs Grand Cross and Dames Grand Cross may bear their Arms with those of the Order in chief. They may further display their Arms on the Badge of the Order.

(c) Knights and Dames, whether "of Justice" or "of Grace," and ministers of the Christian religion placed in the Grade of Chaplain prior to the Appointed Day may display their Arms on the Badge of the Order.

(d) Members of any Grade of the Order other than Grade VI may suspend from their Armorial Bearings the riband and badge of their Grade.

50. Insignia and Robes

The Insignia and Robes of the Order shall be such as may from time to time be specified by Regulations and shall be used and worn as therein provided.

51. Uniform of the St. John Ambulance

Members of the St. John Ambulance so entitled by the appropriate Regulations or Rules shall if so directed and when on duty wear such uniform as is specified in or pursuant to such Regulations or Rules.

52. Medals

(1) The Order may award Medals, Certificates of Honour, and Votes of Thanks in accordance with such provision as may from time to time be made by Regulations.

(2) The award of medals shall be made, in the name of the Sovereign Head, by the Grand Prior on the recommendation of the Grand Council and where appropriate of a Priory Chapter, save that in the case of the Life Saving Medal an immediate award may, where the circumstances so justify, be made by the Grand Prior on the advice of the Lord Prior.

(3) If any person to whom a medal has been awarded shall be deemed by his or her subsequent conduct to have become unworthy of it, his or her name may be erased by the Grand Prior on the recommendation of the Grand Council and where appropriate of a

Priory Chapter from the Register of those upon whom the medal of the Order has been conferred, and he or she shall thereupon cease to be entitled to wear it.

53. Alterations prohibited

No addition to, nor alteration nor modification of the Arms, Badge, Banner, Insignia or Robes of the Order, nor of any other item in these Statutes, may be made by any Priory or Commandery, except that in the case of the Arms of a Priory or a Banner to be used by an Establishment, the Grand Prior may authorise the addition of a suitable distinctive emblem.

54. Emblem Protection

Each Establishment shall use its best endeavours at its own expense to comply with any directions given by the Grand Council for the protection of the Arms of the Order, the Badge of the Order, or the cross commonly known as the Amalfi Cross being a white eight-pointed cross without embellishments.

55. Intellectual Property Rights in respect of the Arms or Badge of the Order or the name St. John

Each Establishment shall use its best endeavours at its own expense to comply with any directions given by the Grand Council with regard to the use and exploitation of intellectual property rights in relation to the Arms of the Order or the Badge of the Order or any variants of them or of the names "St. John" or "St. John Ambulance" with or without additions.

PART FIVE: TRANSITIONAL PROVISIONS

56. Interpretation of Part Five

In this part of these Statutes, unless the context otherwise requires:
>   (a) the expression "appointed day" means 29 April 1974; and
>   (b) the expression "1955 Statutes" means the Statutes annexed to the Royal Charter of 1955 as amended and in force immediately prior to the appointed day.

57. Existing Establishments of the Order

It is hereby declared that the following are the existing Priories and Commanderies of the Order which shall be deemed to be duly and effectively constituted by their existing Instruments and Regulations or Rules under the provisions of Statutes 18, 19 and 20 hereof, that is to say:

(a) The Priory of England and the Islands, the Priory of Scotland, the Priory for Wales, the Priory for South Africa, the Priory in New Zealand, the Priory of Canada, the Priory in Australia, and the Priory in the United States of America; and

(b) The Commandery in Western Australia (dependent on the Priory in Australia) and the Commandery of Ards in Northern Ireland (dependent on the Priory of England and the Islands).

58. Existing St. John Associations

It is hereby declared that the following are the St. John Associations which shall be deemed to be duly and effectively constituted under the provisions of Statute 22 that is to say Antigua & Barbuda, Barbados, Bermuda, Cyprus, Fiji, Ghana, Gibraltar, Grenada, Guyana, India, Jamaica, Kenya, Malawi, Malaysia, Malta, Mauritius, Montserrat, Namibia, Nigeria, Pakistan, Papua New Guinea, St. Kitts & Nevis, St. Lucia, Sierra Leone, Singapore, Solomon Islands, Sri Lanka, Swaziland, Tanzania, Trinidad & Tobago, Uganda, Zambia and Zimbabwe.

59. Instruments of Allocation

It is hereby declared that any instrument having legal force immediately prior to the appointed day by virtue of which any property of the Order is allocated to any Establishment under the provisions of Statute 20 of the 1955 Statutes shall continue to have full force and effect on and after the appointed day as if such instrument had been made under the provisions of Statute 26 hereof until such time as it is varied or revoked thereunder.

60. Foundations

It is hereby declared that there shall be two Foundations of the Order, namely:

(a) The St. John Eye Hospital in Jerusalem; and

(b) St. John Ambulance.

61. Regulations and Rules

Where under powers conferred by any provisions of the 1955 Statutes, any Regulations were made and were in force immediately prior to the appointed day, such Regulations shall be deemed to be duly made under the corresponding provisions of these Statutes and any such Regulations shall be read and construed as Rules if the corresponding provisions of these Statutes provide for the making of Rules for corresponding purposes instead of Regulations.

Order Secretariat

25 St. John's Lane

London EC1M 4 PP

December 2003

APPENDIX F

TYPES OF INSIGNIA OF THE ORDER

Bailiff Grand Cross

Dates Issued	Description
1926-	Star: Eight-pointed cross, gold with white enamel, 92 mm wide, not embellished. Badge: Eight-pointed cross, gold with white enamel, 82 mm wide, embellished (worn on a sash over the right shoulder). Ribbon: Solid black morae 100 mm wide
1871-1888	As current issue, various sizes of insignia, badge was surmounted by a Royal Crown. Before 1926 the ribbon was 76 mm wide.
pre-1871	As current issue, various sizes of insignia, with no embellishment on the star or badge.

Dame Grand Cross (before 1926 known as Dame of the Order of St. John)

Dates Issued	Description
1936-	Star: Eight-pointed cross, gold with white enamel, 92 mm wide, not embellished. Badge: Eight-pointed cross, gold with white enamel, 82 mm wide, embellished (worn on a sash over the right shoulder). Ribbon: Solid black morae 56 mm wide
pre-1936	As current issue, but badge only no star. Before 1936 Dames wore the badge only and no star. Various sizes for the badge are known to exist ranging from 78 mm to 92 mm in width.

Knight of Justice

Dates Issued	Description
1926-	Star: Eight-pointed cross, gold with white enamel, 76 mm wide, not embellished. Badge: Eight-pointed cross, gold with white enamel, 57 mm wide, embellished (worn around the neck). Ribbon: Solid black morae, 50 mm wide.
1912-1926	As current but Star was 63 mm wide and embellished, the Badge was 56 mm wide.
pre-1888	As current, badge surmounted by a Royal Crown. This was likely discontinued before 1901.

Dame of Justice (before 1906 known as Lady of Justice)

Dates Issued	Description
1936–	Star: Eight-pointed cross, gold with white enamel, 82 mm wide, not embellished Badge: Eight-pointed cross, gold with white enamel, 47 mm wide, embellished (worn on the left breast/shoulder) Ribbon: Solid black moare 32 mm wide
pre-1936	As current issue, but badge only no star. Before 1936 Dames of Justice wore the badge only

Knight of Grace

Dates Issued	Description
1926–	Star: Eight-pointed cross, silver with white enamel 76 mm wide, embellished Badge: Eight-pointed cross, silver with white enamel, 56 mm wide (worn around the neck) Ribbon: Solid black moare, 50 mm wide
1912-1926	As current but Star was 63 mm wide and embellished, the Badge was 56 mm wide
pre-1888	As current, badge surmounted by a Royal Crown. This was likely discontinued before 1901

Dame of Grace (before 1906 known as a Lady of Grace)

Dates Issued	Description
1936–	Star: Eight-pointed cross, silver with white enamel 76 mm wide, embellished. Badge: Eight-pointed cross, silver with white enamel, 47 mm wide (worn around on the left breast/shoulder). Ribbon: Solid black moare, 32 mm wide.
pre-1936	As current issue, but badge only no star. Before 1936 Dames of Grace wore the badge only.

Commander

Dates Issued	Description
1991–	Badge: Eight-pointed cross, silver with white enamel, 57 mm wide, embellished. Ribbon: Solid black moare, 36 mm wide (worn around the neck by gentleman and on the shoulder by ladies).
1936-1990	As above for Commander Brothers, the badge worn by Commander Sisters was 47 mm wide, and the ribbon was 32 mm wide. This change was slowly introduced in Canada.
pre-1936	As above, the badge worn by Commander Brothers was 47 mm wide, while that for Commander Sisters was 32 mm wide. Holders of the pre-1936 versions were invited to return them for issue as Officers.

Officer

Dates Issued	Description
1991–	Badge: Eight-pointed cross, silver with white enamel, 45 mm wide, embellished. Ribbon: Solid black morae, 36 mm wide.
1936-1990	Badge: For Officer Brothers same as current, for Officer Sisters 32 mm wide.
1926-1936	Badge: Eight-pointed silver cross, 45 mm wide. This badge was found in both frosted silver and bright polished silver. Ribbon: Solid black morae, 36 mm wide.

Serving Brother/Serving Sister (Serving Member)

Dates Issued	Description
1985–	Badge: Eight-pointed cross, silver, 45 mm wide, embellished. Bright polished silver (rhodium). Both convex and flat issues exist. It appears that the convex version was issued in Canada until 2003. Ribbon: Solid black morae, 36 mm wide.
1980-1984	Badge: Eight-pointed cross, silver, 38 mm wide, embellished, frosted silver slightly convex. Ribbon: Solid black morae, 36 mm wide.
1974-1980	Badge: Circular silver, 36 mm wide insignia containing a flat embellished enamel eight-pointed cross. Ribbon: Solid black morae, 36 mm wide.
1939-1947 "War Economy Issue"	Badge: Circular silver, 36 mm wide, containing an eight-pointed cross embellished. Ribbon: Solid black morae, 36 mm wide.
1892-1939, 1947-1974	Badge: A raised eight-pointed cross, silver with white enamel, embellished superimposed on a circular black enamel background, surrounded by a silver rim, 36 mm wide. Ribbon: Solid black morae, 36mm wide for Serving Brothers and 32 mm wide for Serving Sisters.

Esquire

From 1906 to 1955 there were two types of esquires: Esquires appointed to the Order, and Esquires appointed as Personal Esquires to each Bailiff Grand Cross and each Knight of Justice. These Personal Esquires were admitted to the Order as Officers and wore the insignia of that grade. Bailiffs Grand Cross and Knights of Justice appointed before 1955 were permitted to continue appointing Personal Esquires who were admitted to the Order, however Esquires appointed after 1955 by Bailiffs and Knights of Justice were no longer admitted to the Order, and are simply presented with a lapel badge.

Esquire

Dates Issued	Description
1955-	Badge: A lapel badge measuring 20 mm wide, bearing an eight-pointed cross in white enamel on a circular black field.
1888-1955	Badge: Eight-pointed cross, silver, embellished, 47 mm wide. Ribbon: Solid black morae, 36 mm wide.

Personal Esquire

Dates Issued	Description
1955-	See Esquire
1906-1955	Badge: Eight-pointed silver cross, 47 mm wide. This badge was found in both frosted silver and bright polished silver. Ribbon: Solid black morae, 36 mm wide. Note: same badge as that worn by Officers.

Associate Member

Associate Members were persons who were not members of the Order but had "taken an active part in the establishment and development of the Order's hospitaller work."[3] The Royal Charter of 1926 permitted non-British subjects, or those who were non-Christians to be admitted to the Order as Associate Members. Since 1991 in Canada there is no religious requirement for being appointed to the Order.

Honorary Associate (discontinued 1926)

Dates Issued	Description
post-1926	Honorary Associates were permitted to offered the opportunity to be appointed Officers or Serving Brothers/Sisters.
1869-1926	Badge: Eight-pointed gold cross, with white enamel, 47 mm wide for men, 36 mm wide for ladies. Ribbon: Solid black morae 25 mm wide.

Associate Member (discontinued 1991 in Canada)

Dates Issued	Description
1926-1991	Associates could be admitted to any grade of the Order of St. John, no differentiation was made in their insignia, only in the ribbon that it was hung from. The ribbon featured a thin white stripe down the centre, 1/12th the width of the total ribbon.
1888-1926	Badge: Eight-pointed cross in frosted silver, 47 mm wide for men, and 36 mm wide for ladies. Ribbon: Solid black morae 25 mm wide.

APPENDIX G

AGREEMENT BETWEEN THE ORDERS OF SAINT JOHN IN CANADA, 1992

The Orders of Saint John in Canada

To all and Singular to whom these presents may come

Greeting:

Whereas, there are in Canada three national originations of the Orders of Saint John, namely the Canadian Association of the Sovereign Military Order of Malta, the Priory of the Most Venerable Order of the Hospital of St. John of Jerusalem and the Sub-Commandery of Die Balley Brandenburg des Ritterlichen Ordens Sankt Johannis von Spital zu Jerusalem, each representing the same tradition, pursuing the same ideals, serving the same cause and wearing the same eight-pointed Cross

And Whereas, these three organizations have forged strong bonds with each other in our common service to mankind through charity to our neighbours, especially Our Lords, the Sick and the Poor.

Now know you that, we the signatories to this Accord pledge ourselves to build upon the good will, which has already been forged and further pledge and undertake to realize this aim by mutual collaboration as well as by our own good works.

Given at St. John House in the City of Ottawa this 23rd day of September in the year of our lord 1992, being the 125th year of Confederation

Donald W. Rae
Chancellor of the Priory of the Most Venerable Order of St. John of Jerusalem

John Alexander MacPherson
President of The Canadian Association of the Sovereign Military Order of Malta

Joachim Brabander
Balley delegate in Canada of the Johanniter Orden

PRIORY OF CANADA COMPETITION TROPHIES, PLAQUES, AND CUPS

Throughout the history of St. John Ambulance in Canada the holding of first aid competitions was a significant part of participation in the brigade. Participants were judged and graded along a points system, with the team achieving the highest number of points in each competition being declared the winner. These competitions were particularly effective in recruiting new members and encouraging people to take first aid training, especially in terms of the special centres, where different teams within each special centre would compete, with the best teams going on to enter competition with rival companies. Victory became a matter of company pride, especially with the railroads, where competition between the Canadian Pacific and Grand Trunk/Canadian National was fierce, and often resulted in the winning team being awarded a salary bonus.

At the national level there were the Dominion Competitions, with the Montizambert Trophy being the pinnacle of achievement. There were other named national competitions that took place annually, with named trophies, donated by members of the Order. Specific competitions existed for intermediate first aid, home nursing, junior first aid, standard first aid, and junior home nursing. As programs such as home nursing changed so did the focus of the particular competition. Some trophy competitions were for specific occupations, such as police officers, miners, and railway men. Each provincial council also held provincial competitions. These were preliminary events undertaken before sending a team onto a national competition.

The trophies that were competed for on a national basis were: the Dominion Perpetual Challenge Trophy, donated by the Dominion Bridge Company in 1912 for the top first aid team in Canada; the Wallace Nesbitt Trophy for Railway First Aid, donated in 1914; the Lady Drummond Challenge Cup donated in 1922 and awarded for the Home Nursing Championship; the Coderre Trophy for First Aid in Mining, donated in 1922; the Sherwood Shield Dominion Championship for police teams, established in 1922; the Murray MacLaren Shield for junior home nursing, established in 1926; the Shaughnessy Shield for police teams in Western Canada, established in 1920; the Wallace Nesbitt Dominion Championship in junior first aid, donated in 1926; The Mrs. Lancelot Dent Challenge Bowl, donated by Ms. Dent, lady superintendent of the Brigade Overseas on the occasion of her visit to Canada in 1926; the J.R. Gaunt Shield for intermediate first aid, established in 1928, the Sir George Burnt Women's Dominion Shield, donated in 1928; the Cadet First Aid Championship Shield donated in 1930; the Viscount

Bennett Cup, donated in 1942; the Jim Pembroke Memorial Trophy for Annual Competition of women first aiders, donated in 1941; and the Stanley McKeen Cup donated in 1956 for the top nursing division; Other senior competitions included the Mary Otter Trophy, for the top military team in Canada, the Provincial Military Trophies, the Tyro Trophy, and lastly the Leonard Trophies/Leonard Shields in junior first aid (one per province).

For individual achievement there was the Robina Viscountess Mountgarret first aid trophy, donated in 1935 and awarded to a member of the brigade who was judged to have made the most significant contribution to the work of the brigade over a specific year. The Alice Alberta Ritchie Award was donated in 1953, and is awarded to a specific provincial or territorial council in recognition of exceptional service. It has been awarded continuously since its establishment and remains an active award.

During the two world wars first aid competitions were not held, so resources could be better focused on contributing to the war effort. The frequency of national first aid competitions began to decline after the Second World War, with a near total end to them by the early 1970s. In 1992 a series of new national trophies was inaugurated, better reflecting the different types of first aid training offered by St. John Ambulance. These are the Junior Team, Senior Team, and Open Trophy. In addition to these awards, every four years St. John Ambulance participates in the International Patient Care Competition, the most recent of these occurred in British Columbia in 2004 under the auspices of St. John Ambulance. Another global event is the International Cadet First Aid Competition, which is held each fall. There has been a resurgence in the number of provincial competitions held throughout Canada each year, especially among cadets and crusaders. This once highly important aspect of first aid training may well come back into its element over the coming years as an effective tool to promote first aid education and excellence.

NOTES

Chapter One

1. Jonathan Riley-Smith, *Hospitallers: the History of the Order of St. John* (London: Hambledon Press, 1999), 33.
2. Jonathan Riley-Smith, "The Military-Religious Orders: Their History and Continuing Relevance," *Conference Proceedings* (Cambridge: Emmanuel College, 2005), 17 March 2005, 1.
3. Riley-Smith "The Military-Religious Orders," 1.
4. Sir Edwin King and Sir Harry Luke, *The Knights of St. John in the British Realm: Being the Official History of the Most Venerable Order of the Hospital of St. John of Jerusalem* (London: St. John's Gate, 1967), 7.
5. Riley-Smith, *Hospitallers,* 27.
6. King and Luke, 4.
7. *Ibid.,* 9
8. Guy Stair Sainty, *The Orders of Saint John: The History, Structure, Membership and Modern Role of the Five Hospitaller Orders of Saint John of Jerusalem* (New York: The American Society of the Most Venerable Order of the Hospital of Saint John of Jerusalem, 1991), 2.
9. It is estimated that the garrison at Acre consisted of 14,000 men, 140 Hospitallers, and 240 Knights Templar.
10. Riley-Smith, *Hospitallers,* 74.
11. King and Luke, 98.
12. Sainty, 9.
13. Initially an individual had to serve ten years in the order's infirmary before being issued with a medical licence. This requirement was later modified, to four years of service to become a surgeon and six years to become a physician. Ian Howie-Willis, *A Century for Australia: St. John Ambulance in Australia, 1883–1983* (Canberra: St. John Ambulance, 1983), 68.
14. Riley-Smith, *Hospitallers,* 21.
15. Howie-Willis, 60.
16. H.J.A. Sire, *The Knights of Malta* (New Haven: Yale University Press, 19794), 176.
17. *Ibid.*
18. Riley-Smith, *Hospitallers,* 81.
19. King and Luke, 99.
20. W.K.R. Bedford and R. Holbeche, *The Order of the Hospital of St. John of Jerusalem* (London: F.E Robinson Press, 1902), 46. Also see H.W. Fincham, *The Order of the Hospital of St. John of Jerusalem and its Grand Priory of England* (London: St. John's Gate, 1933), 14.
21. King and Luke, 100.
22. A. Mifsud, *Knights Hospitallers of the Venerable Tongue Of England in Malta* (Valletta: The Malta Herald, 1914), 207.
23. Sainty, 67.
24. King and Luke, 104.
25. *Ibid.,* 107.

26. King and Luke, 110.
27. Sire, 187.
28. King and Luke, 113.
29. H.J.A. Sire, *The Knights of Malta* (New Haven: Yale University Press, 1994), 189.
30. Sire, 189.
31. In 1920 the Swedish branch separated itself from the Johanniter Orden and was founded as Johanniterorden I Sverige under the patronage of the sovereign of Sweden. The Netherlands followed suit in 1945 as the Johanniter Orde in Nederland, under the patronage of the husband of the Queen of the Netherlands. These three orders continue the hospitaller work of their antecedents.

Chapter Two

1. Major F. Duncan "First Aid to the Injured" speech to Social Sciences Congress, Dublin, 4 October 1881. *Annual Report (UK), 1881,* 91.
2. The Order of Malta did not establish a full-fledged association in Canada until 1950.
3. *The Orders of St. John: Report of the Co-operation Working Group,* 20 September 2004, 18.
4. The Alliance of the Orders of St. John of Jerusalem consists of Die Balley Brandenburg des Ritterlichen Ordens Sankt Johannis vom Spital zu Jerusalem (The Johanniter Orden), The Most Venerable Order of the Hospital of St. John of Jerusalem, Johanniter Orde in Nederland, and Johanniterorden I Sverige.
5. *The Orders of St. John; Report of the Co-operation Working Group,* 20 September 2004, 18.
6. *Ibid.,* 19.
7. For an excellent discussion see Sainty, 63.
8. George Thomas Beatson, *The Knights Hospitallers in Scotland and their Priory at Torphichen* (Glasgow: James Hedderwick, 1903), 12.
9. Howie-Willis, 97.
10. Ernle Bradford, The Knights of the Order of St. John: Jerusalem, Rhodes, Malta (Dorset Press, 1972), 214–217.
11. The designation Protector of the Order had previously only been given to Henry VII and Henry VIII of England.
12. Edgar Erskine Hume, *Medical Work of the Knights Hospitallers of Saint John of Jerusalem* (Baltimore: Johns Hopkins Press, 1940), 204–207.
13. Colin Cross, *The Fall of the British Empire* (London: Book Club Associates, 1968), 47.
14. Hume, 206.
15. At this time the colony of Malta became an independent country within the British Commonwealth and would retain The Queen as head of state until 1974.
16. For a discussion of these unrecognized orders of St. John, see Sir Harry Luke, *An Examination of Certain Claims to be an Order of St. John* (London: St. John's Gate, 1965) and Sainty.
17. The refusal of the Pope to appoint a grand master and the appointment of only a lieutenant-master was another indication that the Order had lost much of its status following the flight from Malta. Pope Leo XIII appointed the first grand master of the Order since the loss of Malta in 1879.
18. Sire, 251.
19. *Ibid.,* 250.
20. In 1818 the British established the Most Distinguished Order of St. Michael and St. George, which was used as the local order for Malta and the Ionian Islands until 1868 when it was opened up to the whole British Empire. A number of members of the Order of Malta would be admitted to this order. A.E. Abela, *The Order of St. Michael and St. George in Malta and Maltese Knights of the British Realm* (Valetta: Progress Publishing, 1988), 163.
21. Howie-Willis, 101.
22. Riley Smith, 128.

23. See Sir Edwin J. King, *The Knights of St. John in the British Empire, Being the Official history of the British Order of the Hospital of St. John of Jerusalem* (London: The Order of St. John, 1934).

24. Géraud-Marie Count Michel de Pierredon, *Histoire Politique de l'Ordre Souverain de Saint-Jean-de-Jérusalem (Ordre de Malte) de 1789 a 1955* (Paris: 1963), Vol. 2.

25. See Riley Smith, 129. Equivalent to £55,500,000 in 2006. Lawrence H. Officer, "Five Ways to Compute the Relative Value of a UK Pound Amount, 1830–2005—" MeasuringWorth.com, 2006.

26. Desmond Seward, *The Monks of War: The Military Religious Orders* (London: Penguin Press, 1995), 340–41.

27. King and Luke, 141. Letter of 14 September 1827.

28. Bedford and Holbeche, 108. Also see King, *The Knights of St. John in the British Empire*, 108.

29. Riley Smith, 129.

30. Peat often styled himself "Sir" because he was a member of the Polish Order of St. Stanislas, even though licence for holders of foreign honours to be styled "Sir" came to an end in 1815. Sainty, note 158, 70.

31. None of the grand priors appointed between the granting of the letters patent of Queen Mary and the reactivation of the Order in 1831 were Englishmen, most were Italians and it is doubtful that any of them ever set foot in England.

32. Bedford and Holbeche, 108.

33. Sainty, 71.

34. *Statutes of the Illustrious and Sovereign Order of the Knights Hospitallers of Saint John of Jerusalem, Venerable Langue of England, Comprehending The Grand Priories, Bailiwicks, and Commanderies in England, Scotland, Ireland, Wales. 1849*, 1.

35. *Ibid.*, 2.

36. G.R. Gayre, *The Heraldry of the Knights of St. John*, Allahabad: Garga Brothers Press, 1956), 39.

37. *Ibid.*

38. King and Luke, 143.

39. *Ibid.*, 143.

40. Thomas W. Heyck, *The Peoples of the British Isles* (Belmont: Wadsworth Publishing, 1992), 31.

41. *The Statutes of the Order of St. John of Jerusalem in England 1871* (Worcester: Deighton and Son, 1871).

42. Riley-Smith, *Hospitallers; The History of the Order of St. John* (London: Hambledon Press, 1999), 139.

43. Also known as the Second Schleswig War, or the Danish-Prussian War.

44. Joan Clifford, *For the Service of Mankind: Furley, Lechmere and Duncan, St. John Ambulance Founders* (London: Robert Hale, 1971), 17.

45. *Annual Report (UK)*, 1883, 8.

46. Caroline Moorehead, *Dunant's Dream: War, Switzerland and the History of the Red Cross* (London: Harper Collins Publishers, 1998), 320.

47. Lechmere served as secretary-general from 1866–1888 and later served as chancellor of the Order from 1890–1894.

48. Nigel Corbet-Fletcher, *The St. John Ambulance Association; Its History and Its Part in the Ambulance Movement* (London: St. John Ambulance Association, 1929), 12.

49. John Pearn, "The earliest days of first aid," *British Medical Journal*, 1994, Vol. 309, 1719.

50. Corbet-Fletcher, 10–13. The original dual purposes of the ambulance association were first, the instruction of pupils in first aid treatment of injured persons and second, the spread of useful ambulance material.

51. Pearn, 1718.

52. King and Luke, 180.

53. Corbet-Fletcher, 13.

54. "St. John Ambulance Association," *Woolwich Gazette*, 30 November 1878.

55. Order of St. John of Jerusalem, First meeting of the organization of the St. John Ambulance Association, *Daily Chronicle*, 25 June 1878.

56. Shepherd was killed on 22 January 1879 during the Zulu War, while trying to save the life of a fellow soldier.

57. *The Kentish Independent*, 2 March 1878.

58. Corbet-Fletcher, 20.

59. Hume, 319–24, and King, *The Knights of St. John in the British Empire*, 163–73.

60. Corbet-Fletcher, 25.

61. *Ibid.*, 26.

62. *Ibid.*, 27.

63. Heyck, 41.

64. Corbet-Fletcher, 15.

65. Linda Colley, *Britons, Forging the Nation, 1707–1837* (New Haven: Yale University Press, 1992), 30–33.

66. Stephen Patterson, *Royal Insignia* (London: Merrell Holberton Publishers, 1998), 32. Edward dressed up as grand prior of the Order of Malta in the style of the 16th century for the Devonshire House Ball, 1897, hosted by the Duke and Duchess of Devonshire.

67. *Annual Report (UK)*, 1885, 8.

68. Edward was even responsible for nominating the Duke of Manchester to be appointed to the Most Illustrious Order of St. Patrick, Ireland's national order of the period. Sir Sidney Lee, *King Edward VII* (London: Macmillan, 1925), 210 and 359.

69. King and Luke, 149.

70. Howie-Willis, 113.

71. HRH Princess Louise took a keen interest in nursing and was also awarded the Royal Red Cross. She was elevated to a Lady of Grace 1926 in recognition of her years of service to the St. John Ambulance Association in Britain.

72. King and Luke, 150.

73. The Order of the League of Mercy was founded in 1898 as a single class order, sanctioned by and awarded in the name of the sovereign. The Order was awarded to those who "assisted and supported hospitals." It ceased to be awarded in 1947, although it was revived in 1999 and is now awarded to volunteers who work with the sick, mentally ill, youth at risk, homeless, and elderly. Only awards of the Order made before 1947 are worn in the order of precedence. It was worn after the Service Medal of the Order of St. John.

74. George E. Buckle, ed., *The Letters of Queen Victoria*, Third Series, 1886–1901 (London: John Murray, 1930), 433.

75. Patterson, 32.

76. Declaration between the Sovereign Military Hospitaller Order of St. John of Jerusalem, of Rhodes and Malta and the Grand Priory in the British Realm of the Most Venerable Order of the Hospital of St. John of Jerusalem, signed at St. John's Gate, Clerkenwell, London, 26 November 1963.

77. *Ibid.*

78. *The Orders of St. John: Report of the Co-operation Working Group*, 20 September 2004, 18.

79. The introduction to Chapter Four of *The Orders of St. John: Report of the Co-operation Working Group*, ably notes "It gives no pleasure to record that there have been many instances of mutual suspicion and lack of regard on the part of the Orders and their members. This has often been born of ignorance. We consider the promotion of mutual understanding between members of the Orders is the precondition to substantial co-operation," 15.

Chapter Three

1. G.W.L. Nicholson, *The White Cross in Canada* (Montreal: Harvest Press, 1967), 29.

2. Richard Colebrook Harris, *The Seigneurial System in Early Canada* (University of Laval, 1968), 4.

3. Robert Pichette, *This Honourable Cross; The Orders of Saint John in the New World* (Ottawa: Sovereign Military Order of Malta Canadian Association, 1999). Jean-Claude Dubé, *Le chevalier de Montmagny: Premier gouverneur de la Nouvelle-France* (Montreal: Éditions Fides, 1999).

4. Pichette, *This Honourable Cross*, 15.

5. Joan Dawson, "The Governor's Goods: The Inventory of the Personal Property of Isaac de Razilly," *Nova Scotia Historial Review*, Vol. 5, No. 1, 1985, 100–112.

6. Pichette, *This Honourable Cross*.

7. W.J. Eccles, *Canada Under Louis XIV, 1663–1701* (Toronto: McClelland & Stewart, 1964), 33.

8. *Historical Statistics of Canada*, 1881 Census Data.

9. Peter B. Waite, *Canada 1874–1896: Arduous Destiny* (Toronto: McClelland & Stewart, Toronto 1971), 74.

10. *Ibid.*, 75.

11. *Ibid.*, 74.

12. *Statutes of the Illustrious and Sovereign Order of the Knights Hospitallers of Saint John of Jerusalem, Venerable Langue of England, Comprehending The Grand Priories, Bailiwicks, and Commanderies in England, Scotland, Ireland, Wales. 1849, 5.*

13. Approved by Special Chapter General held at London 16 April 1862, *The Statutes of the Sovereign and Illustrious Order of St. John of Jerusalem, Anglia* (London: John E. Taylor Press, 1862).

14. These appointments came before the Royal Charter of 1888 which made Queen Victoria the sovereign head of the Order and gave the Order official recognition within the British honours system.

15. The Honourable Hamnett Pinhey was listed as a deceased Knight of Grace, having died on 11 August 1857, although like many of the early appointments there are few additional details about this individual. Ryland and Pinhey were appointed Knights of Grace on 8 June 1859.

16. *Dictionary of Canadian Biography*, entry for Hamnett Pinhey.

17. *Ibid.*, entry for Herman Witsius Ryland.

18. Peter A. Russell, *Attitudes to Social Structure and Mobility in Upper Canada, 1815–1840* (Queenstown: Edwin Mellen Press, 1990), 127.

19. *Dictionary of Canadian Biography*, entry for Hamnett Pinhey.

20. Between the months of November and February.

21. *Annual Report (UK), 1883*, 31.

22. *Ibid.*, 9.

23. "First Aid in Canadian Industry," *The St. John Ambulance Gazette*, June 1938.

24. Sir Andrew MacPhail, *The Medical Services* (Ottawa: King's Printer, 1925), 12.

25. *Annual Report (UK), 1883*.

26. *Annual Report (UK), 1884*, 29.

27. *Ibid.*, 8.

28. Howie-Willis, 134.

29. *Dictionary of National Biography* (London: Smith, Elder Company, 1901), Vol, 1, 262.

30. The Brasseys also visited St. Kitts; Port of Spain; Trinidad; and Nassau, Bahamas. *Annual Report (UK), 1884*.

31. Nicholson, *The White Cross*, 29.

32. *Ibid.*, 29.

33. Howie-Willis, 140.

34. *The Halifax Herald*, 24 June 1892.

35. Nicholson, *The White Cross*, 30.

36. In *The White Cross in Canada*, Nicholson notes that in 1895 a Halifax branch of the St. John Ambulance Brigade was established by the same members of the Voluntary Fire Brigade, yet there is no mention of this in the records at St. John's Gate or in the annual report of the ambulance brigade. It is most likely that an unofficial brigade of sorts, made up of volunteer fire fighters, acting in a dual capacity as fire fighters and first aiders was what was established.

37. *Annual Report of the St. John Ambulance Association, Council for the Dominion of Canada* [henceforth *Annual Report (Canadian Branch)*], 1897, 31.

38. The date of 1889 for the establishment of a centre at Halifax is likely an error, given that there is no evidence of anything before 1892.

39. George Sterling Ryerson, *Looking Backwards* (Toronto: Ryerson Press, 1924), 109.

40. *Annual Report (UK), 1896*.

41. Ryerson, 80.

42. *Annual Report (Canadian Branch), 1897*, 11.

43. Ryerson, 106.
44. *Ibid.*, 108.
45. The Permanent Active Militia Army Medical Corps was founded in 1904, and the name was subsequently changed to Canadian Army Medical Corps in 1909. Following the end of the First World War. The corps was honoured by King George V and was designated the Royal Canadian Army Medical Corps (RCAMC). With the unification of the Royal Canadian Navy, Canadian Army, and Royal Canadian Air Force in 1968 the RCAMC simply became the Medical Service Branch of the Canadian Forces.
46. *Dictionary of Canadian Biography,* entry for George Sterling Ryerson.
47. Ryerson also played a leading role in the creation of the United Empire Loyalist Association.
48. Ryerson, 105.
49. *Ibid.*, 109.
50. *Ibid.*, 105.
51. Illuminated address from St. John Ambulance Association to G.S. Ryerson, 22 March 1910.
52. James A Hanna, *A Century of Red Blankets: A History of the Ambulance Service in Ontario* (Erin, ON: Boston Mills Press, 1982), 34.
53. *Annual Report (UK), 1897,* 248.
54. *Ibid.*, 249.
55. *Ibid.*, 248.
56. *Annual Report (Canadian Branch), 1897,* 17.
57. *Annual Report (UK), 1897,* 225.
58. President: Sir George Airey Kirkpatrick. Vice-presidents: Lieutenant-General Montgomery Moore (Halifax Centre), The Honourable A.F. Randolph (Fredericton Centre), Angus W. Hooper (Montreal Centre), F.W. Evans (Westmount Branch); Henry Coby (Belleville Centre), John T. Small (Toronto Centre), J.A. Lampry (Guelph Centre), J.S. Niven (London Centre), Elizabeth Greene (Orillia Branch), T.W. Nisbet (Boy's Brigade Sarnia), Sir James Grant (Ottawa), Senator James Gowan (Barrie), Henry Cawartha (Toronto), and W.R. Brock (Toronto). Members: G.E. Franklyn (Halifax), Ms. Davidson (Fredericton), H.B. Yates (Montreal), James Harrison (Westmount), Arthur McGinnis (Belleville), C.R. Dickson (Toronto), Captain Clarke (Guelph), Ms. Muir (Orillia), Charles F. Complin (London), and W.D. Brydone-Jack (Vancouver). General secretary: George Sterling Ryerson. Assistant general secretary and treasurer: C.R. Dickson.
59. *Annual Report (Canadian Branch), 1897,* 17.
60. In 1898 Brantford offered the women's first aid course to thirty women, of whom twenty-three would go on to receive their certificates.
61. *Annual Report (UK), 1899,* 209.
62. *Ibid.*, 209.
63. *Annual Report (UK), 1901,* 231.
64. The Toronto Centre also reported income of $83.06. *Annual Report (UK), 1907,* 192.
65. *Annual Report (Canadian Branch), 1897,* 17.
66. Nicholson, *The White Cross,* 34.
67. King, *The Knights of St. John in the British Empire,* 151.

Chapter Four

1. MacPhail, 176.
2. Hanna, 36
3. *Annual Report (UK), 1909, 203.*
4. *Annual Report (UK), 1910, 33.*
5. Member of the Royal Victorian Order and Knight of Grace.
6. Lord Grey's presidency of the association was provisional pending the election of a president following the adoption of a constitution for the Canadian branch.

7. Geoffrey Bilson, "Dr. Frederick Montizambert (1843–1929); Canada's First Director General of Public Health," *Medical History,* 1985, Vol. 29, 389.

8. *Annual Report (UK), 1910,* 226.

9. Included with 1919 edition of Constitution and General Regulations of the St. John Ambulance Association Canadian Branch. Similar leaflets and advertisements were included with earlier association publications.

10. Ambulance Department of the St. John Ambulance Association, The Canadian Branch, 1919 Edition of the pamphlet.

11. *Annual Report (UK), 1907,* 192.

12. Corbet-Fletcher, 49.

13. Mentioned in the *Annual Report (UK), 1909.*

14. *Annual Report (UK), 1908.*

15. *Ibid.,* 197.

16. *Annual Report (UK), 1909,* 204.

17. Corbet-Fletcher, 26.

18. *Annual Report (Canadian Branch), 1914,* 65.

19. Nicholson, *The White Cross,* 44.

20. See Pamphlet, "Priory of Canada Golden Jubilee Celebrations, London Ontario 2–4 May 1959," Golden jubilee of the brigade in Canada. A service of thanksgiving was held at St. Paul's Cathedral in London, Ontario, to mark the occasion.

21. Nicholson, *The White Cross,* 44.

22. Hanna, 8.

23. The ambulance divisions were as follows: Forest City No. 1 Ambulance Division, 4 May 1909; Toronto Central Ambulance Division, 30 September 1911; Parkdale Ambulance Division, 23 February 1912; West Toronto Ambulance Division, 1 March 1912; Riverdale Ambulance Division, 25 March 1912; Toronto Corps, 30 June 1912; Hamilton Central Ambulance Division, 1 October 1912; Owen Sound Ambulance Division, 15 November 1912; Fort Gary Ambulance Division, 1 January 1912.

24. *Annual Report of the St. John Ambulance Brigade Overseas* [henceforth *Annual Report (Overseas)*], 1912, 211.

25. It was a persistent cause of confusion that even in Canada the brigade was referred to as the St. John Ambulance Brigade Overseas. Although it was "overseas" from the perspective of officials at St. John's Gate in London it was not "overseas" to Canadians.

26. Copp was found giving first aid instruction to 40 men and joined the association as soon as it was established in Canada, going on to become one of the great builders and supporters of not only the association but also the brigade. Corbet-Fletcher, 49.

27. This would be organized as the No. 3 Fort Garry Ambulance Division in May of 1912.

28. *Annual Report (Overseas), 1912,* 438.

29. Atrill was one of the nurses who ministered to a young Georges Vanier after the amputation of his leg following the battle of Arras. She would later be made a Dame of Grace of the Order for her years of exemplary service.

30. *Annual Report (UK), 1911,* 261.

31. Shaughnessy and Clouston donated $1,000 each, while Manuel and Drummond donated $500 each.

32. Donations ranged from a dollar to $1,000. The total raised in the 1910–11 year was $4,065.38. *Annual Report (Canadian Branch), 1911,* 23.

33. Although Drummond was born into a wealthy family throughout his life he engaged in philanthropic work.

34. *Annual Report (UK), 1911,* 41.

35. *Annual Report (Canadian Branch), 1910,* 35.

36. *Annual Report (UK), 1912,* 277.

37. *Annual Report (UK), 1911,* 285.

38. *Ibid.,* 39.

39. Nicholson, *The White Cross,* 42.

40. *Annual Report (Canadian Branch), 1914,* 46.

41. *Ibid.,* 49.

42. His Majesty King George V to H. Boulton. *Annual Report (Canadian Branch), 1910,* 40.

43. *Annual Report (Canadian Branch)*, *1914,* 23.

44. *Annual Report (UK), 1911,* 280.

45. *Annual Report of the Chief Inspector of Mines for the Province of British Columbia, 1912* (Victoria: King's Printer), 4.

46. *Dictionary of Canadian Biography,* Sir Richard McBride.

47. *Annual Report (UK), 1911,* 261.

48. *Ibid.,* 261.

49. *Ibid.,* 273.

50. The cars would be left in various locations for two-month periods, and instruction was held from 8 a.m. to 10 p.m. and usually conduced before small groups.

51. *Annual Report (Canadian Branch) 1914,* 59.

52. *Annual Report (UK), 1911,* 263.

53. Connaught was appointed grand prior in 1910 by his nephew King George V, who was the outgoing grand prior having recently ascended to throne. He retired from the grand priorship in 1939, three years before his death.

54. *Annual Report (UK), 1911,* 263.

55. *Annual Report (UK), 1912,* 277.

56. John Cowan, *Canada's Governors General* (Toronto: York Publishing Company, 1967), 103 and 106.

57. The commissioner of the Yukon Territory was made vice-patron of the Territorial Council.

58. *Annual Report (Canadian Branch), 1911,* 21.

59. *The Encyclopedia of Saskatchewan,* "Regina Cyclone Entry."

60. *Annual Report (Canadian Branch), 1912,* 10.

61. Parliament of Canada, *An Act to Incorporate The General Council of the Canadian Branch of the St. John Ambulance Association. Act of Incorporation,* 4–5 George V, Chapter 145, 1914.

62. Acts incorporating corporations passed through the Senate without reference to the House of Commons, this practice continues to this day.

63. *Debates of the Senate,* Bill D-3, 373. Also see pages 400 and 458 for 2nd and 3rd readings.

64. *Journals of the Senate,* 1914, 328.

65. Davis was previously premier of Prince Edward Island and would go on to serve as chief justice of the Supreme Court from 1918–1924.

66. The Bylaws had been approved by the Central Executive Committee of the St. John Ambulance Association on 11 December 1913, nearly six months before passage of the act incorporating the Canadian branch of the association.

67. Macpherson would go on to be commissioned as an officer in the Newfoundland Regiment in 1914 and he helped invent a special gas mask to combat the use of mustard gas by the Germans. He survived the war and returned to Newfoundland being made a Companion of the Order of St. Michael and St. George by King George V for his services.

68. Joey Smallwood, ed., *Encyclopedia of Newfoundland and Labrador, Vol. 5* (St. John's: Smallwood Heritage Foundation, 1991), 33.

69. Smallwood, Vol, 1, 40. Also see various editions of the *Newfoundland Quarterly,* 1911–1914.

70. *Annual Report (UK), 1910.*

71. *Annual Report (UK), 1911,* 277.

72. *Annual Report (Overseas), 1912,* 329.

73. An Anglican (Church of England) youth organization established in England in 1891 by Walter Gee. It became popular among Anglican youth in many parts of the British Empire, including Newfoundland and Canada. The St. John's branch of the Church Lad's Brigade was founded on 31 December 1892. Other religious brigades were also present in St. John's. Notable among them were the Catholic Cadet Corps and Methodist Guard. One-fifth of the original membership of the Newfoundland Regiment were members of the Church Lad's Brigade.

Chapter Five

1. Lance Corporal Francis George Bacon; Nurse Grace Errol Bolton; Second Lieutenant Ronald Baines Brookes; Private Joseph Chadwick; Lance Corporal Charles Daintree; Private George Henry Grindley; Private Norman Claude Hain; Private James Harbinson; Private John Harding; Private Frank Higgins; Private Frank Morris Hobden; Sergeant Major Albert Keen; Private George Newburn; Driver Lillian Beatrice Nichols; Private George Noble; Private A. Oates; Sister P. Petrie; Private William Prince; Private Charles Stagg; Nurse Dorothy Pearson Twist; Private George Washington.

2. MacPhail, 12.

3. This would become the Defence Medical Association in 1937. G.W.L. Nicholson, *Seventy Years of Service: A History of the Royal Canadian Army Medical Corps* (Ottawa: Borealis, 1977), 61.

4. Nicholson, *The White Cross*, 55.

5. *Annual Report (UK)*, 1915, 32.

6. *Annual Report (Canadian Branch)*, 1916, 16.

7. *Ibid.*, 22.

8. *Annual Report (Canadian Branch)*, 1915, 34.

9. *Ibid.*

10. *Annual Report (Canadian Branch)*, 1916, 30.

11. *Ibid.*, 18.

12. Ronald G. Haycock, *Sam Hughes; The Public Career of a Controversial Canadian, 1885–1916* (Waterloo: Wilfrid Laurier University Press, 1986), 4.

13. *Annual Report (Canadian Branch)*, 1916, 22.

14. *Annual Report (Canadian Branch)*, 1915, 13.

15. *Annual Report (Canadian Branch)*, 1916, 26.

16. *Annual Report (Canadian Branch)*, 1917, 26.

17. *Annual Report (Canadian Branch)*, 1915, 37–38.

18. This was the forerunner of the International Nickel Company of Canada (INCO).

19. According to the Bank of Canada, one dollar in 1914 has the purchasing power of $17.75 in 2005. *A History of the Canadian Dollar* (Ottawa: Bank of Canada, 2006), 88.

20. *Annual Report (Canadian Branch)*, 1916, 14.

21. *Ibid.*, 12.

22. *Annual Report (Canadian Branch)*, 1915, 19.

23. *Annual Report (Canadian Branch)*, 1916, 25.

24. Linda J. Quiney, *Assistant Angels: Canadian Women as Voluntary Aid Detachment Nurses During and After the Great War 1914–1930*, (unpublished Doctoral Dissertation, University of Ottawa, 2002), see Chapter 3.

25. *Annual Report (Canadian Branch)*, 1916, 25.

26. *Ibid.*, 25.

27. *Annual Report (UK)*, 1917, 14.

28. *Annual Report (Canadian Branch)*, 1918, 18.

29. VAD units in Canada: No. 1 Ottawa; No. 2 Montreal; No. 3 Quebec City; No. 4 Victoria; No. 5 St. John; No. 6 Halifax.

30. St. John National Headquarters Archives [henceforth SJA], VAD Series, Evelyn, Duchess of Devonshire to the Association and Brigade, 14 December 1917.
31. *Annual Report (Canadian Branch), 1915*, 46.
32. Although the 1916 annual report of the Canadian branch of the St. John Ambulance Association makes reference to this donation of 280,000 pairs of socks, the quantity seems unrealistically high and the author believes that this was a typographical error in the original report. A quantity of 2,800 or 28,000 would seem more reasonable.
33. *Annual Report (Canadian Branch), 1916*, 64.
34. *Ibid.*, 41.
35. *Annual Report (UK), 1917*, 24.
36. *Annual Report (Canadian Branch), 1916*, 65.
37. *Annual Report (Canadian Branch), 1917*, 26.
38. *Annual Report (Canadian Branch), 1916*, 57.
39. *Ibid.*, 23.
40. *Annual Report (Canadian Branch), 1918*, 46.
41. Later promoted to Field Marshal and raised to the peerage as 1st Viscount Allenby.
42. The EEF was composed of British, Australian, Indian, New Zealand, and smaller number of other British Empire Forces.
43. Luke and King, 166.
44. *Annual Report (Canadian Branch), 1917*, 14.
45. T.J. Murray, "Medical Aspects of the Disaster: The Missing Report of Dr. David Fraser," *Ground Zero: A Reassessment of the 1917 Explosion in Halifax Harbour,* (Halifax: Nimbus, 1994), 241.
46. *Annual Report (Overseas), 1917*, 42.
47. Neena Abraham, "Medical Memories of the 1917 Explosion," *Ground Zero: A Reassessment of the 1917 Explosion in Halifax Harbour,* (Halifax: Nimbus, 1994), 249.
48. Janet Kitz, *Shattered City: The Halifax Explosion and the Road to Recovery,* (Halifax: Nimbus Press, 2004), 56.
49. *Annual Report (Canadian Branch), 1918*, 34.
50. *Ibid.*, 34.
51. Janice P. Dickin McGinnis, "The Impact of Epidemic Influenza: Canada 1918–1919," *Canadian Historical Association, Historical Papers, 1977,* 128.
52. *Ibid.*, 123.
53. *Ibid.*, 128.
54. Library and Archives Canada [henceforth LAC], Record Group [henceforth RG] 13, series A-2, Vol 228, file 1918–2233, Acting Prime Minister to Deputy Minister of Justice, 12 October 1918.
55. McGinnis, 128.
56. J.M. Gibbon. *The Victorian Order of Nurses for Canada (*Montreal: Southam Press, 1947), 72.
57. *Annual Report (Canadian Branch), 1919*, 13.
58. *Ibid.*, 13.
59. *Annual Report (UK), 1919*, 28.
60. *Annual Report (Canadian Branch), 1918*, 17.
61. *Ibid.*, 20.
62. *Ibid.*, 19
63. House of Commons, *Debates* 14 April 1919, 1441. (W.F. Nickle).
64. *Annual Report (UK), 1919*, 30.
65. This Table does not include those members of the CEF trained by St. John Ambulance during the First World War.
66. Dates of founding for these divisions were; Church Lad's Brigade, Ambulance Division, 7 May 1912; Dalton Ambulance Division, 29 July 1913, No. 4 Ambulance Division, 6 April 1914 and Lady Davidson Nursing Division, 17 September 1914.

67. Cassie Brown, *Death on Ice; The Great Newfoundland Sealing Disaster of 1914*, (Toronto: Doubleday Canada, 1972), 208.

68. Memorial University Archives [henceforth MUA], COLL-002, Macpherson Papers, Dr. Cluny Macpherson to Mr. Carberry, 20 October 1954. Macpherson Notebook 1, 158.

69. *St. John's Daily News*, 1 September 1914.

70. MUA, COLL-002, Macpherson Papers, Macpherson Notebook 2, 126.

71. *Annual Report (UK), 1915*, 55.

72. MUA, COLL-002, Macpherson Papers, Dr. Cluny Macpherson to Governor Sir Walter Davidson, 15 May 1915. Notebook 1.

73. MUA, COLL-002, Macpherson Papers, Notebook 1, 13 July 1940 (Recalling events leading up to development of smoke helmet type of gas mask. Also see "An Episode at the War Office" Macpherson Notebook 1, 128.

74. *Annual Report (UK), 1915*, 55.

75. Provincial Archives of Newfoundland and Labrador, PANL P18-A1.

76. Linda J. Quiney, "Borrowed Halos: Canadian Teachers as Voluntary Aid Detachment Nurses During the Great War," *Historical Studies in Education*, Spring 2003.

77. See Quiney, "Borrowed Halos."

78. *Annual Report (Overseas), 1917*, 18.

Chapter Six

1. This consisted of fourteen ambulance divisions and twenty-three nursing divisions.

2. *Annual Report (Canadian Branch), 1918*, 13.

3. *Ibid.*, 13.

4. *Annual Report (Canadian Branch), 1919*, 11.

5. *Ibid.*, 12.

6. *Annual Report (Canadian Branch), 1924*, 44.

7. *Annual Report (Canadian Branch), 1923*, 14.

8. *Ibid.*, 14.

9. *Ibid.*, 13.

10. On 12 September 1922.

11. *Annual Report (UK), 1922*, 27.

12. *Annual Report (UK), 1938*, 177.

13. "First Aid in Canadian Industry," *The St. John Ambulance Gazette*, June 1938

14. *Ibid.* In 1925 among 4,080 employees there were 302 accidents, or 7.35 percent accident rate. For the next five years there was a gradual decrease, culminating in 462 accidents among 7,392 employees, a 6.26 percent accident rate. From 1929 to 1936 there was a marked reduction. In 1936 among 3,788 (outdoor employees) there were only seventy-eight accidents, a 2.06 percent accident rate. In this twelve-year period, therefore, the reduction in the number of accidents in this company was 70 percent.

15. "First Aid in Canadian Industry," *The St. John Ambulance Gazette*, June 1938.

16. *Ibid.* Hollinger made mining "compulsory for all its underground workers."

17. *Annual Report (Overseas), 1924*, 31.

18. Nicholson, *The White Cross*, 78.

19. See Sir Edwin King, *The Pilgrimage of 1926: Being the Official Journal of the Knights of St. John* (London: St. John's Gate, 1926).

20. *Annual Report (Canadian Branch), 1925*, 15.

21. *Annual Report (Canadian Branch), 1923*, 12.

22. *Annual Report (Canadian Branch), 1926*, 8.

23. *Annual Report (UK), 1921*, 32.

24. Approximately $100 Canadian in 1927. An additional $585 was donated by the commandery in 1938.

25. Constitution of the Canadian Branch of the St. John Ambulance Association, 1914, revised 1933.

26. King and Luke, 159.

27. SJG, Commandery in Canada, Hewett to Sir Percival Wilkinson (Secretary General) 30 October 1933.

28. Dictionary of National Biography, 384.

29. SJG, Commandery in Canada, Hewett to Earl of Scarborugh, 2 November 1933.

30. SJG, Commandery in Canada, Beatrice H. Dent, Lady Superintendent in Chief Brigade Overseas to Colonel Sleeman, 7 July 1933.

31. SJG, Commandery in Canada, C.G. Cowan to Sir Percival Wilkinson, 10 December 1932.

32. The total profit for 1931 was $5,482.22. In 1932 this amount declined by $1,384.93.

33. *Annual Report (Canadian Branch), 1932*, 19.

34. SJG, Commandery in Canada, Scarborough to Sir Malcolm Murray, regarding letter from the Grand Prior, HRH The Duke of Connaught, 27 November 1933.

35. Cowan wrote to St. John's Gate "we are still hoping that Sir John Hewett will be able to pay us the long promised visit in September next." SJG, Commandery in Canada C.G. Cowan to Sir Percival Wilkinson, 9 May 1933.

36. Howie-Willis, 326.

37. Itinerary of Sir John Hewett, 1933–1934

Date	Location
26 October	Arrive at Quebec City
26 October	Ottawa
4 November	Toronto
11 November	Ottawa
17 November	Toronto
18 November to 15 December	Winnipeg
	Regina
	Edmonton
	Victoria
	Calgary
16 December	Montreal
20 December	Toronto
5 January	Sail for Britain from New York

38. SJG, Commandery in Canada, Hewett to Wilkinson, 30 October 1933.

39. SJG, Commandery in Canada, Hewett to Scarborough, 2 November 1933.

40. SJG, Hewett to Pellatt, August 1933. [exact date illegible]

41. SJG, Commandery in Canada. Address by Sir Henry Prescott Hewitt, Bailiff of Egle, on the Venerable Order of St. John of Jerusalem, Montreal, 19 December 1933.

42. SJG, Commandery in Canada, Draft Regulations for the Commandery in Canada, No. 16.

43. SJG, Commandery in Canada, Hewett to Percival, 15 November 1933.

44. Minutes of the meeting of the General Council Canadian Branch St. John Ambulance Association, Ottawa, 15 November 1933.

45. Minutes of the meeting of the General Council Canadian Branch St. John Ambulance Association, Ottawa, 15 November 1933.

46. A full discussion of the honours dimension of the Order is included in Chapters Eleven, Twelve, and Thirteen.

47. SJG, Canada 1934, Full Report of the Delegation to Canada with Appendices.

48. SJG, Commandery in Canada, Cowan to Sir Percival Wilkinson, 8 December 1933.

49. SJG, Canada 1934, Full Report of the Delegation to Canada with Appendices, 29 January 1934.

50. "I agree with your condemnation of separate appeals for the Association and Brigade." SJG, Commandery in Canada, Hewett to Cowan, 21 December 1933.

51. SJG, Commandery in Canada, Cowan to Hewett, 22 December 1933.

52. SJG, Commandery in Canada, Hewett to Percival, 30 October 1933.

53. SJG, Canada 1934, Full Report of the Delegation to Canada with Appendices, 29 January 1934.

54. Provincial Commissioners: Dr. Charles Copp (Ontario District), Dr. E.A. Braithwaite (Alberta); Lieutenant-Colonel R.M. Grosiline (Quebec); A.M. Warner (British Columbia); Reverend C.W. Downe (Saskatchewan); Lieutenant-Colonel George H. Gillespie (Manitoba), Reginald V. Harris (Nova Scotia, appointed 1940); Dr. Gilbert Peat (New Brunswick, appointed 1940); Lieutenant-Colonel Arthur Gaboury (commissioner for French-speaking Divisions in Quebec, appointed 1941).

55. Even such things as placement of the name of the brigade on the annual report would be cause for tension between the brigade and association after the founding of the Commandery in Canada.

56. *Mail and Empire*, 16 February 1934.

57. *Ibid.*

58. *Ibid.*

59. SJA, Commandery Series, Memo, 8 September 1934.

60. SJA, Commandery Series, Major General Sir Percival Wilkinson, Secretary General of the Order, to Colonel J.T. Clarke, Director General of the Canadian Branch of the St. John Ambulance Association, 2 October 1934.

61. See Chapter Eleven.

62. SJA, Commandery Series, Percival Wilkinson to Colonel J.T. Clarke, 28 November 1934.

63. SJA, Commandery Series, Bessborough to Lieutenant-Governor Bruce, 16 November 1934.

64. *Annual Report (Canadian Branch)*, 1932, 51.

65. *Annual Report (Canadian Branch)*, 1928, 15.

66. *Annual Report (Canadian Branch)*, 1923, 42.

67. *Annual Report (Canadian Branch)*, 1929, 18.

68. *Annual Report (Canadian Branch)*, 1928, 15.

69. *Annual Report (Canadian Branch)*, 1934, 18.

70. See Nicholson, 90–91 for a complete discussion of the brigade's activities in Nova Scotia during the 1939 Royal Tour.

71. In response to the "downward trend in home nursing courses" being taken (by women), a special sub-committee was struck to investigate the decline in female participation. *Annual Report of the Commandery in Canada of the St. John Ambulance Association and St. John Ambulance Brigade* [henceforth *Annual Report (Commandery in Canada)*], 1937, 14.

72. *Annual Report (Overseas)*, 1924.

73. *Annual Report (UK)*, 1926.

Chapter Seven

1. J.L. Granatstein and Peter Neary, *The Good Fight: Canadians and World War II* (Toronto: Copp Clark, 1995), 2.

2. Granatstein and Neary, 3.

3. *Annual Report (Commandery in Canada)*, 1938, 18.

4. *Annual Report (Commandery in Canada)*, 1939, 6–9.

5. *Annual Report (Commandery in Canada)*, 1940, 9.

6. *Ibid.*, 9.

7. *Annual Report (Commandery in Canada)*, 1942, 12.

8. *Ibid.*, 12.

9. *Annual Report (Commandery in Canada)*, 1940, 22.

10. *Ibid.*, 22.

11. The conference took place between 14 and 15 May 1942.

12. *Annual Report (Commandery in Canada), 1945*, 22.

13. *Annual Report (Commandery in Canada), 1940*, 17.

14. *Annual Report (Commandery in Canada), 1939*, 20.

15. *Annual Report (Commandery in Canada), 1943*, 21.

16. *Annual Report (Commandery in Canada), 1940*, 8.

17. *Ibid.*, 6.

18. *Annual Report (Commandery in Canada), 1942*, 16.

19. The Victorian Order of Nurses assisted with training St. John instructors from 1942 until the conclusion of the war.

20. *Annual Report (Commandery in Canada), 1942*, 17.

21. *Ibid.*, 33.

22. *Annual Report (Commandery in Canada), 1943*, 23.

23. *Annual Report (Commandery in Canada), 1945*, 37.

24. *Ibid.*, 40.

25. *Annual Report (Commandery in Canada), 1942*, 11.

26. *Annual Report (Commandery in Canada), 1943*, 18.

27. *Annual Report (Commandery in Canada), 1945*, 35.

28. *Annual Report (Commandery in Canada), 1944*, 22.

29. *Annual Report (Commandery in Canada), 1942*, 30.

30. Herbert A. Bruce, *Varied Operation*, (Toronto: Longman's Press, 1958), 306.

31. *Annual Report (Commandery in Canada), 1942*, 28.

32. *Annual Report (Commandery in Canada), 1940*, 17.

33. *Annual Report (Commandery in Canada), 1942*, 25.

34. Nicholson, *The White Cross*, 95.

35. SJA, VAD Series Correspondence, Kay Gilmour to Lady Redfern, 10 August 1943.

36. *Annual Report (Commandery in Canada), 1942*, 12.

37. McKenzie Porter, *To All Men: The Story of the Canadian Red Cross* (Toronto: McClelland & Stewart, 1960), 141.

38. Nicholson, *The White Cross*, 106.

39. *Ibid.*, 106.

40. During the Second World War one name developed for VADs was "Virgins Awaiting Destruction." This has been recounted by a number of surviving VADs who insisted that the author include this so a bit of the "popular history" of the VADs could be preserved.

41. *Annual Report (Commandery in Canada), 1942*, 10.

42. *Annual Report (Commandery in Canada), 1943*, 13.

43. The only province Gilmour did not visit was Prince Edward Island.

44. *Annual Report (Commandery in Canada), 1943*, 22.

45. The other eight were, Elsie Little, Edith Hay, Madeline Cantelon, Beatrice Martin, Ms. Trudeau L. Spencer, Margaret MacLaren, Myra Gold, Ruth Mackenzie, and Amelia Prentice.

46. SJA, VAD Series, Correspondence, circular to Canada from Joint War Origination of St. John Ambulance and the Red Cross, 20 April 1944.

47. *Annual Report (Commandery in Canada), 1944*, 26.

48. King and Luke, 174.

49. *Annual Report (Commandery in Canada)*, 20.

50. 1942 Linen Guild gave $325, which was more than the commandery gave to the hospital ($251). *Annual Report (Commandery in Canada), 1941*, 14.

51. In 1939 the brigade had a total of 2,773 members; by the end of 1945 this had expanded to 8,410.

Type	Divisions	Membership
Ambulance Divisions	113	3,135
Nursing Divisions	158	4,154
Cadet Ambulance Divisions	57	1,121
TOTAL	328	8,410

Chapter Eight

1. The 1945 annual report was slightly alarmist, noting "the Victorious conclusion of World War II had a very marked effect upon Association activities since the fighting ceased." The slump in first aid training was short-lived. *Annual Report (Commandery in Canada)*, 1945, 19.
2. Deena Toxopeus, *The 1951 Agreement Between the Red Cross and St. John Ambulance: A Case Study of the Effect of Civil Defence on Canada's Health Care System* (Unpublished Master of Arts Thesis, University of Ottawa, 1997), 72.
3. Donald Creighton, *Canada 1939–1957; The Forked Road* (Toronto: McClelland & Stewart, 1976), 219.
4. Since Gray's departure chancellors have been elected on a biennial basis with the possibility of a one year extension.
5. *Annual Report (Commandery in Canada)*, 1945, 7.
6. Nominations for appointment were sent to the grand prior through the secretary-general of the Order. The secretary-general was not empowered to pass judgment on the proposed appointments after 1946 and simply acted as a messenger for the Priory of Canada.
7. St. John's Gate Archives [henceforth SJGA], Canada 1934–35, Lord Wakehurst (Sub-Prior) to Priory of Canada, 27 March 1947.
8. *Annual Report of the Priory of Canada, 1947*, 21.
9. *Annual Report of the Priory of Canada, 1949*, 19.
10. *Annual Report of the Priory of Canada, 1946*, 23.
11. For an excellent and exhaustive examination of the agreement see Toxopeus.
12. SJA Red Cross Agreement Series, T.H. Leggett to Dr. W.P Stanbury, 21 March 1949.
13. People at the first meeting of the Joint Committee included Dr. W.P. Warner, Margaret MacLaren, George Craig, W.J. Bennett from St. John, Leopold Macaulay, H.H. Leather, F.F. Huill, and Dr. W.S. Stanbury.
14. SJA, Red Cross Relations Series, Joint Committee 1951, 25 January 1951.
15. Toxopeus, 75.
16. The potential for joint advertising was never fully explored by the Joint Committee.
17. SJA, Red Cross Relations Series, Minutes of A meeting of the Joint Committee, 28 January 1952.
18. SJA, Red Cross Relations Series, W.P. Stanbury (National Commissioner of the Red Cross) to William Warner, 31 December 1952.
19. In 1961 the Red Cross moved its Water Safety Week to the same week that St. John Ambulance had always held its Save-A-Life-Week. This conflict was dealt with by the joint board to the satisfaction of both parties. The Joint Committee continued to operate until 1963, and the agreement continued until 1973, when the Red Cross terminated the agreement and once again entered the field of widespread first aid training.
20. *Annual Report of the Priory of Canada, 1952*, 24.
21. *St. John News,* September 1952, 1.
22. *Annual Report of the Priory of Canada, 1953*, 24.
23. *Annual Report of the Priory of Canada, 1959*, 13.
24. *Annual Report of the Priory of Canada, 1961*, 9.
25. *Annual Report of the Priory of Canada, 1967*, 24.

26. It is estimated that the 1996 Saguenay Flooding cost $1.6 billion, while the 1997 Red River Flood cost $2.0 billion, and the 1998 Ontario-Quebec Ice Storm, $5.25 billion.

27. This would later be replaced by mouth to mouth resuscitation.

28. Rex Wright-St. Clair, *The Order of St. John in New Zealand* (Wellington: Priory of the Order of New Zealand, 1977), 80.

29. *St. John News*, April 1958, 3.

30. *Ibid.*, November 1952, 2.

31. *Ibid.*, November 1953, 2.

32. Quoting Chancellor Molson, *Annual Report of the Priory of Canada, 1960*, 6.

33. *St. John News*, September 1960, 2.

34. Sadly following the sale of St. John House in 2002 and move to an office block the library was boxed up and has largely been forgotten.

35. Prefix to Statutes, 1964–1965, Acts Proclaimed in Force, 13 Elizabeth II, Chapter 77, An Act Respecting The General Council of the Canadian Branch of the St. John Ambulance Association, 77–81.

36. *Debates of the Senate of Canada*, 1964, 65.

37. *Ibid.*, 537.

38. Beament was appointed to the Order of Canada in December 1986. His citation reads:

    This respected Ottawa lawyer has held many positions of national prominence as well as being an ardent supporter of numerous charitable organizations. For some thirty years, he has rendered invaluable services to the Order of St. John of Jerusalem and was elected Chancellor of the Priory of Canada.

    The Order of Canada citations of both Donald Rae and René Marin contain reference to their service to St. John Ambulance.

39. Matheson is the same man who along with George Stanley designed the Maple Leaf Flag.

40. *St. John News*, February 1965, 1.

41. Frances Gregor, "Mapping the Demise of the St. John Ambulance Home Nursing Program in Nova Scotia: 1950–1975," *Canadian Bulletin of Medical History*, Vol. 21:2, 2004, 359.

42. *Annual Report of the Priory of Canada, 1967*, 12.

43. The first concentrated efforts to begin first aid training in the North began in 1949.

44. *Annual Report of the Priory of Canada, 1947*, 54.

45. The Community Chest would become known as the United Way in 1973.

46. *Report of the Chapter General of the Grand Priory of the Most Venerable Order of the Hospital of St. John of Jerusalem, 1950*, 102.

Chapter Nine

1. St. John Ambulance Association, Provincial Executive Committee Meeting, 23 November 1960.

2. Gregor, "Mapping the Demise."

3. *Annual Report of the Priory of Canada, 1968*, 11.

4. Government of Canada Treasury Board Circular 1968/48 of 5 July 1968.

5. *Annual Report of the Priory of Canada, 1968*, 26.

6. *St. John Today*, March-April, 1970, 1.

7. *Annual Report of the Priory of Canada, 1972*, 14.

8. *Annual Report of the Priory of Canada, 1972*, 14; and *Annual Report of the Priory of Canada, 1973*, 14.

9. *Annual Report of the Priory of Canada, 1971*, 26.

10. *Annual Report of the Priory of Canada, 1971*, 23.

11. *Annual Report of the Priory of Canada, 1971*, 27.

12. *Annual Report of the Priory of Canada, 1971*, 10.

13. *St. John News,* September 1974, 5.
14. *St. John News,* March 1973, 1.
15. *Annual Report of the Priory of Canada, 1973,* 15.
16. *Annual Report of the Priory of Canada, 1974,* 23.
17. *Ibid.,* 1974, 14.
18. *Annual Report of the Priory of Canada, 1973,* 24.
19. *Annual Report of the Priory of Canada, 1975,* 22.
20. *Annual Report of the Priory of Canada, 1974,* 23.
21. *Annual Report of the Priory of Canada, 1975,* 11.
22. The Royal Charter was adopted in 1974 but it did not come into force until 1975.
23. *Annual Report of the Priory of Canada, 1976,* 11.
24. Marc Lalonde speaking to an Order of St. John luncheon, 29 October 1976, quoted in *St. John News,* December 1976, 1.
25. *Annual Report of the Priory of Canada, 1976,* 12.
26. *Annual Report of the Priory of Canada, 1977,* 12.
27. The building at 321 Chapel Street was purchased in 1942.
28. *Annual Report of St. John Ambulance Canada, 1979,* 10.
29. *Annual Report of the Priory of Canada, 1979,* 8.
30. *St. John News,* December 1979, 1.
31. *Annual Report of St. John Ambulance Canada, 1980,* 7.
32. *Annual Report of St. John Ambulance Canada, 1983,* 14.
33. *Ibid.,* 1983, 6.
34. This was provided by the Alberta Provincial Council.
35. *Annual Report of St. John Ambulance Canada, 1983,* 7.
36. Since 2004, it has been known as the St. John Eye Hospital.
37. *Annual Report of the Priory of Canada, 1970,* 11.
38. *St. John News,* June 1957, 3.
39. Dr. Lawrence Brierley, Dr. John Harvey, Dr. George Hay, Dr. Harold Climenhaga, Dr. Michael Boyd, Dr. George Beiko and Dr. Mathias Fellenz. Fellenz was the most recent Canadian to serve at the hospital, working there from 1993–1994.

Chapter Ten

1. *Annual Report of St. John Ambulance Canada, 1997,* 3.
2. *Annual Report of St. John Ambulance Canada, 1987,* 12.
3. This decline was been attributed to an aging membership and declining interest in involvement by non-brigade members.
4. *Annual Report of St. John Ambulance Canada, 1989,* 7.
5. *Annual Report of St. John Ambulance Canada, 1992,* 6.
6. *Ibid.*
7. *Annual Report of St. John Ambulance Canada, 1995,* 5.
8. One jurisdiction where St. John Ambulance maintains almost total dominance in the field of ambulatory care is New Zealand, where 85 percent of all ambulance services are provided by St. John Ambulance in that country.
9. *St. John Canada Today,* Vol. 6, No. 2. Autumn 1996.
10. *Annual Report of St. John Ambulance Canada, 1993,* 2.
11. Gentle Jenny was one of thirty dogs use by the Kawartha Great Pine Ridge Corps.
12. This division was originally named The Northwood Therapy Dog Division, and changed to its current designation on 1 June 2007.

13. SJA, SJE File, "Reorganization Community Resource Kit."

14. *Ibid.*

15. *Annual Report of St. John Ambulance Canada, 1998,* 4.

16. SJGA, Canada 1945–1951, Reorganization of the Order of St. John as a Confederation of Priories, 14 April 1947.

17. *Ibid.*

18. The name of the foundation in the Order's statutes was changed from "Ophthalmic" to "Eye" effective January 1, 2004.

19. *Annual Report of St. John Ambulance Canada, 1991,* 4.

20. Kendra Napp, Myrna Hamson, Norma Cochrane, Kristi Nelimarkka, Sherry Weiler, Heidi Bartsch.

21. *Annual Report of St. John Ambulance Canada, 1986,* 18.

22. SJA, Linen Guild Series, Minutes 28 March 1994.

23. SJA, Ophthalmic Hospital Series, Brian Leonard to Alec Harden, 22 August 1997.

24. This grant is broken down into monthly contributions of $10,000.

25. St. John House had previously been located at 321 Chapel Street since July 1942. Before that the national headquarters of St. John Ambulance had been located in Hope Chambers Building at 63 Sparks Street from 1934 to 1941; the Victoria Building on Wellington Street across from the West Block of Parliament from 1930 to 1933; the Plaza Building from 1925 to 1929; and in Room 52 of La Banque National Building from 1920 to 1925. Until the establishment of the Commandery of Canada the brigade headquarters were located in Toronto at 554 1/2 Young Street.

26. Members of the committee included The Honourable René Marin, Roger Lindsay, Leslie Ahlstrom, Richard Bruce, Ian D. Robinson, Logan Stewart, Dr. Keith Anstead, and Daniel Bellemare.

27. *Annual Report of St. John Ambulance Canada, 2003,* 2.

28. *Ibid., 2003,* 3.

29. *Annual Report of St. John Ambulance Canada, 2006,* 13.

Chapter Eleven

1. Effective 1 January 2007 no additional appointments of Esquires as part of the Order will be made, save those approved in 2006. Esquires are appointed to attend upon Bailiffs, Knights and Dames of the Order. No Order insignia is bestowed on Esquires, although they are given a lapel badge to wear, and they are entitled to use the post-nominals Esq.St.J., within the Order.

2. In a number of countries the awards of the Red Cross Society are recognized and included in national honours systems, but this is not the case in Canada, even though the Red Cross possesses a highly regarded three-levelled order. Nevertheless it is conceivable that this situation could change. The Red Cross Society's work in Canada is worthy of such recognition. There has long been a rivalry between the two organizations, which perform different charitable works, and have cooperated in a variety of ways during the two World Wars of the last century.

3. For an extensive discussion of honours in Canada and the development of the modern Canadian honours system please see *The Order of Canada; Its Origins, History and Development* (Toronto: University of Toronto Press, 2005).

4. In 1941 no appointments were made because of war restrictions and rationing of war related materials, which included both precious and base metals.

5. *Annual Report (Canadian Branch), 1919,* 30.

6. Such as the Order of the Star of India or the Order of the Indian Empire.

7. What is essentially modern day Ontario and Quebec, originally know as Upper and Lower Canada and after 1841 known as Canada East and Canada West.

8. *The Statutes of the Sovereign and Illustrious Order of St. John of Jerusalem, Anglia.* Approved by Special Chapter General held at London 16 April 1862 (London: John E. Taylor Press, 1862).

9. These appointments came before the Royal Charter of 1888, which made Queen Victoria the sovereign head of the Order and gave the Order official recognition within the British honours system.

10. The Honourable Hamnet Pinhey was listed as a deceased Knight of Grace, having died on 11 August 1857, although like many of the early appointments there are few additional details about this individual.

11. Women were also encouraged to participate in the work of the Order and St. John Ambulance.

12. LAC, Manuscript Group [henceforth MG] 26 H, Borden Papers, Memo to Borden from the Minister of Justice, 15 September 1919, 1285.

13. *Ibid.*, 1286.

14. Since 1931 appointments to and elevations within the Order have been published in the annual reports, but these have not included a complete register of the membership of the Order. See *St. John Ambulance Association in Canada Annual Reports* for year 1931, 2 March 1932.

15. LAC, MG 26 I, Meighen Papers, Bernard Rose to Meighen, 16 September 1921, 16788.

16. LAC, MG 26 I, Meighen Papers, Memo from the Department of External Affairs to Meighen 15 October 1921, 16791.

17. LAC, MG 26 I, Meighen Papers, Meighen to Bernard Rose, 3 November 1921, 16794.

18. LAC, MG 26 J, Bennett Papers, Memorandum from the Deputy Minister of Justice to the Minister of Justice, 15 September 1919, 235844. Note added to this memo 21 April 1924.

19. *Annual Report (Canadian Branch)*, 1927, 13.

20. LAC, MG 26 J, Mackenzie King Papers, Donald James Cowan to Mackenzie King, 20 January 1929, 147042–43.

21. LAC, MG 26 J, Mackenzie King Papers, Mackenzie King to D.J. Cowan, MP, 29 January 1930, 147944.

22. *The Order of Canada: Its Origins, History and Development* (Toronto: University of Toronto Press, 2005), 59.

23. LAC, MG 26 K, Bennett Papers, Earl of Scarborough to Bennett, 8 October 1939, 235766.

24. LAC, MG 26 K, Bennett Papers, Memo from Scarborough to Bennett, 3 October 1930, 235769.

25. LAC, MG 26 K, Bennett Papers, Bennett to Scarborough, 13 October 1939, 235782.

26. LAC, MG 26 K, Bennett Papers, Scarborough to Bennett, 23 October 1930, 235788.

27. LAC, MG 26 K, Bennett Papers, Bennett to Scarborough, 7 November 1930, 235788.

28. LAC, MG 26 K, Bennett Papers, Secretary General of the Order to Mr. Wallace Nesbitt, 24 February 1931, 235818.

29. *Ibid.*

30. LAC, MG 26 K, Bennett Papers, Scarborough to Bennett, 14 May 1931, 235824.

31. LAC, MG 26 K, Bennett Papers, Bennett to Scarborough, 21 June 1931, 235834-235835.

32. In 1931 a total of sixteen Canadians were appointed to the Order: Two Knights of Grace, five Commanders, eight Officers and one Serving Member.

33. LAC, MG 26 K, Bennett Papers, Scarborough to Bennett, 3 July 1931, 235889.

34. *Annual Report (Canadian Branch)*, 1931, 18.

35. *Annual Report (Canadian Branch)*, 1932, 21. "It is with great pleasure that your Committee records the admission of the Right Honourable R.B. Bennett K.C., P.C., [*sic*] Prime Minister of Canada to the Venerable Order in the British Realm of the Hospital of St. John of Jerusalem as a Knight of Grace."

36. Bennett remained active in the Order until his death in 1941. LAC, MG 26 K Bennett Papers, R.E. Wodehouse to Miss A.E. Millar, 5 June 1939, 612438.

37. SJG, Canada 1934, Full Report of the Delegation to Canada with Appendices.

38. *Ibid.*

39. *London Gazette*, 3 January 1932.

40. *Canada Gazette*, 22 July 1933, published in the *London Gazette*, 23 June 1933.

41. SJA Commandery Series, The Grand Priory of the British Realm of the Venerable Order of the Hospital of St. John of Jerusalem "Distinctions."

42. The publication of Canadian appointments to the various British orders did not take place regularly until 1905. All Canadian honours were gazetted in the *London Gazette* and *Canada Gazette* until the establishment of the Order of Canada in 1967.

43. SJA, Commandery Series, Major-General Sir Percival Wilkinson, Secretary General of the Order, to Colonel J.T. Clarke, Director General of the Canadian Branch of the St. John Ambulance Association, 2 October 1934.

44. SJA Honours Policy, C.A. Gray to Brigadier W.B.G. Barne (Secretary General) 5 November 1947.

45. An increased number of annual appointments were permitted to make up for the decade long absence of Canadian appointments.

46. SJA Honours Policy, C.A. Gray to Brigadier W.B.G. Barne (Secretary General) 5 November 1947.

47. SJA Honours Policy, W.B.G. Barne to C.A. Gray 29 November 1947.

48. SJA Honours Policy, W.B.G. Barne to C.A. Gray 17 December 1947.

49. SJA Honours Policy, Gray to Barne, 24 December 1947.

50. SJA Honours Policy, Gray to Barne, 20 February 1948.

51. This point system was based on population, donations to the Hospital of Jerusalem, members of the association, brigade strength, and cadet strength.

52. SJA Honours Policy Series, 1948 Revised Establishment of Priories, 12 November 1948.

53. SJA Honours Policy Series, Bessborough to Gray, 25 July 1953.

54. This was exactly what Gray has asked for in 1953, with the exception to the Serving Brother/Serving Sister grade, of which he requested an annual allotment of seventy-five. C.T. Evans (Priory Secretary) to W.J. Bennett, 22 February 1954.

55. By 1969–73; 100 Knights/Dames (total), 200 Commanders (total), eighty Officers (per annum), and 160 Serving Brothers/Serving Sisters (per annum).

56. From 1867 to 1972 the responsibility for honours was principally overseen by the Department of the Secretary of State. In 1972 this responsibility was transferred to the Office of the Governor General. Originally called the Honours Directorate, the name was subsequently changed to the Chancellery of Canadian Honours.

57. LAC, RG 2, Cabinet Conclusions, 4 March 1954.

58. *Ibid.*

59. Cabinet Directive 30 allowed Canadian civilians to receive the George Cross and George Medal for "acts of bravery performed at the risk of death or serious injury." Thus, for the most part, the Canadian honours system consisted of bravery awards: The George Cross, the George Medal, and the Queen's Commendation for Brave Conduct. Allowances were also made to permit appointments, for bravery, to the various levels of the Order of the British Empire. Members of the armed forces were still eligible for the various British gallantry awards, although there were no such allowances for meritorious service awards such as the Order of the Bath or the Order of the British Empire.

60. SJA Honours Policy Series, L.H. Nicholson to T.A. Johnson, 7 July 1962.

61. LAC, RG 2, Vol. 7020, Order of St. John of Jerusalem Honours List 1958, 24 January 1958.

62. LAC, RG 2, Vol 7020, Order of St. John of Jerusalem Honours List 1958, Rear Admiral H.S. Rayner, Chair of PMC, 24 January 1958. This listed the awards in the same way that the *London Gazette*.

63. LAC, RG 2, Vol. 7020, Order of St. John of Jerusalem, Brigadier General H.L. Cameron to Chairman of the PMC, 30 June 1955.

64. Order in Council 1972–1206 1 June 1972.

65. Until 1990 the Canadian order of precedence was a blended version of the British and Canadian order of precedence.

66. *Manual of Official Procedure of the Government of Canada, Vol. 1* (Queen's Printer: Ottawa, 1968), 222.

67. Privy Council Office Files, 655-1, 6/11/1990.

68. Only a trickle of Canadian appointments to British honours were made following the end of the Second World War. The last awards were two George Medals in 1964 to Canadians serving with the United Nations in the Congo.

69. PCO File 32000–1 Memorandum "The Order of St. John," January 1990, attached to a letter from James Gervais, Deputy Secretary to Nicole Jauvin, Assistant Secretary to the Cabinet, 8 January 1996.

70. *Ibid.*

71. *Ibid.*

72. The "accolade of the Realm" confers the title "Sir or Dame" upon the recipient. The dubbing occurs when the sovereign taps the recipient on each shoulder with a sword. This is the process followed for persons appointed to the Order of the Garter; Order of the Thistle; as Knight Bachelors or to the top two grades of the Order of the Bath; Order of St. Michael and St. George; Royal Victorian Order; or Order of the British Empire. Appointment to these Orders is only completed when the appointee is dubbed. The "accolade of the Order" confers knighthood upon the recipient, however there is no title associated with this knighthood. The dubbing occurs when the grand prior or his delegate taps the recipient three times on the left shoulder. The act of investiture is the ultimate public award of status as a member of the Order. Appointment to the top two grades of the Order of St. John, unlike other orders, does not require the appointee to attend an investiture.

73. Since 1935, there have existed at the provincial level, honours and awards committees that submit to the national office; then a commandery; today a priory; and nomination lists of those, who at the provincial level, have made a significant contribution to St. John. Since 2004 the nomination forms have been standardized and modelled on that used by the Order of Canada. As the bulk of appointments to the Order emanate from the provincial level, this is one of the most important mechanisms for ensuring a fair distribution of appointments to all regions of the dominion.

74. *Ibid.*

75. Appointments to the various British orders of chivalry and awards of British medals and decorations made before 1972 for services related to Canada are considered "Canadian appointments." Thus a separate order of precedence exists for pre-1972 appointments. The current Canadian order of precedence is confirmed in Order in Council 1990–2307.

76. In the Order of St. John dubbing is not the same as the conferring of a British knighthood. Both include a dubbing ceremony, but after the accolade of knighthood is conferred, the recipient may use the appellation "Sir" or "Dame."

77. *Canada Gazette,* 24 August 1991, 2730.

78. A 1974 augmentation of the Royal Charter removed the terminology "British Realm" from the name of the Order. The Grand Priory in the British Realm of the Most Venerable Order of the Hospital of St. John of Jerusalem was the formal designation given to the Order with the 1955 Royal Charter granted by Queen Elizabeth II. The 1926 Royal Charter granted by King George V carried the designation The Grand Priory in the British Realm of the Venerable Order of the Hospital of St. John of Jerusalem.

79. Order Honours Review Group Report, 14 December 2005.

80. The Review of the Order Honours; Summary of Grand Council Decisions, 9–11 May 2006.

81. 3.1.(a-b) The Review of the Order Honours; Summary of Grand Council Decisions, 9–11 May 2006. This last clause was added in recognition of the fact that the Order of Canada, Order of Australia, and the national orders of a number of other countries are given automatically to the spouse of the governor general, as the Order of St. John has been since Lord Bessborough's time.

82. Statement of Criteria for Admission to and Promotion in the Order, 9 May 2007, 4.

83. In the normal course of volunteering for St. John Ambulance an individual who is appointed to the Order would have been a volunteer for three or more years. Allowances are made for exceptional circumstances, contributions, and exceptional people.

84. Clause II of *The Chivalric Alliance of Orders of Saint John,* 13 June 1961.

85. *Joint Declaration between the Most Venerable Order of the Hospital of St. John of Jerusalem and the Sovereign Military and Hospitaller Order of St. John of Jerusalem of Rhodes and of Malta,* 26 November 1963.

86. Sainty, 111.

87. *The Orders of St. John; Report of the Co-operation Working Group,* 20 September 2004. Chapter One of the Report outlines the milestones in the process: (a) 13 June 1961, Convention by which the Alliance of the Orders of St. John was constituted; (b) 26 November 1963, Declaration of Mutual Esteem by the Sovereign

Military Order of Malta and the Venerable Order; (c) 1974, Formation of the Committee on the Orders of St. John (FOC), then called the False Orders Committee; (d) 14 October 1987, the London Declaration (the first joint instrument of mutual recognition between the five Orders); (e) 9 November 1988, Joint Declaration by the SMOM and the Johanniter Orden of their intention to collaborate; (f) 9 November 1988, Formation of the Liaison Committee between the SMOM and the Alliance Orders; (g) 23 September 1992, Accord between the SMOM, Johanniter Orden and the Venerable Order pledging mutual co-operation in Canada; (h) 26 September 1996, Formation of the Joint Commission on Emblem Protection by the SMOM and Alliance Orders; (i) 18 November 2000, Further Declaration between the SMOM and the Johanniter Orden reaffirming their intention to collaborate.

88. *The Orders of St. John: Report of the Co-operation Working Group*, 20 September 2004, 18.

89. *Ibid.*, 18.

90. King and Luke, 223–224.

91. Robert Pichette, *Historical Sketch and Armorial of the Canadian Association of the Sovereign Military Order of Malta* (Toronto: Pro Familia Publishing, 2003), 38.

Chapter Twelve

1. Beginning in 2006 the chaplain general of the Canadian Forces has served as Chaplain of the Order in Canada. The position of Chaplain of the Priory also existed sporadically beginning in 1946; this has now been replaced with Dean of the Order.

2. *Annual Report (Canadian Branch), 1911*, 11.

3. Elias Ashmole, *The Institution, Laws and Ceremonies of the Most Noble Order of the Garter,* 1672, 54.

4. The sixth level, Esquire, does not confer on the recipient a decoration, just the official designation as an Esquire. There is an official lapel badge that is worn by Esquires.

5. *Illustrious and Sovereign Order of the Knights Hospitallers of Saint John of Jerusalem, Venerable Langue of England, Comprehending The Grand Priories, Bailiwicks, and Commanderies in England, Scotland, Ireland, Wales.* 1849.

6. Sixteen Bailiffs, eighteen Knights Commander, twenty-three Knights of Justice, six Chaplains, six Sergeants-at-Arms/Esquires, ten Ladies, twenty Knights of Grace, one Donat, and one Serving Brother. *The Statutes of the Sovereign and Illustrious Order of St. John of Jerusalem, Anglia*. As passed by the Capitular Commission held at London 3 April 1867 and approved by Chapter General 24 June 1867 (E. Taylor Press, 1867).

7. Charles Tozer, *The Insignia and Medals of the Grand Priory of the Most Venerable Order of the Hospital of St. John of Jerusalem* (London: Hayward and Son, 1975), 19.

8. This grade of the Order does not confer an insignia, just a simple lapel badge. Since 2007 no further appointments to this grade have been made as it is no longer considered a grade of the Order.

9. This does not include the appointment of R.B. Bennett as a Knight of Grace in 1932.

10. Unfortunately records related to the total membership of the Order in Canada for this period are scant and reliable figures are impossible to collate.

11. Between 2000 and 2004 the elevation of three Serving Brothers to the grade of Knight of Grace caused great difficulties and almost lead to a complete breakdown of relations between the Chancellery and the Order of St. John. The standard procedure involving Chancellery officials was not followed and it has taken time to rebuild a healthy working relationship.

12. *Regulations of the Order of St. John of Jerusalem in England*, 1872, 1.

13. *The Statutes of the Sovereign and Illustrious Order of St. John of Jerusalem, Anglia*. Approved by Special Chapter General held at London 16 April 1862 (London: John E. Taylor Press, 1862).

14. In many European countries to this day it is the requirement of the newly appointed member or their sponsor to obtain the insignia from an official supplier.

15. SJGA. Canada 1934–35, W.J. Bennett to Brigadier General W.G.B. Barne, 14 January 1946.

16. Tozer, 34.

17. SJA Commandery Series, Sir Percival Wilkinson (Secretary General) to J.T. Clarke, Director General of the Canadian Branch, 25 April 1934. In 1934 one British pound was worth $4.99 Canadian. Foreign Exchange Rates, 1910–1960, Series H619–630, The Historical Statistics of Canada, 276.

18. In 1959 one British pound was worth $2.69 Canadian.

19. It was only in 1984 when Rideau Ltée began manufacturing the Order of Canada that a Canadian firm became capable of mass producing enamelled insignia. Although Birks and a number of other Canadian Jewellers were in a position to produce small batches of enamelled items, they were not in a position to manufacture large numbers of insignia.

20. This practice came to an end in 1956 at the request of Vincent Massey, the prior, as it was found "to be contrary to the intent of the regulations of the Department of National Revenue." SJA, Commandery Series, A.G. Cherrier to the Secretary General of the Order of St. John, 25 February 1959.

21. In 1995 Joe Drouin Enterprises of Gatineau, Quebec, began making the insignia of all grades of the Order bestowed in Canada. The first batch of Drouin insignia were presented in 1996. An experiment was attempted. The enamel part of the insignia for Officers through to Knights/Dames was made of an epoxy plastic rather than the more toxic lead-based enamel. This was seen as a cost-effective alternative, although the epoxy enamel was abandoned in 2004 when it was found to turn yellow and become soft with time and exposure.

22. Statues of the Grand Priory of the Order of the Hospital of St. John of Jerusalem in the British Realm, 1972.

23. SJGA Canada 1934–35, W.J. Bennett (Priory Secretary) to Brigadier General W.B.G. Barne (Secretary General), 25 January 1950.

24. A King would wear a ribbon 10 cm wide.

25. Protocol for The Chains of Office of the Priory of Canada. Letter from Roger Lindsay to Christopher McCreery, 11 May 2007.

26. Before 2003, Cleave and Company operated as J.R. Gaunt & Son.

27. Alan Mansfield. Ceremonial Costume, Court, Civil and Civic Costume from 1660 to the Present (London: A&C Black, 1980), 46.

28. Tozer, 49.

29. Mansfield, 244.

30. Tozer, 23.

31. G.R. Gayre, The Heraldry of the Knights of St. John, (Allahabad: Garga Brothers Press, 1956), 108.

32. Gayre, 106.

33. Roll of Members and Honorary Associates and Recipients of Awards of Honour, 1902.

34. Tozer, 23.

35. "Order of Wear," Annual Report (UK), 1905, 31.

36. After 1984 the Member 4th Class was designated as lieutenant of the Royal Victorian Order (LVO), while the Member 5th class was designated member of the Royal Victorian Order (MVO).

37. Usually a black round tin box (a skippit) used to contain a wax seal to prevent damage. The College of Arms, London, uses gold coloured skippits on their granting documents.

38. Occasionally the seal was impressed on a maroon coloured legal seal.

39. This new certificate, based on that used by other Canadian orders was designed by the author.

40. SJGA, Draft Regulations of the Commandery in Canada of the Grand Priory in the British Realm of the Venerable Order of the Hospital of St. John of Jerusalem, section 15.

41. SJA Commandery Series, P. Wilkinson to C.A. Hodgetts, 15 March 1932.

42. The Honourable Hewitt Bostock served as Speaker of the Senate from 1922 until his death in 1930. Born in 1844 in England, Bostock immigrated to British Columbia in 1893 after travelling extensively through America, Australia, New Zealand, China, and Japan. After being elected to the House of Commons in 1896 Bostock was summoned to the Senate in 1904 and became leader of the opposition in the Senate, a post he would hold until becoming Speaker. It was during the First World War that Bostock became involved with the work of St. John Ambulance. He was elected president of the St. John Ambulance Association in 1928.

43. Minutes of a special meeting of the Select Vestry of Christ Church Cathedral, 31 January 1940.

44. Thanks is owed to Robert Doyle for his work on the article "The Chapel of St. John of Jerusalem," who undertook the bulk of the research related to the chapel of the Order.
45. SJGA, Canada 1934–35, Brigadier General W.G.B. Barne to W.J. Bennett, 7 January 1949.
46. SJGA, Canada, 1934–35, W.J. Bennett to Brigadier General W.G.B. Barne, 18 December 1948.

Chapter Thirteen

1. The Service Medal was awarded for 15 years of service to members of St. John Ambulance in Britain until 1990 when it was reduced to 12 years. The Service Medal has been awarded for 12 years service in Australia, Canada, New Zealand, and South Africa since its inception. In certain colonies such as Ceylon (Sri Lanka), India, and tropical places the Service Medal was awarded for 10 years of service. This was in recognition of the harsh living conditions people experienced.
2. Tozer, 42.
3. British awards of the Service Medal ceased to be named in 1942.
4. The concept for these commendations was taken from the US Presidential Unit Citation which was approved on 3 November 1966.
5. *Annual Report (Commandery in Canada), 1939,* 10.
6. *Ibid.*
7. Royal Charter of Incorporation 1888, section 38.
8. To this day the Order and the Royal Society coordinate their awards to ensure that there is no overlap. Also see Colin Dawson, "The Medals for Saving Life on Land Awarded by The Order of St. John of Jerusalem in England." St. John Historical Society Proceedings, Vol. 11, 1999, 3.
9. Tozer, 41.
10. Created in 1866 by Queen Victoria, the Albert Medal was originally awarded for the saving of life or attempted saving of life at sea. This criteria was broadened in 1867 to include life saving on land.
11. Royal Warrant constituting the Albert Medal, 12 April 1867.
12. *Annual Report (UK), 1874,* also see Dawson, 1–18.
13. *Annual Report (UK), 1874.*
14. *Annual Report (UK), 1874.*
15. Thomas William Heyck, *The Peoples of the British Isles: A New History, 1688–1870,* (Belmont: Wadsworth Press, 1992), 223.
16. Royal Charter 1888, section 48.
17. The St. John (Order) Regulations, 2003, Appendix III, 7(1), 43.
18. SJGA Canada 1934–35, Major General J.E.T. Younger (Secretary of the Order) to W.J. Bennett, Priory Secretary, 23 August 1948.
19. SJGA Canada, 1934–35, W.J. Bennett to Major General J.E.T. Younger, 7 September 1948.
20. Roll of Members and Honorary Associates and of Recipients of Awards, 1902.
21. Reynolds' Life Saving Medal was the 235th awarded, and is listed in the St. John Life Saving Medal Register. SJGA Life Saving Medal Roll Entries 001–333.
22. Priory of the Order of St. John in Canada, 1946, 10.
23. Royal Charter 1888, section 38.
24. *Annual Report (UK), 1896.*
25. Pichette, *Historical Sketch.*
26. SJGA Canada 1934–35, Thomas Guerin (Quebec Provincial Council) to Brigadier General W.B.G. Barne (Secretary General), 14 September 1947.
27. SJGA Canada 1934–35, Brigadier W.B.G. Barne to Thomas Guerin, 25 November 1947.
28. SJGA Canada 1934–35, Brigadier W.B.G. Barne to Thomas Guerin, 25 November 1947.
29. SJGA Canada 1934–35, Brigadier W.B.G. Barne to Thomas Guerin, 25 November 1947.
30. Barne noted that "a suitable sword—with hilt long enough for it to be carried with both hands by the Sword-

Bearer of the Priory—can be obtained from Messrs Wilkinson of Pall Mall. Direct personal application might be made to the Director of the Firm who is an expert in this and has already supplied similar swords for other priories. Mr. J.W. Latham, Oakley Works, Southfield Road, Acton Green, London W.4." SJGA Canada 1934–35, Brigadier W.B.G. Barne to Thomas Guerin, 25 November 1947.

31. *Annual Report of the Priory of Canada, 1960*, 20.

32. King and Luke, 4. Also see Delaville, *La Roulx, Les Hospitaliers en Terre Sainte,* 37.

33. Mansfield, 241. Ashmole, Elias. *The Institution, Laws and Ceremonies of the Most Noble Order of the Garter,* 1672. 54.

34. Tozer, 17.

35. *Ibid.*

36. *A Short History of The Order of the Hospital of St. John of Jerusalem* (London: St. John's Gate, Clerkenwell) 14.

37. Hypericum Depression Trial Study Group. Effect of Hypericum perforatum (St. John's Wort) in major depressive disorder: A randomized controlled trial. *Journal of the American Medical Association.* 2002; 287(14):1807–1814.

38. *Speaker's Notes; A Guide to the Order of St. John and Its Work Today* (London: St. John's Gate, 1962), 8.

39. *Ibid.*

40. The Royal License, and Authority to use the Royal Crest, 1 February 1926.

41. A.C. Fox-Davies, p. 133.

42. Guy Stair Sainty and Rafal Heydel Mankoo, ed., *Burke's World Orders of Knighthood and Merit* "Heraldic Privilege and the Venerable Order of Saint John—A Canadian Perspective" 1944–1948.

43. *Ibid.*

Appendices

1. What is essentially modern day Ontario and Quebec, originally known as Upper and Lower Canada, and after 1841 known as Canada East and Canada West.

2. *The Statutes of the Sovereign and Illustrious Order of St. John of Jerusalem, Anglia.* Approved by Special Chapter General held at London 16 April 1862 (London: John E. Taylor Press, 1862).

3. Tozer, 38.

BIBLIOGRAPHY

Primary Sources

Library and Archives Canada (LAC).
Memorial University Archives (MUA).
Provincial Archives of Newfoundland and Labrador (PANL).
St. John's Gate Archives (SJGA).
St. John National Headquarters Archives (SJA).

Primary Documents

Annual Report of the Canadian Branch of the St. John Ambulance Association, 1911–1933.

Annual Report of the Commandery of Canada, 1934–1946.

Annual Report of the Priory of Canada, 1947–present.

Annual Report of the St. John Ambulance Association (UK).

Annual Report of the St. John Ambulance Association, of the Council for the Dominion of Canada, 1897.

Annual Report of the St. John Ambulance Brigade Overseas, 1910–1948.

Charter of Incorporation, Amended statues and Supplemental Charter, The Grand Priory of the Order of the Hospital of St. John of Jerusalem in England. London, Charles Cull, 1905.

The Grand Priory of the Order of the Hospital of St. John of Jerusalem in England, Regulations and Bye-Laws. Approved 2 December 1912.

The Grand Priory of the Order of the Hospital of St. John of Jerusalem in England, Supplemental Charter. 22 May 1907. London: Charles Cull, 1907.

Regulations passed by the Capitular Commission held at London 3 April 1867 and approved by Chapter General 24 June 1867. E. Taylor Press, 1867.

Statutes of the Illustrious and Sovereign Order of the Knights Hospitallers of Saint John of Jerusalem, Venerable Langue of England, Comprehending The Grand Priories, Bailiwicks, and commanderies in England, Scotland, Ireland, Wales. 1849.

The Statutes of the Order of St. John of Jerusalem in England 1871. Worcester: Deighton and Son, 1871.

The Statutes of the Sovereign and Illustrious Order of St. John of Jerusalem, Anglia. Approved by Special Chapter General held at London 16 April 1862, London: John E. Taylor Press, 1862.

The Statutes of the Sovereign and Illustrious Order of St. John of Jerusalem, Anglia. Approved by Chapter General 24 June 1862, London: John E. Taylor Press, 1864.

The Statutes of the Sovereign and Illustrious Order of St. John of Jerusalem, Anglia.

Publications

Abela, A.E. *The Order of St. Michael and St. George in Malta and Maltese Knights of the British Realm*. Valetta: Progress Publishing, 1988.

Abraham, Neena. "Medical Memories of the 1917 Explosion," *Ground Zero: A Reassessment of the 1917 Explosion in Halifax Harbour*. Halifax: Nimbus, 1994.

Ashmole, Elias, *The Institution, Laws and Ceremonies of the Most Noble Order of the Garter*. London: Frederick Muller, 1672.

Barber, Malcolm (ed). *The Military Orders: Fighting for the Faith and Caring for the Sick*. Aldershot: Variorum, 1994.

Beaston, George Thomas. The Knights Hospitallers in Scotland and their Priory at Trophichen. Glasgow: James Hedderwick, 1903.

Bedford, W.K.R. and R. Holbeche. *The Order of the Hospital of St. John of Jerusalem*. London: F.E Robinson Press, 1902.

Bilson, Geoffrey. "Dr. Frederick Montizambert (1843–1929); Canada's First Director General of Public Health," *Medical History*, 1985 Vol. 29.

Brown, Cassie. *Death on Ice; The Great Newfoundland Sealing Disaster of 1914.* Toronto: Doubleday Canada, 1972.

Buckle, George E., ed. *The Letters of Queen Victoria*, Third Series, 1886–1901. London: John Murray, 1930.

Cambray, P.G. and G.G.B. Briggs. *Red Cross and St. John; The Official Record of the Humanitarian Services of the War Organization of the British Red Cross Society and the Order of St. John of Jerusalem*. Eastbourne: Sumfield and Day Press, 1949.

Clifford, Joan. *For the Service of Mankind*. London: Robert Hale, 1971.

Colebrook Harris, Richard. *The Seigneurial System in Early Canada*. University of Laval, 1968.

Cole-Mackintosh, Ronnie. *A Century of Service to mankind: A History of the St. John Ambulance Brigade*. Acford Ltd, 1986.

Colley, Linda Colley. *Britons, Forging the Nation, 1707–1837*. New Haven: Yale University Press, 1992.

Cowan, John. *Canada's Governors General*. Toronto: York Publishing Company, 1967.

Cowan, Ian, P.H.R. Mackay, Alan Macquarrie. *The Knights of St. John of Jerusalem in Scotland*. Edinburgh: Scottish History Society, 1983.

Corbet-Fletcher, Nigel. *The St. John Ambulance Association: Its History, and Its Part in the Ambulance Movement*. London: St. John's Gate, 1929.

Cromer, Ruby. *The Hospital of St. John in Jerusalem*. Will Carter Press, 1961.

Cross, Colin. *The Fall of the British Empire*. London: Book Club Associates, 1968.

Dawson, Joan. "The Governor's Goods: The Inventory of the Personal Property of Isaac de Razilly." *Nova Scotia Historical Review*, Vol. 5, No. 1, 1985.

Debates of the Senate of Canada, 1914 and 1964. Ottawa: Queen's Printer.

Dictionary of Canadian Biography. Toronto: University of Toronto Press.

Dictionary of Newfoundland and Labrador Biography. St. John's: Harry Cluff Publishing, 1990.

Eccles, W.J. *Canada Under Louis XIV, 1663–1701*. Toronto: McClelland and Stewart, 1964.

Edgert, Hugh A.R. *Champions of the Cross*. Watton: Rapide Press, 1983.

Edmonds, E. *St. John Ambulance: Aspects of History in Europe and Canada*. Prince Edward Island Council, 1983.

Fincham, H.W. *The Order of the Hospital of St. John of Jerusalem and its Grand Priory of England*. London: St. John's Gate, 1933.

Foster, Benjamin. *Foster's History of Ye Gate of St. John*. London: Gilbert and Rivington, 1851.

Galloway, Strome. *The White Cross in Canada: A history of St. John Ambulance*. Ottawa: Priory of Canada, 1983.

Gayre, G.R. *The Heraldry of the Knights of St. John*. Allahabad: Garga Brothers Press, 1956.

Gibbon, J.M. *The Victorian Order of Nurses for Canada*. Montreal: Southam Press, 1947.

Granatstein, Jack, L. and Peter Neary. *The Good Fight: Canadians and World War II.* Toronto: Copp Clark, 1995.

Gregor, Frances. "Mapping the Demise of the St. John Ambulance Home Nursing Program in Nova Scotia: 1950–1975." *Canadian Bulletin of Medical History,* Vol. 21:2, 2004.

Hanna, James. *A Century of Red Blankets: A History of the Ambulance Service in Ontario.* Erin: Boston Mills Press, 1982.

Haycock, Ronald G. *Sam Hughes; The Public Career of a Controversial Canadian, 1885–1916.* Waterloo: Wilfrid Laurier University Press, 1986.

Heyck, Thomas William. *The Peoples of the British Isles: A New History, 1688–1870.* Belmont: Wadsworth Press, 1992.

Howie-Willis, Ian. *A Century for Australia: St. John Ambulance in Australia 1883–1983.* Canberra: Order of St. John, 1983.

____. *St. John Ambulances and Western Australia: A Centenary Anthology, 1892–1992.*Perth, 1992.

Hume, Edgar Erskine. *Medical Work of the Knights Hospitallers of Saint John of Jerusalem.* Baltimore: Johns Hopkins University Press, 1940.

King, Sir Edwin and Sir Harry Luke. *The Knights of St. John in the British Realm: Being the Official History of the Most Venerable Order of the Hospital of St. John of Jerusalem.* London: St. John's Gate, 1967.

King, Sir Edwin J. *The Knights of St. John in the British Empire, Being the Official History of the British Order of the Hospital of St. John of Jerusalem.* London: The Order of St. John, 1934.

____. The *Pilgrimage of 1926: Being the Official Journal of the Knights of St. John.* London: St. John's Gate, 1926.

Kitz, Janet. *Shattered City: The Halifax Explosion and the Road to Recovery.* Halifax: Nimbus Press, 2004.

Land, R.E.A. *Fifty Years in the Malta Order: Being Data Dealing with the Foundation of the Ancient Order, Its History, Constitution and Ritual Including the Grand Priory of the Sixth Langue, Especially in Scotland, Together with a Complete History of the Regular Order of the Same Name in America.* Toronto: Privately Published, 1928.

Lee, Sir Sidney. *King Edward VII.* London: MacMillan, 1925.

Luke, Sir Harry. *An Examination of Certain Claims to be an Order of St. John.* London: St. John's Gate, 1965.

McCreery, Christopher. *The Canadian Honours System.* Toronto: Dundurn Press, 2005.

____. *The Order of Canada: Its Origins, History and Development.* Toronto: University of Toronto Press, 2005.

McGinnis, Janice P. Dickin. "The Impact of Epidemic Influenza: Canada 1918–1919," *Canadian Historical Association, Historical Papers, 1977.*

MacPhail, Sir Andrew. *The Medical Services.* Ottawa: King's Printer, 1925.

Mansfield, Alan. *Ceremonial Costume, Court, Civil and Civic Costume from 1660 to the Present.* London: A&C Black, 1980.

Members of the Order of St. John on the Roll of the Priory for Canada, 1956.

Mifsud, A. *Knights Hospitallers of the Venerable Tongue Of England in Malt*a. Valetta: The Malta Herald, 1914.

Moorehead, Caroline. *Dunant's Dream: War Switzerland and the History of the Red Cross.* London: Harper Collins Publishers, 1998.

Murray, T.J. "Medical Aspects of the Disaster: The Missing Report of Dr. David Fraser," *Ground Zero: A Reassessment of the 1917 Explosion in Halifax Harbour.* Halifax: Nimbus, 1994.

Nicholson, G.W.L. *The White Cross in Canada; A History of St. John Ambulance.* Montreal: Harvest Press, 1967.

O'Malley, Gregory. The Knights Hospitaller of the English Langue, 1460-1565. Oxford: Oxford University Press, 2005.

Patterson, Stephen Patterson. *Royal Insignia.* London: Merrell Holberton Press, 1998.

Pearn, John. "The Earliest Days of First Aid," *British Medical Journal,* 1994, Vol. 309.

Pichette, Robert. *Historical Sketch and Armorial of the Canadian Association of the Sovereign Military Order of Malta.* Toronto: Pro Familia Publishing, 2003.

____. *This Honourable Cross: the Order of St. John in the New World.* Sovereign Military Order of Malta, Canadian Association, 1999.

Porter, McKenzie. *To All Men: The Story of the Canadian Red Cross*. Toronto: McClelland and Stewart, 1960.

Quiney, Linda. *Assistant Angles: Canadian Women as Voluntary Aid Detachment Nurses During and After the Great War 1914–1930*. Unpublished Doctoral Dissertation, University of Ottawa, 2002.

____. "Bravely and Loyally they Answered the Call: St. John Ambulance, the Red Cross, and the Patriotic Service of Canadian Women During the Great War." *History of Intellectual Culture,* Vol. 5, No. 1, 2005.

Rees, William. *A History of the Order of St. John of Jerusalem: In Wales and on the Welsh Border*. Cardiff: Western Mail, 1947.

Riley-Smith, Jonathan. *Hospitallers: the History of the Order of St. John*. London: Hambledon Press, 1999.

____. "The Military-Religious Orders: Their History and Continuing Relevance," *Conference Proceedings.* Cambridge: Emmanuel College, 2005.

Royal Charter of the Grand Priory in England of the Venerable Order of the Hospital of St. John of Jerusalem, 1888.

Royal Charter of the Grand Priory in the British Realm of the Venerable Order of the Hospital of St. John of Jerusalem, 1926.

Royal Charters of the Most Venerable Order of the Hospital of St. John of Jerusalem, (1955 and 1974). Statutes and Regulations, 1981 edition, 1985 edition.

Russel, Peter A. *Attitudes to Social Structure and Mobility in Upper Canada, 1815–1840*. Queenstown: Edwin Mellen Press, 1990.

Ryerson, George Sterling. *Looking Backward*. Toronto: Ryerson Press, 1924.

Sainty, Guy Stair and Rafal Heydel Mankoo, eds. *Burke's World Orders of Knighthood and Merit*. London: Burkes Peerage, 2006.

Sainty, Guy Stair. *The Orders of Saint John: The History, Structure, Membership and Modern Roles of the Five Hospitaller Orders of Saint John of Jerusalem*. New York: The American Society of the Most Venerable Order of the Hospital of Saint John in Jerusalem, 1991.

Seward, Desmond. *The Monks of War: The Military Religious Orders*. London: Penguin Press, 1995.

Sire, H.J.A. *The Knights of Malta*. New Haven: Yale University Press, 1994.

Smallwood, Joey, ed. *Encyclopedia of Newfoundland and Labrador, Vol. 5*. St. John's: Smallwood Heritage Foundation, 1991.

St. George Saunders, Hilary. *The Red Cross and the White; A short history of the joint war organization of the British Red Cross Society and the Order of St. John of Jerusalem during the war, 1939–1945*. London: Hollis and Carter, 1949.

St. John Councils, (General) Regulations, 1975.

St. John Historical Society Proceedings.

The Priory of Canada of the Most Venerable Order of the Hospital of St. John of Jerusalem. Priory Rules 1991.

Thourot-Pichel, Charles Louis, *History of the Sovereign Order of Saint John of Jerusalem: Knights of Malta, 1048–1970*. Shickshinny PA, 1970.

Toxopeus, Deena. *The 1951 Agreement Between the Red Cross and St. John Ambulance: A case study of the effect of Civil Defence on Canada's Health Care System*. Unpublished Master of Arts Thesis, University of Ottawa, 1997.

Tozer, Charles. *The Insignia and Medals of the Grand Priory of the Most Venerable Order of the Hospital of St. John of Jerusalem*. London: Hayward and Son, 1975.

Wright-St. Clair, Rex. *The Order of St. John in New Zealand*. Wellington: Priory of the Order of New Zealand, 1977.

____. *St. John in New Zealand, 1885–1985*. Wellington: Millwood Press, 1985.

Waite, Peter B. *Canada 1874–1896: Arduous Destiny*. Toronto: McClelland and Stewart, Toronto 1971.

Friends of the Maple Leaf and the White Cross

A project of this magnitude requires a significant amount of support and resources to make it a reality. The publication of this national history chronicling one of the nation's longest-serving charitable organizations would not have been possible without the financial contributions by members and friends of the Order of St. John, St. John Ambulance volunteers, and St. John Councils across Canada. Through your support, our long history of volunteerism and philanthropy is enhanced and maintained.

Sincere thanks are extended to the following Friends of the Maple Leaf and White Cross:

Full Name	City	Prov
LCol. Leslie E. (Lee) Ahlstrom, KStJ, CD, QC	Sherwood Park	AB
Mrs. Marilyn Alberti, OStJ	Ottawa	ON
Mr. Douglas Anthony Alberts, SBStJ	Port Elgin	ON
Ms. Mary J. Aldum, DStJ	Winnipeg	MB
Mr. Thomas E. Allan, KStJ	Hamilton	ON
Saint John Ambulance Division 280	Saint-Hyacinthe	QC
Mr. L. Ross Andrews, OStJ	Straffordville	ON
Dr. Borden Bachynski, KStJ, CD	Regina	SK
Mr. Harry D. Barons, SBStJ	Orillia	ON
LCol. (Ret'd) Eric L. Barry, GCStJ, CD	Oakville	ON
Capt. Peter Beatty, SBStJ, CD	Orleans	ON
Mrs. Madeleine R. Bédard, OStJ	Quebec	QC
Mr. Ian Bennett	Kanata	ON
Mr. Daniel A. Bellemare, KStJ, MSM, QC	Ottawa	ON
Capt. Samuel W. Billich, OStJ, CD	North York	ON
Mr. Allan Bird	Manotick	ON
Cdr. John Blatherwick, CM, CStJ, CD	New Westminster	BC
Capt. Jack Boddington, KStJ	Edmonton	AB

Full Name	City	Prov
CWO Arthur H. Boon, MMM, SBStJ, CD	Stratford	ON
Mr. Roman Borysko, OStJ	Saskatoon	SK
Mr. Robert A. Brathwaite, KStJ, CD	Toronto	ON
Mr. F. Hugh Brennan, KStJ, CD	Toronto	ON
Mr. Joseph-Hyacinthe Breton, SBStJ, CD	Lévis	QC
Mrs. Euphemia Bridges, OStJ	Downsview	ON
Sgt. Anthony G. Bruce, CStJ, CD	Montreal	QC
Mr. F. Richard Bruce, MOM, CStJ	Brandon	MB
Mr. J. Bruce Buchanan, CM, CStJ	West Vancouver	BC
Miss Sylvia Burkinshaw, DStJ	Kingston	ON
Mr. Randall E.G. Burtch	Cookstown	ON
HCol. Robert V. Cade, CStJ, CD	Regina	SK
Mr. Brock Cairns, KStJ	Calgary	AB
LCol. Jeffrey R. Cairns, OStJ, CD, AdeC	St. Catharines	ON
Dr. Bevan J.M. Carrique, SBStJ	Barrie	ON
Ms. Marjorie A. Carroll, OStJ	Ottawa	ON
Cst. Adam J.D. Carter, OStJ	Fenwick	ON
Mr. Michael Cava, SBStJ	Edmonton	AB
Mr. Garry Chandler, CStJ, CD	Borden	ON
& Mrs. Donna Chandler, SSStJ		
Maj. Richard Choquette, OStJ, CD	Laval	QC
Mrs. Claudette Chrétien, CStJ	Matane	QC
Maj. (Ret'd) Roman J. Ciecwierz, CStJ, CD	Waterloo	ON
Mr. Berthier Cimon, SBStJ	Mont-Joli	QC
Dr. Alexander M. Clark, SBStJ	Pubinco	NS
Dr. Wendy A. Clay, CMM, OStJ, CD	North Saanich	BC
Mr. J. Stuart Clyne, CStJ, QC	West Vancouver	BC
Mr. James E. Cooper, KStJ	Pembroke	ON
Mr. Robert Côté, SBStJ	Port-Cartier	QC
Col. Jean-Louis Cousineau, KStJ, CD, ADC	Pointe-Claire	QC
Mr. Sidney A. Crow, KStJ	Vineland	ON
A/Commr. Patrick M. Cummins, OStJ	Ottawa	ON
Supt. W. Ulysses Currie, MOM, SBStJ	Edmonton	AB
Mrs. Barbara A. Davis, DStJ	St. John's	NL
Mr. Shawn G. Davis	Windsor	ON
Mr. Lannon de Best, OStJ	New Westminster	BC
Col. (Ret'd) Leslie K. Deane, OStJ, CD	Burnaby	BC
Supt. (Ret'd) Clarence J. Dent, KStJ	Dartmouth	NS

Full Name	City	Prov
Col. Jacques Duchesneau, CM, KStJ	Ottawa	ON
Mrs. Sharon Ann Dufton, SSStJ	Kitchener	ON
Dr. John M. Dugan, CStJ	Red Deer	AB
Dr. Elizabeth C. Eaton, OStJ	Shediac	NB
Mrs. Kathaleen Eaton, DStJ	Ottawa	ON
Mr. Lynn Edwards, SBStJ	Edmonton	AB
Mr. Peter B. Edwards, CStJ, CD	Toronto	ON
C/Cst. Derek C. Egan, OStJ	Victoria	BC
Mrs. Eleonore E. Erber, OStJ	Scarborough	ON
Ms. Deanna M. Fakeley, SSStJ	Elk Point	AB
Dr. Louis Hugo Francescutti, OStJ	Sherwood Park	AB
Mr. Ian A. Fraser, SBStJ	Sherwood Park	AB
Mr. R. Graeme Fraser, KStJ	Ottawa	ON
Cpl. William Allistair (Al) Fraser, MOM, KStJ	Sherwood Park	AB
VAdm. James A. Fulton, OMM, OStJ, CD	Mahone Bay	NS
Mr. Claude Gagnon, KStJ	Trois-Rivières	QC
Mr. Jeffrey G. Gilmour, KStJ, CD	Calgary	AB
Dr. Anne Kathleen Ritchie Gilmour-Bryson, SSStJ	North Vancouver	BC
Dr. Christopher Gordon-Craig, KStJ	Edmonton	AB
Mrs. Anne M. Graham, CStJ	Peterborough	ON
Dr. James H. Haldane, MC, KStJ	Halifax	NS
Ms. Katharine Harapniuk, DStJ	Edmonton	AB
Mrs. Joyce Hart, CStJ	Botwood	NL
Their Honours John Harvard, PC, KStJ, OM & Lenore Berscheid, OStJ	Winnipeg	MB
Capt. (Ret'd) Gary Hayes, CD & Mrs. Carole Hayes	Kingston	ON ON
BGen. John C. Hayter, KStJ, CD	Barrie	
Mr. Melvin G. Hazlewood, SBStJ	St. Marys	ON
Ms. Diane Hébert, SSStJ	Montreal	QC
Dr. Kenneth H. Hedges, CStJ	Washago	ON
Mr. Paul R. Herbert, CStJ	Welland	ON
Mr. Herman H.C. Ho, CStJ, ADC	Vancouver	BC
Mr. Edward David Hodgins	Edmonton	AB
Mr. John Hodgson	Darwell	AB
Hong Kong Chapter of the Ontario St. John Fellowship	Toronto	ON
Mr. David J. Hook, CStJ	Edmonton	AB

Full Name	City	Prov
Mr. R.J. (Sam) Houston, OMM, OStJ, CD	Ottawa	ON
CPO2 Charles Hurst, OStJ, CD	Victoria	BC
Mr. Kevin Hutchings, KStJ, ADC	St. John's	NL
Mrs. S. Oriel Jackson, SSStJ	Ottawa	ON
Mr. John E. James-Davies, CStJ	Calgary	AB
Mr. Brent D. Johnson, OStJ	Calgary	AB
LCol. (Ret'd) Arthur R.W. Jordan, CStJ, CD	Kingston	ON
Mr. Bill Jordan, OStJ & Mrs. Leta Jordan	Tottenham	ON
Ms. Patricia K. Kearney	Ottawa	ON
LCol. (Ret'd) Evelyn A. Kelly, SSStJ, CD, AdeC	Toronto	ON
Mr. Mark L. Kennedy, CD	Kingston	ON
Maj. (Ret'd) A. Charles King, CStJ, CD	Ottawa	ON
Ms. Barb King	St. Albert	AB
Mr. William Douglas Kirkwood, KStJ	Oakville	ON
Mr. Robert A. Klassen, CStJ	Abbotsford	BC
Mr. Terrence C. Ko, SBStJ	Vancouver	BC
Mr. William Kwok-Keung Ko, SBStJ	Thornhill	ON
Mr. Vicken Koundakjian, SBStJ	Ottawa	ON
Mr. Leopold Kurcz, OStJ	Calgary	AB
Ms. Margaret Kury, SSStJ	Maple Ridge	BC
Mr. George Kutash, SBStJ	St. Paul	AB
Ms. Lily Kwan	Coquitlam	BC
Col. (Ret'd) Terence D. Lafferty, CStJ, CD	Orleans	ON
Mrs. Beverly Lafortune	Sherwood Park	AB
Ms. Kim Laing, OStJ	Monarch	AB
LCol. (Ret'd) Fung Fai Lam, KStJ, AdeC	Unionville	ON
Ms. Jennifer Lavoie	Ottawa	ON
Dr. Thomas M. Lawley	Fort McMurray	AB
Col. Georges Letourneau, OStJ, CD	Sutton	QC
Mr. Steven Shufan Leung, CStJ	Markham	ON
Mr. Roger Alexander Lindsay of Craighall, KStJ, AdeC	Toronto	ON
Mrs. Queenie Little, CStJ	Innisfil	ON
Ms. Jacqueline Loignon, SSStJ	Orleans	ON
Mr. W. Paul Loofs, OStJ, CD	Victoria	BC
Mr. Edwin Lorenz, SBStJ	Brampton	ON
Mr. Geoffrey Lougheed, KStJ	Sudbury	ON
Dr. Marie A. Loyer, DStJ	Ottawa	ON

Full Name	City	Prov
Capt. A. David Luker, SBStJ	North Sydney	NS
Col. The Hon. Alfred G. Lynch-Staunton, KStJ, ED, CD	Qualicum Beach	BC
Dr. Ian M. MacDonald, CM, OStJ	Edmonton	AB
LCol. Daniel Sutherland Campbell Mackay, OMM, CStJ, CD	Ottawa	ON
Ms. Alice MacKinnon, DStJ	Edmonton	AB
Mr. R. Gordon M. Macpherson, KStJ	Burlington	ON
Mr. John C. Mah, KStJ, CD, QC	Edmonton	AB
Mr. Charles R. Maier, CStJ, CD	Ottawa	ON
The Hon. Gary Mar, SBStJ, QC	Calgary	AB
The Hon. Justice T. David C. Marshall, SBStJ	Cayuga	ON
Dr. Markus C. Martin, OStJ, CD	Montreal	QC
Mr. Carl Reginald Mason, KStJ	Barrie	ON
Mr. Pierre Masse, KStJ	Joliette	QC
Mr. Charles H. Mattila	Thompson	MB
Maj. (Ret'd) John A. McDonald, OStJ, CD	Mitchell	ON
HCol. John R. McDougall, OStJ, CD	Edmonton	AB
Mr. John D. McDowell, OStJ	Woodstock	ON
Mrs. Margaret A. McGee, OStJ	Ottawa	ON
Mr. John C. McKinnon, KStJ	Winnipeg	MB
The Hon. Hugh H. McLellan, SBStJ, CD	Saint John	NB
LCol. (Ret'd) John W. McNeil, KStJ, CD	Whitehorse	YT
Dr. Charles McVicker, SBStJ	St. John's	NL
Cpl. Lawrence J. Mercer, OStJ, CD	Middle Sackville	NS
Dr. Helen K. Mussallem, CC, DStJ	Ottawa	ON
Mr. Gordon Neill, SBStJ, QC	Regina	SK
Lt(N) Scott E. Nelson, SBStJ, ADC	Halifax	NS
Miss Esther I. Nicholas, DStJ	Brantford	ON
MGen. (Ret'd) Francis John Norman, CStJ, CD	Kingston	ON
Mr. William Oleksy, SBStJ	Lethbridge	AB
Ms. Alicia D. Osepchuk	Edmonton	AB
Mr. Renald Parent, CStJ	St-Georges de Beauce	QC
Mrs. Ilmi Peltola, OStJ	Thunder Bay	ON
Mr. Daniel Pépin, KStJ	Montreal	QC
Mr. Denis Perrier, OStJ, CD	St-Jean-sur-Richelieu	QC
Miss Diane Perry, DStJ	Winnipeg	MB
Mr. Robert Pichette, CStJ, ONB	Moncton	NB

Full Name	City	Prov
Capt. Richard D. Pihlaja, SBStJ, CD	Sault Ste. Marie	ON
Mr. Francis Pitre, KStJ, CD &	Bathurst	NB
Mrs. Brenda Pitre, CStJ		
Ms. Alvine Poitras, SSStJ	Edmonton	AB
Dr. James R. Popplow, SBStJ, CD	Winnipeg	MB
Mr. Percy L. Price, OStJ, CD	Ottawa	ON
LCol. Ross A. Purser, CStJ	Sherwood Park	AB
Miss Marjorie J. Reed, DStJ	Winnipeg	MB
LCdr. Darin E. Reeves, CStJ, CD	Yellowknife	NT
LCol. (Ret'd) Colin W. Reichle, CStJ, CD	St. Albert	AB
Mr. Jordy Reichson, OStJ	Côte Saint-Luc	QC
Col. (Ret'd) Gary H. Rice, SBStJ, CD	Carleton Place	ON
Ms. Dawn Roach	Ottawa	ON
Mr. Donald T.H. Roach	Kingston	ON
Mr. Dany Robert, SBStJ	Saint-Hyacinthe	QC
PO2 Edward C. Roberts, OStJ, CD	Bath	ON
The Hon. Edward M. Roberts, KStJ, QC	St. John's	NL
Mrs. Ruth M. Robinson, SSStJ	Bedford	NS
HLCol. Solomon (Sol) Rolingher, CStJ, QC	Edmonton	AB
Mr. Edward W. Routledge, CStJ	Uxbridge	ON
Col. (Ret'd) Edgar H. Rowe, OMM, KStJ, CD	Sault Ste. Marie	ON
Mrs. Anne Rudiak, SSStJ	Calgary	AB
Dr. William B. Sara, SBStJ	Crowsnest Pass	AB
Sceptre Investment Counsel Ltd.	Toronto	ON
Mrs. Jean Schimnosky, OStJ	Saskatoon	SK
Maj. Justin Schmidt-Clever, OStJ, CD	Kanata	ON
Mr. Orest Semenuik, KStJ	Edmonton	AB
Mr. Ron S. Seney, SBStJ	Meisner's Section	NS
Mrs. Virginia G. Shyluk, DStJ	Calgary	AB
LCol. Harriet J. Sloan, CM, CStJ, CD	Ottawa	ON
Mr. Wade Smith, SBStJ	Markland	NL
Maj. (Ret'd) Douglas J.G. Soper, SBStJ, CD	London	ON
Mr. Anthony Sosnkowski, OStJ	Charlottetown	PE
Mr. Rod Sparks, SBStJ	Selkirk	MB
Mr. Lyle E. Sproat, KStJ, CD	St. Albert	AB
St. John Ambulance Council for Alberta	Edmonton	AB
St. John Ambulance Council for Manitoba	Winnipeg	MB
St. John Council for Federal District	Ottawa	ON

Full Name	City	Prov
Mr. Grant D. Stange, OStJ	Red Deer	AB
Mr. David Steeves	Mississauga	ON
Miss H. Faye Stephenson, SSStJ	Hamilton	ON
Mr. Rick L. Stewart	Edmonton	AB
Capt. Jean St-Laurent, KStJ, CD, ADC	Baie-Comeau	QC
Mrs. Lucette St-Laurent, OStJ	Baie-Comeau	QC
Mr. Peter Tang, SBStJ	Vancouver	BC
Mr. Andrew Tay Teng Yew	Singapore	BC
Mr. Aurélien Tremblay, KStJ	Chicoutimi	QC
Mrs. Joyce Trimmer, SSStJ	Alliston	ON
Mrs. Jeanie S. Tronningsdal, SSStJ	Creston	BC
Mr. Neil Tull, OStJ & Mrs. Elizabeth Tull	Aylmer	ON
Col. (Ret'd) Roger W. Turnell, OStJ, CD	Edmonton	AB
Dr. Kenneth R. Turriff, OStJ	Bridgewater	NS
Mr. David P.J. Tysowski, CStJ, CD, AdeC	Ottawa	ON
Dr. John E. Udd, SBStJ	Ottawa	ON
Ms. Doreen I. Van Eaton, SSStJ	Athabasca	AB
Dr. Vincent Van Hooydonk, CStJ	Tillsonburg	ON
Mr. Robert H. Vandewater, OStJ	Winnipeg	MB
Mr. Roy J. Verbrugge, KStJ	Winnipeg	MB
Maj. (Ret'd) Eric J. Vincent, OMM, KStJ, CD	Saskatoon	SK
Mr. Derek Vollrath	Ottawa	ON
Mrs. Patricia Colleen Vousden, CStJ	Scarborough	ON
BGen. H. Ovas Wagg, CM, KStJ, CD	Collingwood	ON
Mr. Sid R. Wallace, KStJ, CD	Calgary	AB
Mr. Terrence Wardrop, SBStJ	Burlington	ON
Mr. Robert White, SBStJ	Brooklin	ON
Mr. George Boyd Whitefield, CStJ, CD	Thunder Bay	ON
Mr. John L. Williamson, KStJ	Fredericton	NB
Mr. Cyril Woods of Slane, KStJ & Mrs. Lorna Woods, SSStJ	Ajax	ON
Mr. Joe Zasada	Beaumont	AB

Thank you

PHOTO CREDITS

INDEX